MW01156555

BEFORE BIOETHICS

BEFORE BIOETHICS

A HISTORY OF AMERICAN MEDICAL ETHICS FROM THE COLONIAL PERIOD TO THE BIOETHICS REVOLUTION

ROBERT BAKER

OXFORD
UNIVERSITY PRESS

OXFORD
UNIVERSITY PRESS

Oxford University Press is a department of the University of Oxford.
It furthers the University's objective of excellence in research, scholarship,
and education by publishing worldwide.

Oxford New York
Auckland Cape Town Dar es Salaam Hong Kong Karachi
Kuala Lumpur Madrid Melbourne Mexico City Nairobi
New Delhi Shanghai Taipei Toronto

With offices in
Argentina Austria Brazil Chile Czech Republic France Greece
Guatemala Hungary Italy Japan Poland Portugal Singapore
South Korea Switzerland Thailand Turkey Ukraine Vietnam

Oxford is a registered trademark of Oxford University Press in the UK and
certain other countries.

Published in the United States of America by
Oxford University Press
198 Madison Avenue, New York, NY 10016

© Oxford University Press 2013

All rights reserved. No part of this publication may be reproduced, stored in a
retrieval system, or transmitted, in any form or by any means, without the prior
permission in writing of Oxford University Press, or as expressly permitted by law,
by license, or under terms agreed with the appropriate reproduction rights organization.
Inquiries concerning reproduction outside the scope of the above should be sent to the Rights
Department, Oxford University Press, at the address above.

You must not circulate this work in any other form
and you must impose this same condition on any acquirer.

Library of Congress Cataloging-in-Publication Data
Baker, Robert, 1937– author
Before bioethics : a history of American medical ethics from the
colonial period to the bioethics revolution/Robert Baker.
p. ; cm.
Includes bibliographical references and index.
ISBN 978–0–19–977411–1 (hardcover : alk. paper)
I. Title.
[DNLM: 1. Ethics, Medical—history—United States. 2. History, 18th Century—United States.
3. History, 19th Century—United States. 4. History, 20th Century—United States. W 50]
174.2—dc23
2013001404

To my wife
Arlene
Without her patience and support, this project
would never have been completed.

TABLE OF CONTENTS

PREFACE

History is philosophy teaching by examples.

Attributed to Thucydides (c. 460–400 BCE)

Prefaces are places where authors directly address their readers to explain why they wrote the book that follows, to justify the author's presumption in asking readers to spend time reading the book, and to thank those who helped in the writing of the book. This book began decades ago as a very different project. A joint NEH-NSF program, Ethics and Values in Science and Technology (EVIST), awarded me a grant to explore the moral methodologies of intensive care units (ICUs). At the time, I thought that emerging medical technologies in ICUs created what the philosopher Ludwig Wittgenstein characterized as "a form of life." My theory was that a novel technology-driven ethics had been created to suit a special form of moral life arising from ICU technology. So I spent eighteen months living in ICUs, interviewing clinicians, patients, and families, attempting to discern the evolution of moral notions and decision-making methodologies integral in the form of life evolving around critical care technologies.

Few things are more disheartening to the life of the mind than having a recalcitrant fact undermine a favored theory. I came across such a fact in a 1794 book, *Medical Jurisprudence,* by British physician Thomas Percival. On page after page, Percival described the same decision-making process that I thought had evolved in twentieth-century ICUs. Evidently, ICU clinicians had not created a new form of life; they were adopting older forms to novel circumstances. Reviewing my data, it appeared that ICUs had experimented with a variety of approaches in coping with how and whether to discontinue apparently futile life support and that the real issue was how some particular approach came to be valorized and legitimated as morally appropriate—and, as I argue in this book, that is something that occurs outside of critical care units.

So I discarded the first version of this book, returned to teaching philosophy, to launching a hybrid online/onsite graduate program that made graduate training in clinical ethics consultation and research ethics accessible for working healthcare professionals, to helping to professionalize the field of bioethics, and to writing about codes of medical ethics past, present, and future. Nonetheless, the issues that prompted my earlier research still haunted me. Why should philosophers, practitioners of an arcane intellectual art who are generally given little or no respect in ultra-pragmatic American society be accorded authority on issues of medical ethics? Why should lawyers and philosophers be working in hospitals to address the moral distress of families forced to face such questions as whether or not to continue life support? Shouldn't physicians, social workers, and nurses be doing this job? The usual answer is that lawyers and philosophers are somehow ideally suited to this job. My answer is that we were never trained to do this job; however, for complex historical reasons explained in this book, American medicine was unable to respond to the ethical and moral challenges posed by emerging medical technologies, research ethics scandals, and even the AIDS epidemic of the 1980s—so the job of bioethicist was invented by default, and we filled the vacancy.

This book could never have been written without extensive assistance from archivists, staff, friends, and colleagues at the American Medical Association (AMA) and its Institute for Ethics, which also assisted me by appointing me Visiting Senior Scholar. I would like to single out for special thanks Linda Emanuel, former director of the Institute (now at Northwestern's Feinberg School of Medicine); Steven Latham, former director of Ethics Standards at the AMA (now Director of Yale's bioethics center); and Matthew Wynia, director of the AMA's Institute of Ethics. Arlene Shaner, curator of the Rare Books Collection and librarian at the New York Academy of Medicine, and a volunteer archivist at the Academy, Dorothy Truman, also provided invaluable assistance. Arlene guided me through the collection, and Dorothy assisted with the records of the Medical Society of the County of New York. A shout out to Scott Podolsky and Jack Eckert of Harvard's Countway Library of Medicine for their assistance in making available to me a rare book, Julius Homberger's flyting pamphlet *Batpaxomyomaxia: a fight on "ethics."* At my home institutions, I owe a great debt to Union College's Humanities Faculty Development Fund for supporting travel to archives and libraries and to the William D. Williams bequest that funds the professorship that I hold. Special thanks to Union College and Union Graduate College staff and students who assisted me with researching and correcting drafts: Amy Bloom, Tammy Curtis, Jennifer Granina, Najiba Keshwani, Randall Miller, Mylenne Salinas, Marianne Snowden, Katelyn Staring, Salman Syed, Chandni Vaid, and Cara Rose Zimmerman—and thanks to Alexandra Chico for helping prepare the bibliography, to Mylenne Salinas for her assistance with indexing, and to Daniel Pallies and Remy Ravitzka for aid in copy editing.

Among the many colleagues in bioethics and the history of medicine whose comments assisted me along the way was my colleague, collaborator, fellow bioethicist-historian, and friend, Larry McCullough. Their advice and comments made this a much better book. I am also grateful to Oxford University Press reviewers, especially George Annas, who unblinded himself to me; and to my editor at Oxford University Press, Peter Ohlin, for his gracious, cheerful, and patient support. The final word of thanks is to my wife Arlene, for repeatedly reminding me that I owed it to myself to complete this book, and so to address issues that haunted me for years.

Bob Baker
Schenectady, New York
December 22, 2012

1

INTRODUCTION: ON MEDICINE, ETHICS, AND MORALITY

> You ever wonder what a Martian might think if he happened to land near an emergency room? He'd see an ambulance whizzing in and everybody running out to meet it, tearing the doors open, grabbing up the stretcher, scurrying along with it. "Why," he'd say, "what a helpful planet, what kind and helpful creatures." He'd never guess that we are not always that way; that we had to, oh, put aside our natural selves to do it.
>
> *The Accidental Tourist*, Anne Tyler[1]

Medical ethics is a hearty perennial these days, a media staple that reliably commands the attention of a large popular audience. Yet, for most of nineteenth and twentieth centuries, the public treated the ethical pronouncements of medical practitioners as parochial affairs, of interest primarily to medical practitioners. Only three new books addressing medical ethics were published in nineteenth-century America, an 1849 critique of quackery by Yale professor Worthington Hooker (1806–1867) that also discussed the American Medical Association's (AMA) 1847 Code of Ethics[2] and two commentaries on the AMA code of ethics, which were published in the 1880s.[3] These books attracted little public notice, and the subject retained this parochial status through the first six decades of the twentieth century.

Perhaps not surprisingly, the only history of American medical ethics written in the twentieth century, a monograph by Donald Konold, published in 1962 by the academic press of the State Historical Society of Wisconsin,[4] also met with little public fanfare.[5] Ironically, some historians mark that same year as a turning point in public interest in professional medical ethics.[6] In May 1962, the *New York Times* covered the story of Dr. Belding Scribner (1921–2003), a Seattle physician who had invented a device called a "shunt," a small Teflon tube used to connect an artery to a vein. Before Scribner's invention, nine out of ten long-term dialysis patients died. Scribner's shunt reversed the mortality of the disease so that only one in ten long-term dialysis patients died. Medical miracles are seldom an unmixed blessing: the cloud surrounding the silver lining was the increasing numbers of survivors who soon overwhelmed the limited supply of dialysis machines. So, Scribner set up an allocation committee of lay people and professionals to decide which patients should have access to long-term dialysis machines. He also alerted the media to the problems confronting him in an effort to solicit funds to buy more dialysis machines.

Public interest in the problem was stirred when, in 1962, reporter Shana Alexander characterized Scribner's selection committee as a "God Committee." NBC followed up in 1965 with a television documentary *Who Shall Live?* The media coverage caught the eye of two experts, lawyer Jesse Dukeminier (1925–2003) and psychiatrist David Sanders, who wrote an article in the University of California, Los Angeles (UCLA) law review criticizing the Seattle "God Committee" for middle-class "prejudices and mindless clichés that pollute the committee's deliberations" on determining access to dialysis machines. Characterizing the decision-making process as "the bourgeoisie sparing the bourgeoisie," they quipped that, "the Pacific Northwest is no place for a Henry David Thoreau with bad kidneys."[7]

Prose as memorable as this commanded the attention of other experts. Media and public interest in the ethics of dialysis was roused further by dramatic testimony offered before the House Ways and Means committee, on November 4, 1971, by Charlotte and Shep Glazer, members of the National Association of Patients on Hemodialysis (NAPH).[8] Shep dialyzed himself in front of the congressional committee, letting some blood drip to the floor as he disconnected a tube. He reportedly exclaimed, "If you don't fund more machines, you'll have this blood on your hands."[9] Within a year, Congress passed the End-Stage Renal Disease Act (ESRDA) extending Medicare (a federal national health insurance program intended for seniors) to fund access to dialysis for patients of all ages.

After passage of ESRDA in 1972, patient activism, combined with government funding of expensive new medical technologies, made media coverage of professional debates over medical ethics inevitable. As medical ethics came out of the closet, it acquired a new name, "bioethics."[10] Under that rubric, the Library of Congress canonized "bioethics" as an official category in 1974, the literature formerly known as "medical ethics" was catalogued under the rubric "bioethics," and a *Bibliography of Bioethics* (1975) and comprehensive *Encyclopedia of Bioethics* (1978) soon followed. By the end of the twentieth century, five new books had been written on the history of bioethics[11]—but not a single new book was published on the prior history of American medical ethics.

WHY THE HISTORY OF AMERICAN MEDICAL ETHICS MATTERS

Yet the history of American medical ethics before the advent of bioethics matters, if for no other reason than to illuminate the nature of bioethics itself. Is bioethics merely a stylishly attractive, media-friendly makeover of medical ethics—just a new way of talking about an old subject, so to speak? Or, is bioethics, as most bioethicists and some historians contend, something else? Is it, perhaps, a revolutionary rejection of the parochialism and paternalism of traditional medical ethics? If so, did it arise as American society drew on a broader spectrum of expertise in response to the ethical challenges posed by new medical technologies like Dr. Scribner's shunt? And, one might ask, if bioethics really is a revolt against some received order of things, some *ancien régime*, some entrenched constellation of power and thought known as traditional medical ethics, then why was there a revolt, and what was revolutionized? Did the revolt consist, as some historians have suggested, of strangers claiming a place at the bedside and benchside,[12] or was the bioethics revolution a fundamental transformation in the way that physicians and biomedical scientists thought about ethics in medicine and the biomedical sciences? And, if it was a revolution, how much changed? Did everything change? Or did bioethics assimilate some conceptions and presumptions from traditional medical ethics? Might it be that the so-called bioethics revolution was, as the French say, *plus ça change, plus c'est le même chose*, a change that left everything more or less the same? Was it perhaps, as bioethicist Leon Kass once remarked, an attempt "to improve our deeds [that] if truth be told, has, at best improved our speech."[13] None of these questions can be addressed without an understanding of what happened previously—without an appreciation of the history of American medical ethics prior to the 1970s.

MEDICAL ETHICS AND MEDICAL MORALITY: THE CASE OF THE ERRANT INTERN

Another reason for assessing the history of traditional American medical ethics is that it remains a source of the moral sensibility that still governs the day-to-day world of the American clinic. As novelist Anne Tyler astutely observed in the passage that opens this chapter, healthcare professionals put aside their natural selves when they function professionally. To understand the unnatural selves that people become as they put on the role of physician, one must be cognizant of two related but distinct notions: "medical ethics" and "medical morality." By medical ethics, I mean articulated, often formal, statements about standards of character or conduct to which someone, a patient, a politician, a philosopher—or a physician—believes healthcare practitioners *ought* to be held accountable. Medical morality, in contrast, refers to standards of conduct or character, often unarticulated and informal, to which a community of healthcare practitioners *actually* holds *itself* accountable.[14] To paraphrase Kass, ethical ideals may not be copacetic with those deeds a profession actually condones or condemns.

An incident that occurred some years ago will help to clarify the distinction that I am drawing between medical ethics (how someone claims practitioners ought to conduct themselves) and medical morality (the standards of conduct practitioners actually commend and condemn). One July, I visited a large academic teaching hospital in a major urban center, which I shall call "City Hospital." July is generally considered the worst time of the year to be a patient at an academic medical center. I once overheard a nurse telling a friend, "Never become a patient in July! Everyone has a new job." The reason is that, in July, medical students are promoted to first-year postgraduate students (interns); interns are promoted to junior residents; junior residents, in turn, become senior residents; and senior residents are promoted to fellows. Thus, in the knowing words of this nurse, "No one knows what they're doing in July!"[15]

The young intern who is the focus of this incident, call her N, was a quintessential neophyte, a newlywed suburbanite educated in college towns, new to the city—call it Metropolis—new to City Hospital, newly an intern, and new to the newborn intensive care unit (NICU) where this incident occurred. N's suburban rearing and college-town education had ill prepared her for Metropolis. Confounded by the city's size, its utter indifference to her and her husband, and its exorbitant expensiveness, she and her husband found themselves struggling to establish the minimal requisites of existence: apartment, utilities, bank account. Their savings and credit limits were exhausted, and they were counting on her first paycheck to get them through the long Fourth of July weekend and the week following. So, on Friday, the day before the holiday began, N felt it imperative to pick up her paycheck from City Hospital's payroll office.

Like the other interns at the NICU that Friday morning, N was assigned a series of tasks related to the newborns placed under her care. After completing her assignments, she took an early lunch hour and rushed to the payroll office. To her chagrin, two notes were posted on the payroll office door. One said "Out to Lunch." The other announced that the office would close at 4:00 PM and would not reopen until Tuesday at 9:00 AM.

On returning to the NICU, intern N was assigned to cover a "transport," a newborn infant who had been transferred to City from the hospital in which she was born because of her extreme prematurity and suspicion of seizure activity. Among N's assignments was taking this patient to radiology for a precautionary computed tomography (CT) scan. Like every other service at City, however, a skeleton crew would staff radiology over the three-day holiday weekend. Precautionary scans had to be performed before 3:30 on Friday, or they would wait until Tuesday morning. The schedule made it unlikely that N could both cash her paycheck and take her patient for a scan. N felt she had to choose between her paycheck and her patient. She chose the paycheck, but, after picking it up, she dashed back to the NICU in a desperate albeit unsuccessful attempt to get the newborn to radiology.

Patient rounds are held at least twice daily in most units of academic teaching hospitals. At rounds, the physician in charge of the unit, known as the "attending physician," systematically reviews patients' health status and treatment plans, using the occasion to discuss cases and to teach various aspects of healthcare. Reports on a patient are usually initiated by the nurses and interns charged with that patient's care. When intern N reported on her patients, however, she omitted any mention of the CT scan for the transported newborn. Off-handedly, the attending physician inquired about the results of the scan. Intern N replied with vague words to the effect that scheduling had been problematic. Puzzled, the attending physician began to probe more incisively. The intern reluctantly related her decision to cash her paycheck instead of taking her patient for a CT scan. The intern insisted that, given her family's desperate need for cash and the merely precautionary nature of the scan, she had made a reasonable decision.

After these remarks, the attending physician's demeanor changed. She began to pace the staff room, hurling interrogatives at the intern. "Had you intended to inform us about this matter... *Doctor*? Or did you intend to keep the matter to yourself... *Doctor*? Tell me, *Doctor*... do you intend to make a practice of abandoning your patients... *Doctor*? What level of personal inconvenience justifies deserting a patient... *Doctor*? Do you intend to desert your patients when you are double-parked... *Doctor*?" And so it went, the attending physician pacing back and forth, pausing only to hurl a question at the intern. Each question ended with an emphatic pronouncement of the title, "Doctor." The intern stood in stunned silence, seeming to shrink before our eyes, shuddering each time the attending pronounced the title, "Doctor."

The public excoriation of intern N before the assembled nurses and her fellow interns and residents lasted almost two minutes––more than ninety very long seconds. On Tuesday, a CT scan was performed. It was negative (normal). Nonetheless, the attending physician was unrelenting. As she remarked when I interviewed her about the incident, "she proved untrustworthy, so I never trusted her with another baby." This decision not to entrust intern N with additional patients was as devastating as the two-minute tongue-lashing. Status among interns and residents is determined in part by their ability to recount their experiences. They strive to impress each other by holding "counting conversations," in which they enumerate how many patients or procedures of a certain type they had dealt with. Alone among the interns at the NICU, N had nothing to relate. Even though the NICU was perpetually short-handed, N was always assigned tasks in tandem with someone else, typically a nurse. When N reported at rounds, the attending physician turned to this companion for confirmation. After that memorable tongue-lashing, the attending physician was always exquisitely polite to intern N, but everyone on the NICU, including N, was acutely aware that she was considered irredeemably untrustworthy. N had been shamed. She had no standing on the NICU.

There is nothing unique about the attending physician's treatment of N. Although this was a particularly dramatic instance, incidents like this occur with a fair degree of regularity in academic medical contexts. They are part of what is sometimes characterized as the "hidden curriculum," the informal ways in which experienced clinicians impart to neophytes the traditional practices and morality of the clinic. The vehemence with which the attending physician chastised intern N—the emphatic iteration of the title "doctor"—was precipitated by N's defense of her decision to prioritize her paycheck over her patient as reasonable, or at least, as excusable. To the attending physician, this meant that N did not understand what was morally required of someone playing the role of doctor. What followed was a lesson in the role morality of the American clinic.

ON ROLE MORALITY

The idea that roles dictate ethics and morality dates to Roman times, when it was articulated by the philosopher Marcus Tullius Cicero (106–43 BCE) in *De Officiis* (On Duties), a book of advice written for his son in what turned out to be the last year of Cicero's life, 44 BCE. (Cicero, a defender of the Roman republic, was executed that year on the order of Mark Antony.) In advising his son on how to be an upright Roman gentleman, Cicero lays out what classicist Ludwig Edelstein (1902–1965) characterized as an implicit "program of professional ethics."[16] Using the example of a judge required to pass judgment on a friend, Cicero observes that "an upright man will never for a friend's sake do anything in violation of his country's interests... *for he lays aside the role of a friend when he assumes that of judge*."[17] Edelstein offers a different translation of the italicized line: "for he lays down the role (or mask) of the friend when putting on that of the judge."[18] The reference here is to Roman theater, in which an individual actor would play several different characters, changing masks (roles) to indicate which character he was playing at a given moment. For Cicero, each role/mask one dons carries with it duties that override normal obligations. When one dons the mask/role of judge, one's duties as judge override one's duties as friend; or, to return to the case of errant intern N, when she donned the role/mask of doctor, she was expected to put aside her role as wife. The exigencies of a situation, "expediency," seldom serve as an acceptable excuse for abandoning role-related duties. To quote Cicero, "for what is there that your so-called expediency can bring you that will compensate for what it can take away, if it steals from you the name of a 'good man.'"[19]

ON TRUTH AND FORGIVENESS IN CLINICAL CONTEXTS

Cicero's characterization neatly encapsulates the dynamics underlying the punishment of intern N. Having prioritized personal expediency, "the paycheck," over being a good doctor, intern N had lost her "good name" as a physician. She demonstrated that she did not know how to play the doctor role properly—or that, as the attending physician put it, she was "untrustworthy," and so she was never again entrusted with the care of another NICU patient. The N incident also illustrates the specific role-generated standards of character and conduct—the *moral norms*—whose violation prompted N's chastisement. As the transcription of the attending physician's questions reveals, N was accused of violating a moral norm of truthful information sharing about patient care (Had you intended to inform us about this matter?), a moral norm of nonabandonment (Do you intend to make a practice of abandoning your patients?), and a moral norm of fidelity to the patient, valuing patient care above personal concerns (What level of personal inconvenience justifies deserting a patient? Do you intend to desert your patients when you are double-parked?). This last norm lies at the core of clinical morality (the norm of nonabandonment is effectively an extension). To quote the perceptive ethnographer Charles Bosk, "When making decisions, the surgeon—any physician, in fact—is expected to bracket all systems of relevance to him as an actor in his other social roles .... Fatigue, pressing family problems, a long queue of patients waiting to be seen, flu—all the excuses that individual's routinely use in everyday life, are inadmissible."[20]

The moral norm of truthful information sharing about patient care is a constituent of the remarkable system of "forgive-and-remember" accountability found in American teaching hospitals. This system, which is documented in detail in Charles Bosk's classic 1981 study, *Forgive and Remember*, is a response to the iterative nature of error in healthcare settings. In the memorable words of the younger Seneca, *errare humanum est*: to err is human. All human systems are error prone, and healthcare is no exception[21]—which means that every healthcare system must have some way of dealing with errors. At one extreme, an indifferent system might leave errors unremarked and uncorrected. At the other extreme, one can imagine a system of absolute accountability in which any error effecting a patient's death, or even any instance of medical ineffectiveness, is considered a capital crime. A Turkish Pasha, for example, is said to have executed an eminent Italian renaissance physician, Gabrielle Zerbi (1445–1505), because Zerbi failed to cure the Pasha of an ailment.[22] Because any such draconian system would soon lack practitioners, functional healthcare systems develop ways of dealing with errors that lie somewhere between these extremes.

The American way of addressing medical error is characteristically complex. On the one hand, we have a system of malpractice laws that, although milder than the Pasha's system of executing errant physicians, is nonetheless the most draconian system of legal accountability for medical error in the developed world. On the other hand, we have complex institutional systems of quality assurance and continual quality improvement. Error, however, is an integral part of learning. So, American academic medical centers employ a different system of accountability in dealing with students and physicians-in-training ("house staff"), like intern N. Recognizing that all physicians make errors and that novice physicians and physicians-in-training, like intern N, are the most error prone of all, attending physicians can be remarkably generous in offering forgiveness, especially to physicians-in-training.

Forgiveness, however, is conditional. The first condition that physicians-in-training must satisfy to earn a supervising physicians' forgiveness is to forthrightly account for the care they delivered to their patients. If this account reveals that the physician-in-training has erred in some way, the physician-in-training is required to acknowledge the error of her or his ways, apologize, and commit her- or himself to never repeat the error. Intern N violated all of these conditions. Instead of forthrightly reporting on her actions, she obfuscated, attempting to hide her failure to obey her supervisor's instructions. When the attending physician penetrated the fog of obfuscation and discovered the intern's failure to obtain a CT scan, the intern defended her actions instead of admitting her failings—and, finally, she never apologized or made a declaration of future diligence in performing her duties to her patients. Intern N violated all of the conditions required to attain forgiveness, so her acts were unforgiven—her character was viewed as flawed, and she became a pariah.[23]

The case of the errant intern illustrates the concept of medical morality. Forgive-and-remember morality is an unwritten standard. It is not documented in any oath, code, or official statement issued by a medical society. Unlike the standards of medical ethics formalized in oaths and codes, the moral standards that medical practitioners embrace and to which they actually hold each other accountable—their medical morality—is often undocumented, unstated, and accessible only to trained ethnographers (like sociologist Charles Bosk). Reprimands to novices can bring these norms to the surface by forcing experienced clinicians to articulate standards. Thus, in judging the conduct of intern N, the attending physician articulated such norms of medical conduct as truth telling, nonabandonment, and fidelity; moreover, the attending physician expressly justified these norms in terms of a conception of good doctoring. The attending physician furthermore interpreted intern N's conduct in terms of these norms, judged her in violation, rejected her excuses, and held her accountable by meting out a punishment—revealing, in so doing, the medical morality of the clinic.

The five elements evident in the case of intern N—norms, justifying/organizing concepts, interpretation, adjudication, and enforcement—are characteristic of any complex system of behavioral norms (a normative framework). What makes this normative framework and these norms moral, rather than institutional or legal, is that they are justified in terms of a moral concept—good doctoring—not by appeals to institutional policy, legal authority, or concepts. Thus, although N's actions violated organizational rules, and although they could have resulted in a malpractice lawsuit (had the baby suffered neurological damage attributable to the delayed CT scan), in chastising intern N the attending physician mentioned neither institutional policy nor the law. Instead, her chastising tirade focused solely on expectations for good doctoring—on the moral norms expected of someone playing the role of doctor well. And so the emphasis at the end of every interrogative was not "employee" or "citizen"—the constantly reiterated word was "doctor." This was not a lesson about obeying hospital rules or being mindful of malpractice laws, it was a lesson in medical morality designed to explain and instill basic precepts of good doctoring into the mind of a terrified intern that was conducted before (and for the benefit of) an audience of the assembled house staff—and, as it happened, a visiting bioethicist.

THE SOCIAL HISTORICAL CRITIQUE OF TRADITIONAL HISTORIES OF MEDICAL ETHICS

The distinction that I draw between medical morality and medical ethics, and the broad evidentiary basis that I draw on to narrate a history of American medical ethics, is testament to the work of generations of social historians of medicine.[24] These historians have exposed the inadequacy of histories of medical ethics that treat the formal ethics of oaths and codes as the primary basis for constructing histories of medical ethics. The social historians' critique is twofold. By focusing primarily on what *doctors* have said about the ethics of doctoring, traditional histories of medical ethics have ignored the views of patients, the public, philosophers, theologians, and others who have views on how healthcare providers ought to behave. Second, and just as important, by focusing on what doctors have *said* about ethics, traditional histories have tended to ignore the question of whether practitioners have actually enforced the standards that they proclaim. To put the point differently, histories of medical ethics often conflate what I characterize as practitioner's medical ethics, by which I mean formal statements characterizing how practitioners ought to conduct themselves if they are to be deemed ethical, with medical morality; that is, the norms of character and conduct actually enforced—commended and condemned—by practitioners. Ethics is thus the norms formalized in oaths and codes; morality is the norms people actually accept and enforce. Sometimes the two coincide; sometimes they do not.

To appreciate the social historian's critique of traditional histories of medical ethics, consider, as an illustrative example, how a social historian of medicine might analyze the earliest known American medical society statement on medical ethics. In 1766, America's first medical society, the New Jersey Medical Society, was founded. In its foundational document, Instruments of Association, the colonial New Jersey doctors pledged "never [to] enter any house in quality of our profession, nor undertake any case, either in physic or in surgery, but with the purest intention of giving the utmost relief and assistance that our art shall enable us, which we will diligently and faithfully exert for that purpose."[25] The New Jersey physicians also pledged to share their medical knowledge and skills with each other, to maintain the dignity and harmony of the profession, and to attend to the medical needs of the poor "readily and cheerfully."[26]

A traditional history of medical ethics might focus on these lines, remarking, for example, on their similarity to certain lines in the ancient Greek Hippocratic Oath. A typical social historian's account, in contrast, would attempt to discern the standards to which the New Jersey practitioners actually held their peers accountable. They would, for example, examine the context in which the Instruments were drafted. As it turns out, the document was drawn up in Duff's Tavern, in New Brunswick, at a meeting called to organize a society for the "Advancement of the Profession."[27] This society aimed, among other things, to "establish necessary regulations respecting the admission of candidates [to medicine and surgery] and [to develop a common fee scale of] the due rewards for practitioner's services."[28] Examination of the minutes of the founding meeting, moreover, show that instead of discussing "entering houses" with the "pure intention of giving the utmost relief and assistance that [their] art shall enable [them]," the assembled practitioners grumbled about "the expense of answering calls in the country" and that much of the discussion focused on establishing "uniform fees."[29] With this evidence in hand, a social historian might challenge the "purity" of the New Jersey practitioners' intent because, as the minutes of the meeting seem to indicate, the real aim of the Instruments of Association appears to have been the creation of a monopoly on medical practice in New Jersey by controlling entry into medical fields, fixing prices, and elevating fees for distant house calls. The altruistic ethical rhetoric in the text of the Instruments would thus appear to be less a statement of intent than verbiage designed to distract attention from the monopolizing ambitions of the new organization.[30]

Another precept of the social history of medicine is to look beyond the voices of practitioners, to seek other perspectives on events. As it turned out, the New Jersey colonists initially rejected the New Jersey physicians' Instruments of Association, "clamoring against the Society, accusing it of [being] an unjust scheme to [bilk] the public."[31] New Jersey physicians responded by launching a public relations campaign to persuade colonists "that their Scheme is design'd to be of Public Utility."[32] In deploying the ethical components of the Instruments for public relations purposes, the New Jersey physicians' actions again suggest that ethical rhetoric served to distract public attention from their self-serving actions. If, as Samuel Johnson famously remarked, patriotism is the last refuge of scoundrels,[33] appeals to ethics have always been their first refuge.

THE ROLE OF OATHS AND CODES IN THE CONSTRUCTION OF HISTORIES OF MEDICAL ETHICS

Pendulums naturally swing beyond the center. In their justified zeal to probe the more venial economic motivations underlying oaths and codes, social historians sometimes ignore the commitments made in these texts or dismiss them as empty verbiage—without ascertaining whether professionals actually abided by the duties laid out in them; that is, without analyzing the extent to which medical ethics and medical morality coincide. Yet the question of whether practitioners' medical morality actually coincides with their medical ethics is empirical. On this point, the case of intern N is again instructive. She not only violated a moral norm accepted by clinical practitioners—fidelity to patients—she also violated an ethical norm propounded in every oath or code of medical ethics issued by an American medical society.

More to the point, intern N violated an oath that she herself had sworn, not once, but twice. Like most American medical students, N swore a version of the Hippocratic Oath at a white coat ceremony that she attended on entering medical school; she swore it a second time at her medical school graduation ceremony.[34] The particular oath that N swore was a variant of the Declaration of Geneva (1948) that specifically affirms a duty of fidelity—"the health of my patient will be my first consideration"[35]—which, in turn, traces to the classic Hippocratic oath of ancient Greece. Thus, in memorably explaining to intern N how this moral norm was interpreted in the NICU, the attending physician not only enforced norms of American medical morality, she also enforced ethical standards proclaimed by American medical societies—norms of medical ethics pronounced at least twice by intern N. Intern N apparently treated the words of her oath as merely symbolic. In this, she erred. So, too, to return to the point of this discussion, do historians of medicine who dismiss the texts of oaths and codes as empty verbiage: these texts are more than empty words, they often formalize medical morality.

Oaths and codes are also invaluable to historians of medical ethics because by formally stating ethical norms and their justifying concepts they provide a documentary record of normative stability and change. As will become evident from the history of midwives' oaths analyzed in Chapter 2, ethical norms can remain remarkably stable through periods of radical change. The "stickiness" of ethical norms conserved over time, or "norm conservation," is a phenomenon documentable by an analysis of oaths, codes, and similar formal materials. Oaths and codes also provide documentary evidence of changes in justifying conceptions and on the process of ethical and moral reform and revolution; that is, on the process by which ethical ideals and norms of one era can sometimes be accepted or rejected as the operant morality of medical practice in later eras.

For example, when Manchester physician Thomas Percival (1740–1804) published *Medical Ethics* in 1803, he offered a vision of how medical practitioners ought to behave in clinical contexts. To ensure forthright disclosure of opinions, he recommended a procedure for rounds in which physicians report on cases in inverse order of seniority that is still followed in ICUs even today.[36] He also recommended a personalized version of forgive-and-remember accountability:

> XXVIII. At the close of every interesting and important case . . . a physician should trace back, in calm reflection, all the steps which he had taken in the treatment of it. . . . This review of the whole curative plan [is important]. . . . But it is in a moral view that the practice is here recommended; and it should be performed with the most scrupulous impartiality. Let no self-deception be permitted in the retrospect; and if errors, either of omission or commission, are discovered; it behooves that they be brought fairly and fully to the mental view. Regrets may follow, but criminality will thus be obviated. For good intentions, and the imperfection of human skill which cannot anticipate the knowledge that events alone disclose, will sufficiently justify what is past, provided the failure be made conscientiously subservient to future wisdom and rectitude in professional conduct.[37]

As the case of intern N illustrates (and as Bosk's classic study confirms) Percival's nineteenth-century ethical ideals have been realized in the operant medical morality of twentieth-century American academic medical centers. Rounds reports are typically delivered in inverse status-seniority order, so that novices must forthrightly declare their treatment of patients to supervising physicians. More intriguing still, if one substitutes the notion of a *public* statement at rounds for a *personal* review, the system of forgive-and-remember ethical accountability that Percival envisioned in 1803 became standard moral practice in twentieth-century American academic medical centers. Physicians are not held culpable by their clinical peers for committing unintended medical errors; as Percival put it, "criminality will be obviated" *if* they were motivated by good intentions and by a resolution to avoid repetition of the admitted error. In Percival's words, errors can be forgiven provided that when "errors, either of omission or commission, are discovered... they be brought fairly and fully to... view," and made "conscientiously subservient to future wisdom and rectitude in professional conduct."

At some point, Percival's ethical vision of inverted-status reporting at rounds and forgive-and-remember accountability transitioned from an ethical ideal of a single medical practitioner to become the operant everyday morality of American academic medical centers. This process of change—the transition from reformist ethics to everyday morality—is integral to the history of medical ethics. Insofar as historians neglect to analyze codes, they lose the ability to document the transformative impact of medical ethics on medical morality. To discount the texts of oaths and codes is to blind oneself to important data about transitions and to the ethical and moral changes that lie at the core of the history of medical ethics and medical morality.[38]

AN OVERVIEW OF *BEFORE BIOETHICS*

As its subtitle indicates, *Before Bioethics* narrates the four-century-long history of American medical ethics and morality from the colonial and postcolonial period of the seventeenth and eighteenth centuries, through the antebellum period and post-Civil War eras, to the Progressive and interwar eras of the twentieth century, culminating in the ongoing bioethics revolution that can be dated from the 1970s—when the term "bioethics" was coined. As any history of ethics should, this narrative will analyze the transformation of ethical and moral concepts and norms. It will, for example, document how the notion of fidelity to crown and church was transformed into the concept of fidelity to the body of the sick, which in, in turn, evolved into the concept of fidelity to the patient—one of the norms violated by errant intern N. Encompassing people as well as periods and concepts, the narrative will naturally devote space to such eminent physicians as Edinburgh-educated Benjamin Rush (1745–1813), whose influential lectures on medical ethics in the years of the early republic should guarantee him a place in any history of American medical ethics. But it will also spotlight Rebekah Chamblit (ca. 1706–1733), an unwed mother executed in Puritan Massachusetts for concealing the dead body of her newly born child. Chamblit deserves attention because her gallows speech reveals the impact of Puritan ethics on unwed mothers and testifies to the morality of midwives—like the midwife who informed on Chamblit, thus setting in motion the events that placed Chamblit on the gallows.

The history of Anglo-American midwives' oaths is the subject of Chapter 2. Prefacing the chapter are two midwife's oaths—one English; the other, American—to graphically attest to the English ethical heritage evident in American midwives' oaths. Curiously, these oaths are not mentioned in the few histories that deal with American medical ethics. One historian, for example, opens a chapter dealing with the history of American medical ethics with the remark that "[t]wo men of medicine came over on the *Mayflower*. One of them, Dr. Samuel Fuller [1612–83] stayed.... But there was nothing recognizable as a medical profession in the colonies until well along in the [19th] century [when] a medical society in Boston... began to proclaim the need to regulate the practice of medicine in the public interest."[39] Dr. Fuller's wife, Bridget, however, was a practicing midwife. Unlike her husband, she did bring with her traditions of regulating medicine in the public interest: traditions that, for example, led a midwife to report to authorities that Rebekah Chamblit had given birth secretly. Moreover, this tradition was formalized in oaths, and some of these oath texts are available for analysis. Yet discussion of American midwives' oaths is strikingly absent from histories of American medical ethics.

Historians' neglect of midwives' oaths might raise the question of whether these oaths hold anything other than antiquarian interest. Do they matter? Obstetricians would ultimately eclipse midwives in the American childbirth chamber; so, does it matter that some obsolete practitioners swore an oath irrelevant to the main line of development of American medical ethics? It matters because these English-, French-, Spanish-, and Latin-language oaths are the oldest known medical ethics texts in North America; because they formulate resolutions to fundamental issues of obstetrical ethics, including maternal-fetal conflict, abortion, and infanticide; and because their centuries-long history offers a documentary basis for analyzing stability and change in ethical and moral norms. They are such an important resource, in fact, that it is astonishing that any history of American medical ethics actually ignored them. Such expressions as "*men* of medicine" suggests that, perhaps, a male-orientated perspective might have obscured the significance of *female* midwives to medical ethics in the eyes of earlier historians.

Like colonial midwives, colonial and postrevolutionary physicians and surgeons imported a British conception of medical ethics and morality. Yet, unlike midwives, they turned away from Mother England and looked instead to another people colonized by the English for inspiration—the Scots. Scottish ideals and practices in medical education, medical ethics, and medical morality dominated American medical thought and practice from the colonial period through the early republic and the antebellum period. Attesting to Scottish influence, Chapter 3 opens with a trio of oaths—one from Edinburgh, two from New York—that graphically illustrate the Scottish influence on American conceptions of medical ethics. These oaths attest to the interconnected tales of two firsts: the first British medical school to require graduates to swear a medical ethics oath and the first formal statement of medical ethics by any American medical society. The American society, moreover, appropriated the Scottish oath for the same reason that motivated the Scots to draft such an oath: a concern to fend off governmental control by asserting the moral autonomy of medicine in the name of a duty of fidelity to the sick.

Chapter 4 explores the role of the medical college of Edinburgh University as schoolmaster and role model for American physicians. It analyzes a 1769 commencement address by Samuel Bard (1742–1821) and the lectures that Benjamin Rush delivered in 1789 and from 1801 to 1811. Striking similarities in language and themes among these lectures and those that Edinburgh faculty member John Gregory (1724–1773) delivered in the 1770s illustrate how medical ethical ideals of the faithful, humane, sympathetic, and cautious physician originating at the Edinburgh medical college were disseminated to American medical students. Rush, however, rebelled against the Edinburgh virtue of caution, embracing in its place the ideal of the *bold*, or, as it later would be called, the "heroic" physician: a paternalistic dictatorial figure committed to a highly interventionist medicine and dedicated to the preservation of human life at all costs. American medicine in the nineteenth century could be understood as the unfolding of the tension between Bard's conservation of the Edinburgh ideals of practicing medicine cautiously and Rush's medical ethics of boldly heroic medicine.

The traditional subject of code formulation is the focus of Chapter 5, which traces the challenges facing American medical societies in the antebellum period, including their attempts to develop common standards of practice, differentiate between legitimate and quack physicians, and develop common fee scales. It also examines the impact of these struggles on municipal, county, and state medical societies' codes of ethics, and the use of language and concepts borrowed from the writings of Thomas Percival in these codes. Part of the appeal of Percival's rules lay in their perceived utility in addressing a dark side of the Scottish heritage—*flyting*. Flyting is a form of disputation in defense of one's status, reputation, and honor in which perceived affronts are disputed until one side or the other either secures an apology or demonstrates to an audience that the opponent is somehow contemptible or dishonorable. Eighteenth- and nineteenth-century American medicine and medical societies were plagued by gentlemanly flytes—some even rising to the status of formal duels. The chapter also deals with medical societies' efforts to address another feature of the darker side of the Scottish medical-moral heritage—body-snatching and grave robbing by medical students, with the complicity of the faculty. In reaction to this conduct, there was a doctor's riot in New York City: not a riot by doctors, but a riot against physicians and medical students suspected of grave robbing. These protests are medical ethics in its rawest form, but they are nonetheless properly included in a historical narrative of American medical ethics. The conflict culminated in a social compromise enacted in the form of anatomy laws, which, in turn, set a precedent for laws involving informed and presumed consent.

Starting in 1820, municipal, county, and state medical societies convened regular regional and national meetings to explore solutions to such shared problems as developing a standard formulary (standard ways of preparing medications and measuring doses), so that a patient suffering from some ailment, say an irregular heartbeat, would receive the same formulation of a prescription for a standard medication, such as foxglove/digitalis, when traveling from one community to another. Such a formulary would also distinguish effective and safe drugs from quack medicines. Drawing on the precedent set by the national meetings to establish standard formularies, in 1846, another national meeting was called to address the absence of common standards: in this case, uniform standards for premedical and medical education. The meeting was about to end in deadlock when, seeking to snatch something of a success from looming failure, a motion was passed to replace these numerous ad hoc national conferences on various subjects with one annual conference at which representatives from all American medical societies would meet to deal with the full range of issues confronting American medicine. This annual conference would deal with standardization issues: from standardizing formularies, to standardizing medical education, to standardizing codes of medical ethics.

To arrange these annual conferences, a national medical confederation was formed that, in the next year, 1847, was named the American Medical Association. As initially conceived, the AMA was a confederation of state and local medical societies, medical schools, hospitals, asylums, and other medical institutions formed to convene annual meetings that would address standardization and other issues facing American medicine. At its founding meeting, the AMA adopted a standard national code of medical ethics that distinguished between standard or "regular" practitioners and "irregularly" educated practitioners (e.g., homeopaths and Thomsonian botanical physicians) who were excluded from membership. By 1855, this code became binding on every "regular" medical society, medical institution, and medical practitioner in America.

The story of the creation of a national medical society and a national code of medical ethics is narrated in Chapter 6. The role played by four key actors, Nathan Smith Davis (1817–1904), John Bell (1796–1872), Gouverneur Emerson (1796–1874), and Isaac Hays (1796–1879), is explored in some detail. So too is the drama of the Kappa Lambda Society of Hippocrates, a fraternity that became America's first national medical society and a direct precursor to the American Medical Association. It was through Kappa Lambda that Bell, Hays, and Emerson began a decades-long process of adapting Percival's code of medical ethics, originally formulated for British physicians and surgeons, to the needs of American practitioners. In the end, Bell, Hays, and Emerson refashioned Percival's code of medical ethics as an explicit social contract between physicians, their patients, their fellow practitioners, and society. The AMA adopted the resulting four-chapter, eleven-article, fifty-section social contract as its official Code of Ethics in 1847. In this code, the formerly prevalent discourse of gentlemanly character and honor (discussed in Chapter 3) is replaced by a discourse of professional duties.

Chapter 7, "Professional Medical Ethics: Abortion, Exclusion, and Inquisition," focuses on a series of decisions made by the AMA by which it introduced content into the yet-to-be defined concepts of "professionalism" and "professional ethics" that it inherited when it adopted Percival's language for its code of ethics. After examining the scientific, moral, and social basis of the AMA's campaign to criminalize prequickening abortion, the chapter explores the decisions by which the AMA interpreted what it meant by a "professional." As it turned out, the AMA interpreted the new concept of a professional in terms of traditional ideals of gentlemanly honor, creating a conception of a professional who, like an honorable gentleman, was engaged in a noncommercial, secular enterprise dedicated to high ideals of science and health, and who, again like the traditional gentleman, was white and male. In the post-Civil War period, this reading of professionalism and of the AMA's code of ethics became a lightning rod for controversy and an instrument of exclusion, wielded not only against "irregulars" but also against African-American and female physicians—and specialists (whose advertisements were deemed commercial, misleading, and unfair).

Chapter 8, "Anti-Ethics Revolution and Laissez Faire Medical Ethics," opens with a little-known phenomenon that recontoured the shape of American medical ethics: a counterrevolution, a revolt within the AMA, in which sanitarians (as public health practitioners were called at the time), scientists, and specialists, chafing at the constraints imposed by the 1847 AMA Code of Ethics, broke from AMA. They later rejoined the organization to stage a coup d'état, taking leadership positions to rewrite the AMA code of ethics as a set of laissez faire principles that substitute individual practitioner's conscience for the ethics of a social compact.

Chapter 9, "American Research Ethics 1800–1946," traces the development of the ethics and morality of American medical research through the nineteenth and twentieth centuries. It focuses on the use of servants and slaves as human subjects by such medical luminaries as U.S. Army surgeon, William Beaumont (1785–1853), whose reputation as the "Father of Gastric Physiology" rests on experiments that he conducted on his servant, Alexis St. Martin (1794–1880). It also discusses the research of James Marion Sims (1818–1883), in whose honor a statue was erected in New York City's Central Park in 1894, commemorating his perfection of a gynecological operation that he developed by experimenting on unanesthetized female African-American slaves. The chapter also examines the 1900 Walter Reed Yellow Fever experiments, which paved the way for a newer model of research ethics based on "volunteerism" and informed consent contracts. Yet, because laissez faire ethics limited the prerogatives of the AMA, Walter Bradford Cannon (1871–1945), president of the AMA in 1914, failed to convince the organization to adopt the principle that experimenting on humans without their consent was unethical and to prohibit the publication of unconsented research. When the AMA refused to take a stand on the ethics of research, ceding the protection of human subjects to the conscience of the researchers themselves, it paved the way for decades of human subjects abuse.

As I show in Chapter 10, the AMA's failure to address not only the ethics of human subjects research but a host of other ethical issues confronting post-World War II American medicine, created the conditions for the emergence of a new paradigm of the relationship between physicians and patients, and medical researchers and their subjects—"bioethics." Current accounts of these research scandals proffer a sequence of events as if it were an explanation of this phenomenon. They detail *what* happened, *when*, *where* and *how*, *who* was involved, and what motivated people to become bioethicists. Missing, however, is a pivotal question essential to transforming an essentially journalistic account into a historical analysis—*Why*? Why couldn't American governmental agencies and professional societies expand government regulation and professional ethics to provide human subjects protections without engendering a bioethics movement? Britain and continental Europe managed to address the issue of protecting human research subjects without launching a bioethics movement. Why was America different? Why did Americans invent a new field, bioethics? Part of the answer is that American medical societies had embraced a laissez faire ethics in which individual practitioners' consciences substituted for authoritative ethical policymaking. This ethos created a vacuum of authority with respect to medical ethics policymaking. Consequently, when individual conscience proved inadequate to prevent ethics scandals in research or to resolve ethical issues surrounding emerging medical technologies, American society sought an alternative source of ethical guidance—and bioethics was born of necessity.

2

MIDWIVES' OATHS OF FIDELITY AND DILIGENCE

That she shall be diligent and ready to help any woman in labor, whether she be poor or rich; that in time of necessity she will not forsake the poor woman and go to the rich; that she will not cause or suffer any woman to name or put any other father to the child, but only him which is the true father thereof, indeed, according to the utmost of her power; that she will not suffer any woman to pretend to be delivered of a child who is not, indeed, neither to claim any other woman's child as her own; that she will not suffer any woman's child to be murdered or hurt; and, as often as she may see any peril or jeopardy, either in the mother or child, she will call other midwives for council; that she will not administer any medicine to produce a miscarriage; that she will not enforce a woman to give more for services than is right; that she will not collude to keep secret the birth of a child; will be of good behavior; and will not conceal the birth of bastards.[1]

Midwives' Oath, New York City, 1716

I Eleanor Pead admitted to the office and occupation of a midwife, will faithfully and diligently exercise the said office according to such cunning and knowledge as God hath given me.

And that I will be ready to help and aid as well the poor as the rich woman being in labor and travail of child, and will always be ready both to poor and rich, in exercising and executing of my said office.

Also, I will not permit, or suffer that women being in labour or travail shall name any other to be the father of her child, than only he who is the right and true father thereof; and that I will not suffer any other body's child to be set, brought or laid before any woman delivered of child in the place of her natural child, so far forth as I can know and understand.

Also, I will not use any kind or sorcery or incantation in the time of the travail of any woman, and that I will not destroy the child born of any woman, nor cut or pull off the head thereof, nor otherwise dismember or hurt the same, or suffer it to be hurt or dismembered, by any manner of ways or means.

Also, that in the ministration of the sacrament of the baptism in the time of necessity I will use apt and the accustomed words of the same sacrament, that is to say, these words following, or to the like effect; "I christen thee in the name of the Father, the Son, and the Holy Ghost."

And that in such time of necessity, in baptizing any infant born, and pouring water upon the head of the same infant, I will use pure and clean water.

And not any rose or damask water, or water made of any confection or mixture: and that I will certify the curate of the parish church of every such baptism.[2]

Eleanor Pead's Oath, Canterbury, England, 1567

THE ENGLISH HERITAGE OF AMERICAN MIDWIVES' OATHS

Res ipsa loquitur is a Latin expression still used by lawyers to capture the insight that some things speak for themselves. The parallelism between the two oaths prefacing this chapter, the eighteenth-century colonial American oath, sworn before a municipal official in New York City and the sixteenth-century English oath sworn before the Archbishop of Canterbury or a church official, speaks for itself. These oaths belong to the same tradition. That tradition is evident in North American midwives' oaths in English, French, Latin, and Spanish and constitutes the oldest documented form of European medical ethics evident in the colonial Americas. It traces to continental Europe, where these oaths date to at least 1365 in France[3] and as early as 1452 in Germany.[4] The English-language tradition dates to at least the 1550s, when Edmund Bonner (c. 1500–1569), Roman Catholic Bishop of London under "Bloody" Queen Mary I (1516–1558, reigned 1553–1558), introduced the practice of having midwives police the birth chamber in England.[5]

He also initiated a traveling inquisition that visited local parishes, interrogating midwives with a standard set of questions known as the Articles of Visitation. Midwives were questioned about whether their sister midwives were faithful, discrete, sober, and diligent; were ready to help all who seek their assistance; or practiced witchcraft,[6] sorcery, incantations, or manifested "any other disorder or evil behavior,"[7] such as administering emergency baptismal rites not approved by Roman Catholic church.

In 1555, Bishop Bonner supplemented the Articles of Visitation with an oath that midwives had to swear in order to receive a license to practice:

> Ye shall n[ei]ther cause no[r] suffer any woman to nayme or put other father to the chylde but only hym that ys the verey father in dede thereof.
>
> Item, Ye shall not suffer any woman to pretend, fane, or surmyse herself to be delivered of chylde which is not in dede [hers]; n[ei]ther to name any other woman's chylde for her own.
>
> Item, ye shall not suffer any chylde to be murdered, maymed, or otherwise hurtydem as nygh—
>
> Item, ye shall not in anywyse use or exercise anye manner of wytchcrafte, sorcerye, invocations or other prayers than may stand with Godde's lawes and the kynge's!
>
> Item, Ye shall have perfectly the woordes appointed for baptysme of children, and use noone other but the same, that ys to say, "I chrysteyn thee N," &c.
>
> Item, When of necessitie ye shall chrystyn any chylde, ye shall use pure and cleane water, nother mixt with rose water, damaske water, or otherwise altered or confected.
>
> Item, ye shall not ynforce any woman by paynes, or by any other ungodly wayes or meanes, to give you any more or greater reward for bryngying her a beede than she would otherwise doo.
>
> Item, ye shall never consent nor agree that any woman be delivered secretly, but in the presence of two or three lyghtes, if she do travell by nyght.
>
> Item, If eny chylde be dead borne, ye shall see yt buried in such secrete place as nother hogge, nor dogge, nor any other beast may come to yt; and ye shall not suffer eny such chylde to be cast into the jaks, or yn eny other inconvenient place or unhonest place, &c.[8]

Rendered into twenty-first-century English, Bonner's oath could be transliterated as:

- You shall not cause or permit any woman to name a man as her child's father unless he is actually the child's [biological] father.

- You shall not permit any child to be murdered, maimed, or otherwise harmed.
- You shall not in any way use or exercise any form of witchcraft, sorcery, invocation, or other [forms of] prayer, except those permitted by God's laws and the king's.
- You shall memorize the official words for baptizing children and only use these words [in baptizing them], i.e., "I christen thee N…"
- When it is necessary to perform [an emergency] christening of a child, you shall use pure and clean water, not water mixed with rose water or otherwise contaminated.
- You shall not extort higher fees for your services from any laboring woman by making her suffer [unnecessary] pain or by any other ungodly means.
- You shall neither consent nor agree to a secret delivery by any woman; and if she travels by night two or three lights must illuminate her route. [NB: public streetlights were introduced to London in 1807, prior to that servants carrying torches or lamps aided nighttime travel.]
- If a child is born dead you shall ensure that it is buried in a secure place so that neither hogs, nor dogs, nor any other beast may uncover its [body], and you shall not permit the corpse of any such child to be cast into any outhouse [jaks] or in any other out of the way or dishonest place.

One out-of-context feature of Bonner's oath is that it opens and closes on a theme absent from similar continental midwives oaths[9] and from the earlier Articles of Visitation: the paternity and treatment of bastard and stillborn infants. Since this oath was designed as part of Queen Mary's campaign to purge the English Church of Protestantism and of pagan religious practices, the preoccupation with bastardy, paternity, and stillborn infants seems out of place. Bishops on the European continent introduced no comparable clauses about midwives' obligations to determine the paternity of bastards,[10] so one might wonder why bastardy, paternity, and stillborn infants hold such a prominent place in the British oath.

A straightforward explanation for Bishop Bonner's preoccupation with bastardy is found in his biography. He was a bastard. Bonner is generally acknowledged to have been the bastard son of a parish rector, George Savage, who arranged to have the boy's mother marry a local carpenter, Edmund Bonner.[11] One need not probe too deeply into Bonner's psyche to speculate that by insisting that midwives force mothers to reveal the true paternity of their bastard children, by requiring them to protect living bastards against harm, and by demanding that dead bastards be given a decent burial—so neither "hogge, nor dogge, nor any other beast may come to yt; and ye shall not suffer eny such chylde to be cast into the [outhouse], or yn eny other… unhonest place"[12]—he was mindful of his own bastardy and sought to protect the lives, dignity, and immortal souls of fellow bastards, newborn and stillborn.[13]

As an agent licensed by and answerable to the ecclesiastic authority of the official state religion, the midwife was also committed by Bonner's oath to survey, report, and prevent any improprieties in christening, any misrepresentation of births and deaths, and any abuse of infants, living or dead. She was further obligated to interrogate unmarried women during labor about the true paternity of their child. These obligations of interrogation, surveillance, reporting, and protection placed midwives in a position of dual loyalty comparable to that of the modern social worker[14]—except that the licensing authority in 1555 was actively engaged in burning heretics at the stake. By placing the interests of the church and the crown above those of the women who called midwives to the birth bed, Bonner's oath challenged any expectations of confidentiality between midwives and laboring women.[15]

SEVENTEENTH-CENTURY PURITAN OATHS

Bonner was removed as bishop of London in 1560, at about the same time that Calvinist reformers known as "Puritans" rose to parliamentary power, acquiring influence in the Church of England under Elizabeth I (1533–1603, reigned 1558–1603) and James I (1566–1625, reigned 1603–1625). Puritan bishops retained the practice of oath swearing, perpetuating the tradition of dual loyalties that Bonner had initiated and retaining with it Bonner's preoccupation with bastardy. By the mid-seventeenth century, Anglican midwives were swearing a full-blown Puritan oath:

> You shall swear first, that you shall be diligent and faithful and ready to help every woman laboring of child, as well the poor as the rich; and that in time of necessity, you shall not forsake the poor woman, to go to the rich.
>
> Item. You shall neither cause nor suffer any woman to name, or put any other father to the child, but only him which is very true father thereof indeed.
>
> Item. You shall not suffer any woman to pretend, fain, or surmise herself to be delivered of a child who is not indeed; neither to claim any other woman's child for her own.
>
> Item. You shall not suffer any woman's child to be murdered, maimed, or otherwise hurt, as much as you may; and so often as you shall perceive any peril or jeopardy, either in the woman or in the child, in any such wise, as you shall be in doubt what shall chance thereof, you shall thenceforth in due

time send for other midwives and expert women in that faculty, and use their advice and counsel in that behalf.

Item. You shall not, in any wise, use or exercise any manner of witchcraft, charms or sorcery, invocation or other prayers than may stand with God's laws and the King's.

Item. You shall not give any counsel or minister any herb, medicine or potion, or any other thing, to any woman being with child whereby she should destroy or cast out, that she goeth withal before her time.

Item. You shall not enforce any woman being with child by any pain, or by an ungodly ways or means, to give you any more for your pains or labor in bringing her abed, than they would otherwise do.

Item. You shall not consent, agree, give, or keep counsel that any woman be delivered secretly of that which she goeth with, but in the presence of two or three lights ready.

Item. You shall be secret and not open any matter appertaining to your office in the presence of any man, unless necessity or great urgent cause to constrain you so to do.

Item. If any child be dead born, you yourself shall see it buried in such secret place as neither hog nor dog, nor any other beast may come unto it, and in such sort done as it be not found not perceived, as much as you may; and that you shall not suffer any such child to be cast into the jaques [i.e., the outhouse] or any other inconvenient place.

Item. If you shall know any midwife using or doing anything contrary to any of the premises, or in any other wise than shall be seemly and convenient, you shall forthwith detect open to show the same to me [i.e., the bishop who administers the oath] or my Chancellor for the time being.

Item. You shall use yourself in honest behavior unto the woman, being lawfully admitted to the room and office of midwife in all things accordingly.

Item. That you shall truly present to myself, or my chancellor, all such women as you shall know from time to time to occupy and exercise the room of a midwife within my diocese and jurisdiction of _______, without my license and admission.

Item. You shall not make or assign any deputy or deputies to exercise or occupy under you in your absence the office or room of a midwife, but such as you shall perfectly know to be of right honest and discreet behavior, as also apt and able and having sufficient knowledge and experience to exercise the said room and office.

Item. You shall not be privy, or consent that any priest, or other party, shall in your absence, or in your company, or of your knowledge or sufferance, baptize any child by any Mass, Latin service or prayers than such as are appointed by the laws of the Church of England; neither shall you consent that any child, born of any woman, who shall be delivered by you, shall be carried away without being baptized in the parish by the ordinary minister where the said child is born, unless it be in case of necessity, baptized privately, according to the Book of Common Prayer: but you shall forthwith upon understanding thereof, either give knowledge to me the said bishop, or my chancellor for the time being.

All which articles and charge you shall faithfully observe and keep, so help you God, and by the content of this book [the Holy Bible].[16] (Puritan-Influenced Anglican Oath, 1649)

As is evident from the last Item, this Puritan adaptation of the Anglican midwife's oath continues the baptismal wars, expressly prohibiting the rituals of the Roman Catholic Church and mandating baptism according to Anglican rites. Thus, midwives are not to be "privy [to], or consent that any priest, or other party, shall in your absence, or in your company, or of your knowledge or sufferance, baptize any child by any [Roman Catholic] Mass, Latin service or prayers." The midwife was also to ensure that an ordinary Anglican minister employed the rituals "of the Church of England" in baptizing the child. Should a midwife need to perform an emergency baptism, she was to follow the rituals in the Anglican Book of Common Prayer (established 1549), then inform either the bishop or his assistant.[17]

The oath also reflects the Puritan values and their emphasis on honesty, requiring midwives to conduct themselves "in *honest* behavior unto the woman," and to employ assistants "know[n] to be of right *honest* and discreet behavior, as also apt and able and having sufficient knowledge and experience."[18] Puritan influence is also evident in the exclusion of males from the birth chamber and in its insistence that a midwife must "be secret and not open any matter appertaining to your office in the presence of any man" except for surgeons, and even then only when "necessity or great urgent cause" makes their service essential.[19] Men were also excluded from childbirth if they "presum[ed] to act the part of midwife."[20]

The most strikingly Puritan provision of the 1649 oath is the requirement that, "You shall not give any counsel or minister any herb, medicine or potion, or any other thing, to any woman being with child whereby she should destroy or cast out, that she goeth withal before her time."[21] Until the end of the nineteenth century, neither the Anglican nor the Roman Catholic Church prohibited what would later be characterized as first trimester "abortions." Like its Anglican sister, the Roman Catholic Church recognized a distinction between the moral status of the inanimate (first-trimester) fetus and the animated or "quickened" fetus (i.e., a fetus considered ensouled because it was capable of initiating movement and was thus animated or "quickened"). Thus, neither Anglican nor Roman Catholic theology classified the intentional termination of pregnancy prior to quickening as homicide.[22] Not surprisingly, therefore, neither Bonner's Roman Catholic oath (1555) nor the later Anglican oaths sworn by Eleanor Pead (1567) and Mary Cooke (1713) prohibit the intentional termination of pregnancy or mention abortion; they only prohibit harming or "destroy[ing] the child *born* of any woman."

Seventeenth-century Puritans, in contrast, declined to recognize any distinction between the quickened and prequickened fetus. Hewing to Calvin's view that the fetus at any stage of development is already a human being, they condemned as sinful and treated as homicidal *any* attempt to terminate a pregnancy. John Calvin (1509–1564) had expressly stated that the "foetus, though enclosed in the womb of its mother, is already a human being.... If it seems more horrible to kill a man in his own house than in a field, because a man's house is his place of most secure refuge, it ought surely to be deemed more atrocious to destroy a foetus in the womb before it has come to light."[23] Not surprisingly, in Puritan Massachusetts, intentional termination of a pregnancy was a sin and an indictable criminal offense.[24]

The Puritan-influenced Anglican oath also incorporates the interrogatories of Bishop Bonner's Articles of Visitation, reparsing them as items of the oath. Like the oaths sworn by Pead and Cooke, it opens with a line from the Articles asserting the midwife's obligation to attend and to "be diligent and faithful and ready to help every woman laboring of child," specifying this obligation as applying "as well [to] the poor as the rich" and adding with even more specificity "that in time of necessity, you shall not forsake the poor woman, to go to the rich."[25] Following the path laid out by the Articles of Visitation, the Puritan oath also obligates midwives to police the ethical conduct of their peers by reporting to authorities the presence of unlicensed midwives and to bring to their attention any dishonest, indiscrete, or incompetent conduct by fellow midwives, licensed or unlicensed. Like Bonner's oath and the Canterbury oath, the Puritan oath obligates midwives to enforce the state religion, conduct surveillance on pregnant women and their families, and report to the bishop all suspicions of misconduct.

THE MEDICAL ETHICS AND MORALITY OF COLONIAL AMERICAN MIDWIVES

England's North American colonies originated as European enclaves on the continent's eastern seaboard. The few trained medical practitioners in these early colonies were mostly midwives. The first midwife known to have settled in New England was Bridget Fuller (fl. 1633–1663), who, as noted in Chapter 1, came over in 1623 on the ship *Anne* to join her husband, a surgeon who had arrived on the *Mayflower* three years earlier.[26] As a Pilgrim who belonged to a Calvinist group that considered the Anglican Church impure, Bridget would *not* have sworn an

Anglican oath. The Puritan midwives who settled the Massachusetts Bay Colony (established 1629–1630), however, were Calvinists and, although some historians hold that they swore an oath like the Canterbury oath, the only documented text of a colonial American midwife's oath is the New York oath prefacing this chapter, which hews closer to the English Puritan oath.[27]

Colonial Massachusetts and colonial New York, although geographical neighbors, were worlds apart socially. The Massachusetts settlements were Pilgrim-Puritan theocratic societies predicated on "veridical" visions of Christian community. Tolerance of dissenting religious voices was minimal: so, for example, Roger Williams (1603–1683) was exiled from Massachusetts for preaching such heresies as the need for a wall of separation between church and state. Mercantile New York, in contrast, was an island of tolerance. Founded as New Amsterdam (1614–1674), a trading center for the Dutch colony of New Netherlands, it inherited traditions of religious freedom and separation of the church from civil governance under the Dutch constitution. So, New Netherlands provided a safe haven for religious exiles from theocratic Massachusetts, such as the midwife Anne Hutchinson (1591–1643).[28]

The Dutch tradition of religious tolerance survived the 1674 English conquest of New Netherlands and the subsequent renaming of both the colony and its capital city, "New York," in honor of the Duke of York. A body of law known as the Duke of York's laws of 1665 and 1675 applied to all three Northeastern British settlements: New Jersey, New York, and Massachusetts (and its territories, including Rhode Island and Providence Plantations).[29] Among these laws was a provision restricting entry into the medical occupations of midwifery, surgery, and physic to those approved by experienced practitioners.[30] Following English practice, applicants for a midwife's license had to provide an ecclesiastical authority with testimonials from more experienced practitioners and/or from the women whom they assisted in the birthing process (typically, under supervision of more experienced midwives) attesting to the length and success of their experience as midwives. These testimonials attested to the applicant's "imployment [as] midwife twenty or thirty years past with good success," or state that she is "apt, able, cunning, expert."[31] Acting on such testimonials, an ecclesiastical authority might approve a license for midwifery, which would be granted upon paying a fee and swearing an oath that the applicant either signed or swore to verbally.[32]

THE MEDICAL MORALITY OF MIDWIVES

Historian Doreen Evenden documents consonance between midwives' actual conduct and the conduct required in their oaths, which is to say that midwives' medical morality was, for the most part, consonant with that required by the ethics of their oaths. Thus, Evenden cites as an example a 1664 incident in which an English midwife

> Mary Franck… refused to cooperate in the unorthodox baptism of an infant without godparents since "shee Could no admitt ye child to bee baptised after that way it being contrary to her Oath." [Furthermore, to cite another incident] Sarah Fish, an elderly gentlewoman of Enfield was well aware of the [oath's requirement to be diligent and faithful and ready to help every woman laboring of child] when [she]… sought [to be] excused from taking the oath in 1697… [because she] "being aged is loth to be hurryed in ye night and in bad weather [for deliveries] to ye prejudice of her health."[33]

Aspiring midwife Sarah Fish and midwife Mary Franck took the precepts of the oath seriously: the latter affirming their importance by seeking to be excused from the onerous duty of attending to *every* delivery for which her services would be requested, irrespective of the time of day or the inclemency of the weather, the former by enforcing the baptismal rules imposed by the oath. In these cases, the medical ethics of the midwife's oath defined everyday medical morality as these midwives understood it.

Although the formalized ethics of oaths and codes is usually more readily documented than evidence of practitioners' medical morality, at present we know more about the standards to which New England Puritan midwives were held accountable than about the text of any oaths sworn by midwives.[34] One resource is diaries. The dairy of Maine midwife Martha Ballard (1735–1812), for example, indicates that she followed the fundamental precepts of the midwife's oaths by attending to *everyone* who called on her services, irrespective of their ability to pay—although, like all American practitioners, she still expected payment, if not in cash then in notes of credit or in goods or services.[35] More dramatically, founding governor of the Massachusetts Bay colony, John Winthrop (1588–1649), describes the sad case of twenty-one-year-old Mary Martin. A married man "soliciting [Mary's] chastity, obtained his desire, and having divers times committed sin with her. [Mary ran away and] put herself in service [as a maid]; and finding herself to be with child, and not able to bear the shame of it, she concealed it."[36] Acting in accordance with the obligation of surveillance stipulated in midwives' oaths, "a midwife in the town, having formerly suspected [Mary of being pregnant] coming to her again, found she had been delivered of a child, which upon examination, she confessed, but said it was stillborn, and so she put it in the fire. But search being made it was found in her chest… a surgeon, being called to examine the body of the child, found a fracture in the skull."[37]

Precepts found in midwives' oaths were also enforced in the Massachusetts colony through an "Act to prevent the destroying and murthering of bastard children" that was passed by the English Puritan Parliament of 1624 and adopted by Puritan Massachusetts in 1696.[38] The reasons for the act are quite explicit:

> WHEREAS, many lewd women that have been delivered of bastard children, to avoid their shame and to escape punishment, do secretly bury and conceal the death of their children, and after, if the child be found dead, the said women do alledge, that the said child was born dead; whereas it falleth out sometimes... that the said child or children were murthered by the said women, their lewd mothers, or by their assent or procurement....
>
> For the preventing therefore of this great mischief, be it enacted... That if any woman... be delivered of any issue of her body, male or female, which being born alive, should by the laws of this realm be a bastard, and that she endeavor privately, either by drowning or secret burying thereof, or any other way, either by herself or the procuring of others, so to conceal the death thereof, as that it may not come to light, whether it were born alive of not, but be concealed: in every case the said mother so offending shall suffer death as in the case of murther, except such mother can make proof by one witness at least, that the child (whose death was by her so intended to be concealed) was born dead.[39]

In other words, any woman found with the dead body of a newborn infant will be presumed to have committed infanticide unless she can prove "by one witness at least" that the child was stillborn. This law thus treats concealment of a crime as presumptive evidence of commission of said crime. Anglo-American law, however, typically separates and distinguishes acts of concealment from acts of commission because embarrassment and fear of public censure may motivate people to conceal things, even if they have not done anything criminal.[40] Consequently, to use the words of the act, although it may "falleth out *sometimes*" that lewd women found with dead infants are guilty of infanticide, it may also falleth out that lewd women found with dead babies *are innocent* because their child was stillborn. This law thus presumes that it is better to execute lewd women who are sometimes innocent rather than let any infanticidal lewd woman go unpunished—lewdness seems to deprive these women of the presumption of innocence.

New England Puritans invoked the 1696 law to pronounce guilty of infanticide an unmarried Boston mother, Rebekah Chamblit, on the grounds that she had attempted to hide her baby's corpse. In a gallows "confession," transcribed on the day of her execution, September 27, 1733, Chamblit protested that "in all which time [of her pregnancy] I am not sensible I [f]elt any Life or Motion in the Child within me [i.e., there were no signs of quickening]; when, the Tuesday the Eighth Day of *May,* I was D[e]liver'd when alo[n]e of a Male Infa[n]t; in whom I did not perceive Life." "BEING under the awful Apprehension of my Execution now in a few Hours; and being desirous to do all the Good I can, before I enter the Eternal Worl[d]," Chamblt confessed that although "[st]ill uncertain of Life [i]n [i]t, I threw it into the Vault about two or three Minutes after it was born, [uncertain], I say, whether it was a living or dead Child." Chamblit concluded reluctantly that, "I confess [it] probable [that] there was Life in it."[41]

Midwives were inextricably ensnared in the spinster mother's dilemma: their testimony would either condemn the woman to public censure or consign her to the gallows. A midwife who would not violate her oath-sworn duty thus inevitably became complicit in the single mother's damnation and possibly her death. The Puritan law punishing "lewd" women made midwives both protectors of bastard infants' lives and guardians and guarantors of Puritan sexual morality. By the late eighteenth century, Puritan influence in Massachusetts was waning, and, in 1784, Massachusetts repealed the act to prevent the destroying and murdering of bastard children. Spinster mothers in Massachusetts, like Rebekah Chamblit, would no longer be at risk of the death penalty because they attempted to hide the corpse of their stillborn babies—and midwives would no longer be complicit in their censure or execution.

THE MEDICAL ETHICS AND MEDICAL MORALITY OF NEW YORK MIDWIVES

None of the tragedy played out in Massachusetts unfolded in its multireligious, multiethnic neighbor, New York. An 1818 attempt to prosecute a single mother, Clarissa Davie, on the grounds that she had attempted to hide the corpse of her stillborn baby, was unsuccessful.[42] New Yorkers had always had a more secular conception of the role of midwife. In July 1716, when New York City alderman passed new regulations governing the licensing of medical practitioners, it accommodated and secularized its English heritage by requiring midwives to swear the oath that prefaces this chapter.[43] What is striking about the New York Midwife's oath is that it appears to be a civic incarnation of the Puritan oath of 1649—from which the provisions dealing with baptism, witchcraft, and burial have been excised.

The New York oath retains the Puritan requirement that midwives be diligently ready to assist any woman in labor, poor or rich. It also requires fidelity to patients in not forsaking a poorer woman for a richer one. Midwives, moreover, are obligated to ascertain truthful paternity, truthful maternity, and to report and not to be complicit in infanticide or child abuse. Midwives are to consult with each other to protect the life and health of mother and child, and they may not overcharge their patients nor collude with them to keep the birth of a child secret or conceal the birth of bastards. Significantly, the New York oath preserves the Puritan oath's prohibition against abortion, but this provision has been updated and secularized to read, "she will not administer any medicine to produce a miscarriage."[44] In 1731, another uniquely Puritan tenet, the exclusion of men from the childbirth chamber, was added to the New York oath.[45]

It is impressive that the New York City oath shares with its Puritan prototype a vision of midwifery as an occupation demanding skill, knowledge, and moral integrity. These oaths envision a practice of midwifery that transcends commercial interests, pledging midwives to fidelity to both mother and child—not to abandon the poor woman for the rich one, not to take bribes to hide the birth of bastards, and not to permit a fee-paying mother to harm her child. The oaths also offer ethical guidance for the complex and tragic circumstances of unmarried pregnant women seeking to terminate their pregnancies, of newly delivered mothers who will not name the men who fathered their babies, and of women so desperate to keep their reputations, or so desperately poor,[46] that they attempt to murder their newborn babies and hide the bodies. Midwives witnessing these tragedies were torn between conflicting loyalties to the mother, to the child, and to society. Like its Puritan precursor, the New York City oath demanded loyalty first to the community, then to child, and last to the mother—albeit the interests of mothers trumped midwives' financial interests, since they could not abandon the poor for more lucrative attendance on the rich.

Although the secular New York midwife was not required to interrogate single mothers to reveal the paternity of their bastard children, she was still obligated to reveal secrets about paternity, prohibited from inducing miscarriages or from assisting or covering up infanticide. Miscarriages, births, and paternity were to be truthfully and publicly declared to officials. The all-male alderman of New York City, unequivocally sympathetic to the fatherly interests of fellow males, had fashioned a code of ethics for the all-female practitioners of midwifery that protected the paternal rights of fathers by continuing the tradition of stripping women of any right to confidentiality with respect to their honorable reputation, the paternity of their children, or stillbirths.

THE DECLINE OF MIDWIFERY AND MIDWIVES' OATHS

A careful study of midwifery in London found that "by 1720, the licensing system had begun to break down"[47] because the Church of England, triumphant in the baptismal wars, was losing interest in regulating the conduct of midwives. Exacerbating this loss of interest was the displacement of female midwives by man-midwives or "obstetricians" (to use the Latinate name coined in the mid-eighteenth century to describe the surgeon who stands opposite to the laboring woman). English midwives had always called on surgeons to assist them during difficult pregnancies, but the surgeon's role began to change in the 1750s when Scottish surgeon William Smellie (1697–1763) published a series of books that included an anatomical atlas accurately illustrating fetal development and depicting the proper use of the obstetrical forceps.[48]

An American surgeon, William Shippen Jr. (1736–1808), offered the first American lectures on the new midwifery practices in Philadelphia, in 1765. Although (male) medical students could audit the course, Shippen's lectures were directed to the practitioners most likely to deliver babies in Philadelphia: female midwives "who have virtue enough to own their ignorance and apply for instruction."[49] Following Shippen's precedent, his student, New York physician Valentine Seaman (1770–1817) also offered lectures to educate female midwives in New York in 1799. Similarly, in 1807–1808, the Edinburgh-educated New York physician Samuel Bard wrote a *Compendium of the Theory and Practice of Midwifery* designed for the use of (female) midwives—although later editions of the book indicate that it was actually reaching an audience of more affluent and literate male physicians rather than less affluent and often illiterate female midwives.

Despite these and other efforts to offer instruction on the latest medical advances in midwifery practice to female midwives, few female midwives enrolled in these lectures. As the eighteenth century drew to a close, American women in urban areas like New York City and Philadelphia increasingly began to send for obstetricians or family physicians, rather than for female midwives. The female midwife was losing her place as the preferred medical practitioner in the American childbirth chamber. New York City enacted the last version of the Midwife's Act and the last version of the Midwife's Oath in 1763. Foreshadowing future developments, just three years earlier, in 1760, the first New York City law calling for a licensing board to examine physicians and surgeons was passed. For the first time in the history of New York City, midwifery was not accorded that hallmark of professional status—examination and licensing. Only physicians and surgeons were to be licensed, although, from at least 1808, the Medical Society for the County of New York provided certificates for midwives, effectively licensing them but marking their role as subservient to physicians.[50] Some outlying jurisdictions, most notably Albany (not yet New York state's capital city), attempted to regulate male midwives in the manner of female midwives. A 1773 ordinance, modeled after the 1731 New York City midwives act, applied the same regulations to male and female midwives, requiring both to swear a version of the New York City midwife's oath.[51]

NORM CONSERVATION DURING TWO CENTURIES OF ANGLO-AMERICAN MIDWIVES' OATHS

The record left by these oaths attests to an extraordinary stability in ethical expectations for midwives' conduct, a phenomenon that can be characterized as *norm conservation* (i.e., the preservation of norms of character and conduct through other changes). To appreciate the extent of norm conservation in Anglo-American midwives' oaths, one needs to distinguish between religious and ethics themes: religious themes address the relationship between divinity and humanity, or between ecclesiastical institutions, officials, and rituals and the laity. Bishop Bonner's 1555 oath, for example, used religiously themed language to address the relationship of midwife, mother, and child to God and the church. Midwives are forbidden to engage in "anye manner of wytchcrafte, sorcerye, invocations or other prayers than may stand with Godde's law," and they are instructed about proper ritual ("the woordes appointed for baptysme of children") and the purity of the christening ritual ("ye shall use pure and cleane water"). In keeping with the conceptual framework of the era, the midwife's relationship with the laboring woman is also characterized in religious language: extorting high payments for care is condemned as "ungodly wayes or meanes."[52]

Ethical language, in contrast, relates to people's more mundane ideals of midwives' relationships to society, to each other and to themselves. Intriguingly, Bonner uses ethical language only in the items relating to the midwife's relations to bastards. The prohibition that "ye shall not suffer any chylde to be murdered, maymed, or otherwise hurtydem,"[53] for example, omits any mention of evil or sin. Even burial instructions requiring that "ye shall not suffer eny such [bastard] chylde to be cast into the jaks [outhouse], or yn eny other inconvenient place or unhonest place, &c,"[54] is characterized ethically as "unhonest" rather than "unholy." The relationships between midwife, mother, and child, including the honest naming of a child, the determination of its paternity, the dishonest feigning motherhood, and issues of battery and infanticide are always characterized in the person-to-person language of ethics, not in religious language.

Norms characterized in ethical language in midwives' oaths tend to be conserved and remain stable even as the religious-themed language changed in the context of two centuries of radical, sometimes bloody, sociopolitical and religious changes from Catholic to Protestant to Puritan to secular. More specifically, although the religious-themed language of midwives' oaths changes markedly and is ultimately secularized, once an ethical norm was added to the midwives' oaths, it tends to stick (i.e., to be conserved—although sometimes specified or elaborated—through religious and antireligious change, except insofar as there was a clear external reason to expunge it). Thus, discussions of baptismal rituals change from Catholic to Protestant to Puritan and are ultimately deleted from the secular New York municipal oath. In contrast, the 1567 oath's provision, "I will be ready to help and aid as well the poor as the rich woman being in labor and travail of child"[55]—part of Bonner's Catholic inquisitorial Articles of Visitation, originally a tactical requirement of the baptismal wars—was parsed in ethical language in the text of the Protestant Canterbury oath. The commitment sticks through later oaths: the norm is conserved, and a variant of this line is added to all known successor Anglo-American oaths, including the 1649 Puritan oath, and the 1716, 1763, and 1773 New York City and Albany oaths. In these later oaths, the ethical language conserves the moral norm: "That she shall be diligent and ready to help any woman in labor, whether she be poor or rich; that in time of necessity she will not forsake the poor woman and go to the rich."[56] All that changes is that the obligation was specified (initially in its 1649 Puritan formulation) to indicate that obligations of diligence and fidelity apply not only in responding to calls for assistance from poor and rich alike, but in delivering care to poor and rich equally. Similarly, Bonner's highly personal norm of protecting bastards' lives and patrimony, which is also parsed in ethical language, is conserved in all later oaths, even though others had no reason to share Bonner's psychological motives.

Another example of ethical norm conservation is the Puritan extension of protection from the newborn to the unborn. Initially framed in ethical rather than religious language as "You shall not give any counsel or minister any herb, medicine or potion, or any other thing, to any woman being with child whereby she should destroy or cast out, that she goeth withal before her time," the norm survived secularization even in the cosmopolitan cultures of New York City and Albany, where midwives' oaths obligated them " not [to] administer any medicine to produce a miscarriage." These examples suggest that once an ethical norm (or at least a norm formulated in ethical language) is introduced into a formal statement of ethics of the sort articulated in oaths, it will tend to be "sticky," enduring through changes in justifying conceptions and different formulations unless there is some pressing reason to remove it. Thus, Bonner's concerns about bastardy survive to secular New York, even though they probably originated from his personal concerns. Puritan prohibitions against males in the birth chamber are similarly sticky through secularization—removed only with the coming of the man-midwife/obstetrician. Most notably, the originally Puritan Calvinist prohibition against induced abortions is conserved through the secularization of midwives' oaths—although, here again, the obsolescence of midwives and their oaths by less constrained, man-midwife/obstetricians reintroduces the practice of inducing abortions, thereby setting up the American abortion debate of the nineteenth century.

REFLECTIONS ON THE HISTORY OF MIDWIVES' OATHS

By the end of the eighteenth century, the trend line was obvious: the era of female midwives dominance in English and American childbirth chambers was drawing to a close. As midwives retired from the birth chamber, the remarkable centuries-long documentary history of Anglo-American midwives' oaths also came to a close. Commencing with Bonner's oath of 1555, through two centuries of religious conflict, and despite secularization in New York, the ethical norms of Anglo-American midwives' conduct were conserved, leaving the ethics of midwifery remarkably stable. Placing communal interests and values above personal interests, midwives were to diligently and faithfully serve all laboring women alike, at all times, and in all types of weather, irrespective of whether the woman was poor or rich. They were to value the lives and health of the newborn as equal to the health and lives of their mothers, protecting the health and lives of mother and child alike, protecting newborns' patrimony and bodies against abuse and infanticide by desperately poor or desperately proud mothers. All the available evidence indicates that colonial American midwife morality lived up to the ethical expectations set out in their oaths.

One might presume that, unlike seventeenth- and eighteenth-century midwives, Anglo-American physicians of this period prioritized fidelity to their patients over fidelity to the church and state and that any oaths that they swore would reflect these priorities. History has a way of confounding expectations. As it happens during these centuries, the ethics detailed in the oaths of Anglo-American midwives is more sophisticated, articulate, and comprehensively developed than the ethics of other medical practitioners. Indeed, as we shall see in the next chapter, with one singular but important exception, seventeenth- and eighteenth-century physicians' oaths committed medical practitioners to loyalty to crown and church and said nothing whatsoever about fidelity to patients or providing for their care.

3

THE MEDICAL ETHICS OF GENTLEMANLY HONOR

I, A. B., do solemnly declare, that I will honestly, virtuously, and chastely, conduct myself in the practice of physic and surgery, with the privilege of exercising which profession I am now to be invested; and that I will, with fidelity and honour, do every thing in my power for the benefit of the sick committed to my charge.[1]

Oath of the Medical Society of the State of New York, 1807

I, A. B., do solemnly declare, that I will at all times hereafter pay due consideration and respect to this Society from which I derive this privilege to exercise the profession of a Physician or Surgeon; *that I will chastely, virtuously and honestly, conduct myself in the practice of physic and surgery, that I will, with fidelity and honor, do every thing in my power for the benefit of the Sick committed to my charge*, and recommend to them if necessary the best medical advice and I do further declare that I will consider all persons who are licensed to practice Physic or Surgery by this Society or any other incorporated Society of this State as Brethren of the same profession with which I am now invested and I will on no occasions wantonly attempt to injure their Medical Reputation.[2]

Oath of the Medical Society of the County of New York, 1806

Tum porro artem medicam caute, caste, probeque excercitaturum, et quoad portero omnia ad aegrotorum corporum salutem conducentia cum fide procuraturum quae denique inter medendum visa vel audita silere convenit non sine gravi causa vulgaturum. Ita presens spondenti adsit numen.

[*I A. B. do solemnly declare that I will] practice physic cautiously, chastely, and honourably; and faithfully to procure all things conducive to the health of the bodies of the sick*; and lastly, never, without great cause, to divulge anything that ought to be concealed, which may be heard or seen during professional attendance. To this oath let the Deity be my witness.[3]

Edinburgh University Medical Oath, Circa 1732–1735 onward

As the case of errant intern N from Chapter 1 reminds us, oaths are distillations of the ethical ideals of a community. The three oaths prefacing this chapter are significant by virtue of the ethical sensibilities they distill and their influence on those who swore them. The English-language oaths presented here are the earliest known North American physicians' medical ethics oaths. For most of the nineteenth century (from 1807 until at least 1880), every physician receiving a medical doctorate and/or a license to practice medicine in New York State had to sign the first oath. The New York State oath, in turn, is a version of the oath adopted in 1806 by the Medical Society of the County of New York, which, in turn, is a version of an older oath sworn by every physician graduated from the medical college of the University of Edinburgh from around 1730 through the twentieth century. Every American contributor to eighteenth-century American medical ethics signed a version of these oaths.[4] And, although it would be an exaggeration to suggest that physicians' ethics in America descends from these oaths, it is also unlikely that American physicians' ethics would have assumed its current form had it not been for these oaths and their influence.

The narrative that unfolds in this chapter explores the historical background of these oaths as well as the medical ethics and morality that Edinburgh-educated physicians transmitted to colonial and postcolonial America. It does so in a suitably eighteenth-century fashion: leisurely combining diverse elements into a complex story. The narrative line opens by discussing the role of oaths as instruments of religious and political repression at Edinburgh University. It then turns to the medical faculty's rebellious creation of an alternative oath and continues by exploring the origins and implications of this oath and its importation by Americans. As in any good eighteenth-century tale, the narrative takes a few detours: a comparison with other repressive oaths, a discussion of the absence of an occupational medical ethics before the Edinburgh oath, the evolution of the physician–patron/patient/sick person relationship, an exploration of gentlemanly honor and virtue, and a discussion of the hidden curriculum of the Edinburgh medical college. Along the way, we chat about some nasty pocky leprous whores, a hanging, body snatching, a riot, a flyte, and a famous duel. These seeming digressions provide the background needed to appreciate the development of American medical ethics, from its eighteenth-century Scottish roots to its creation of the world's first national code of medical ethics in the nineteenth century.

THE ATTRACTION OF EDINBURGH

Edinburgh attracted colonial- and postcolonial-American physicians because, unlike Cambridge, Oxford, and most Continental universities, daily lectures were delivered in plain English rather than in Latin, although, as Samuel Bard complained in a letter to his father, doctoral defenses still involved "exercises [that] were not only written in Latin but required [one] to defend them [orally] in the same language; not.... being allowed to speak a work of English."[5] A sojourn in Edinburgh also appealed to American colonials because the city's clubs and coffeehouses were the capital of the Scottish Enlightenment that "for.... nearly half a century.... ruled the Western intellect."[6] Among the coffee-sipping Scottish intelligentsia were philosopher and historian David Hume (1711–1776); moral philosopher and economist Adam Smith (1723–1790); the founder of modern geology, James Hutton (1726–1797); and the engineer whose steam engines would power the industrial revolution, James Watt (1736–1819). Drawn to this environment, young physicians from colonial and postcolonial English-speaking America who had the means to travel would supplement their medical training as apprentices in the colonies[7] with a stint in the Scottish-run anatomy schools of London, followed (or preceded) by a course of formal study at the University of Edinburgh.[8]

The medical curriculum at Edinburgh involved courses in anatomy, botany/*materia medica*, chemistry, mathematics, natural philosophy (biology), physics, physiology, and the theory and practice of physic (internal medicine). Supplementing these lectures were programs of dissections, vivisections, laboratory demonstrations, and clinical teaching at Edinburgh's dispensaries and hospitals. The faculty was world-renowned: the Monro family of anatomists; James Watt's teacher, Joseph Black (1728–1799), the pioneering chemist who discovered latent heat and carbon dioxide; and the physician and nosologist, William Cullen (1710–1790). Moreover, from time to time, medical students were invited into faculty homes for social events or dinner. Some found themselves, in Samuel Bard's words "happ(ily) in the Personal acquaintance of the Principal, and most of the Professors of the university" and "particularly intimate" with "some of the younger faculty."[9] This experience indelibly imprinted itself on the minds of the Americans. Benjamin Rush mentioned in his autobiography that "The two years

I spent in Edinburgh, I consider as the most important in their influence on my character and conduct of any period in my life."[10]

On returning to America, these young physicians tried to replicate Scottish institutions in the colonial or postcolonial context. Thus, after receiving his doctorate in 1762, William Shippen (1736–1808) returned to Philadelphia to offer a course of lectures on anatomy. The young Samuel Bard was jealous, as he confessed to his father,

> You perhaps are not acquainted with the whole of that scheme; it is not to stop with anatomy, but to found.... a medical college.... Mr. Morgan, who is to graduate next spring.... intends to lecture on the theory and practice of physic..... I wish, with all my heart, they were at New York, that I might share amongst them, and assist in founding the first medical college in America.... I am afraid that the Philadelphians, who will have the start of us by several years, will be a great obstacle [to starting a college in New York].... I own that I feel a little jealous of the Philadelphians, and should be glad to.... see the college of New York at least upon an equal footing with theirs.[11]

As Bard feared, in 1765, Philadelphians John Morgan (1735–1789) and William Shippen founded America's first medical college—which they modeled on the one in Edinburgh—at the College of Philadelphia (now the University of Pennsylvania).[12] Emulation of the Edinburgh medical college ran so deep that Edinburgh's logo, the thistle, was inscribed on the seal of the new medical college. This medical college became the first in England's American colonies to offer doctoral degrees in medicine based on an Edinburgh-style education: basic sciences and medical theory taught didactically but supplemented by dissections, laboratory demonstrations, and hands-on medical training in a hospital—and dissertations written in Latin.[13] With the assistance of his father, Bard soon replicated their achievement in New York, founding an Edinburgh-style medical college at King's College (now Columbia) two years later, in 1767.

In combination, the idea that a "regularly educated" physician had either studied in Edinburgh or in an Edinburgh-model American medical school meant that, by the end of the eighteenth century, virtually every physician with a medical degree in Philadelphia had either studied in Edinburgh or under someone who had studied there. Much the same was true in New York City.[14] Turning southward, about 230 Virginia physicians studied at Edinburgh between 1765 and 1800, approximately half receiving formal degrees (the others typically studied between one and four years without receiving a degree[15]). Although the number of irregularly trained medical practitioners exceeded these "regulars" even in New York, Pennsylvania, and Virginia, it was the degree-holding Edinburgh-style "regularly educated" physicians, the "regulars," as they referred to themselves, who created mainstream American medical ethics and who are the focus of this chapter and this book.

THE IMPORTANCE OF OATHS IN THE EIGHTEENTH CENTURY

The American physicians who graduated from Edinburgh signed or affirmed the Latin oath prefacing this chapter. Like errant intern N, contemporary readers might regard such oath signings as merely ceremonial and therefore of little significance. In the eighteenth century, however, oaths were an important part of public life. This was as true in colonial and postcolonial America as it was in Britain: thus, General George Washington's order of May 7, 1788 required officers in the Revolutionary Army to take an oath renouncing loyalty to King George III, and the very first law passed by the U.S. Congress, on June 1, 1789 (chap. I, statute 1), regulated the time and manner of administering official oaths.[16] During this period, swearing an oath meant signing a written promise made before a witness or witnesses, often in a ceremonial context. Oaths use specifically performative language such as "'I swear," "I affirm," or their equivalent, so the act of signing the oath ceremonialized one's commitment, thereby differentiating this act from ordinary acts of writing or speaking. The ceremonial power of oath signing was so great that Quakers and other devout Christians refused to partake in oath signings, believing, as Benjamin Rush argued, that they undermine faithful Christians' commitment to honor their word, irrespective of an accompanying signature.[17]

As a likely author of the Edinburgh oath wrote[18] about taking oaths, "Every Man can only with a safe conscience make a declaration of what he judges to be truth, or promise to perform what he believes to be just, if he acts otherwise he is a bad man."[19] As he wrote elsewhere, "Whoever knowingly errs against Truth commits what is morally Evil, and the Crime is greatly aggravated, if the God of Truth is appealed to when a Lye is told [as in a] false Oath."[20] One's reputation and character rested on one's honor, and no honorable person would sign or attest to an oath falsely. Oaths were taken so seriously that signing a loyalty oath was taken as sufficient evidence of loyalty and could even secure pardons. Conversely, refusal to sign a loyalty oath was tantamount to treason and grounds for punishment. The power accorded to oaths made them effective mechanisms of political and religious control used by kings, bishops, generals, and priests to verify loyalty and to root out and destroy disloyalty and dissent.

Oaths were also used to test religious faith. This practice was so deeply despised by the founders of the American republic that, in 1787, when drafting a constitution for the new nation, the founders expressly protected citizens against it. Article VI, Section 3 of the United States Constitution forbids inflicting religious tests—that is, a religious oath—on candidates for public office. To understand why religious tests came to be despised and to appreciate the significance of the Edinburgh oath, one needs to understand the inquisitional use of academic oaths against faculty and, more specifically, against the medical faculty at Edinburgh University. A brief history follows.

THE SCOTTISH *SPONSIO ACADEMICA* AND ACADEMIC FREEDOM

The academic loyalty oath, the *sponsio academica*, was introduced to Britain in 1587 when King James VI (1566–1625, reigned 1567–1625) required the first students to graduate from Edinburgh University to sign an oath pledging loyalty to Scotland's official church and to him as sovereign.[21] James had good reason for his actions. In the culmination of the religious-political Catholic-Protestant struggle (discussed in the previous chapter), James's Roman Catholic mother, Mary Stuart, Queen of Scots (1542–1587, reigned 1542–1567), had just been beheaded by order of a Protestant monarch, Queen Elizabeth I of England. Elizabeth, by the way, was so impressed by James' *sponsio academica* that she imposed a similar oath on the English universities of Cambridge and Oxford—where the practice continued until being repealed by an 1859 Act of Parliament.[22]

When Elizabeth I died in 1603, James inherited the English throne, thereby uniting the kingdoms of England and Scotland. Attempting to unify the national churches of his two kingdoms, James commissioned a common English-language bible, known as the King James Bible (1611), and, in 1616, launched a campaign to Anglicize Scottish culture and religion, banning the use of Scotland's native language, Gaelic (*Gàidhlig*), and introducing Anglican precepts into Scottish religious worship. The Scots protested. In an effort to silence these protests, the English imposed new loyalty oaths on the universities. Over the course of two centuries, a series of religious and cultural Anglicization campaigns were launched, typically meeting with often-violent protests. These led to, among other things, new loyalty oaths imposed on Scottish universities and purges of dissident faculty and students.

To prevent further Anglicization of their culture and religion, in 1638, the Scots created a National Covenant in which they pledged loyalty both to the *English* crown and to *Scotland's* traditional national religion, Presbyterianism. In effect, the National Covenant pledged political loyalty in exchange for religious and cultural autonomy. It thereby imposed a single national culture and religion on Scotland, and any dissent from the universities, whether perceived or actual, created an excuse for additional oaths and inquisitions on university faculty and students. Thus, in the name of Scottish national culture and religion, university students swore an oath obligating them to spy on each other, on the faculty, and on the administration and to report "un-Christian" conduct to the authorities.[23] Faculty members who refused to take a loyalty oath were dismissed.[24]

In 1688, Presbyterians seized control in Edinburgh, and a committee of inquisition was formed to purge Edinburgh University of "Papists, deists, and atheists."[25] The inquisition immediately targeted the university's Episcopalian principal, Andrew Monro (1648–1698, principal 1685–1690) who was suspect because he had liberalized the *sponsio academica*,[26] changing its wording to open the college to Christians of any denomination, including non-Presbyterians.[27] Also targeted were those faculty members hired to initiate medical education at the university: physician-botanist Sir Robert Sibbald (1641–1722) and physician-anatomist Archibald Pitcairne (1652–1713).

At the center of the inquisition was the charge that Principal Monro had permitted Dr. Pitcairne to give a lecture at which "the existence of God [was] impugned, without Answer or Vindication."[28] Doctor Pitcairne was charged with atheism,[29] and Principal Monro with promoting it—both hanging offenses. Monro responded in Pitcarine's defense and his own that:

> Doctor [Pitcairne] did not Impugn the Existence of a Deity,[30] he endeavoured fairly, like a True Philosopher, to load some Propositions in the *Thesis* with this Absurdity.... The most Sacred Fundamentals in Religion are thus disputed in the Schools, not with a design to overthrow them (as [my accuser] ignorantly fancies) but to establish and set them in their true light, that they may appear in their evidence.... Yet I foresaw that some Ignorant or Malicious People would misrepresent this Argument, and therefore I desired the *Doctor* to let it fall, [i.e., stop lecturing] and without any more [discussion] he did so.[31]

Monro's defense rescued him and Doctor Pitcairne from the gallows, but it did not save their jobs. Principal Monro resigned,[32] and Pitcairne departed Edinburgh to take a professorship at Leiden—returning later to marry and, as a matter of self-preservation, signing the required public oaths.[33]

Dr. Pitcairne's discretion was well advised. In 1696, the Privy Council passed an act "against the Atheistical Opinions of the Deists," setting the stage for "blasphemy trials."[34] An Edinburgh student, Thomas Aikenhead (1676–1697), son of a surgeon-apothecary, was charged for an offhand observation that, by 1800, Christianity "would be utterly extirpat[ed]" (i.e., surgically removed).[35] "The sum of this confused discourse," prosecutors alleged, "which probably he learned from Hobb[e]s, amounts to this: God had no law to our moral actions, by which they are regulated. Those, which are called moral laws, are only the determinations of government, or.... of men, concern what they think meet to be done for their own endes."[36] Convicted of blasphemy on Christmas Eve 1696, Aikenhead issued a famous gallows statement championing the right to seek the truth. "The Aikenhead case" one historian wrote, "inaugurated a battle for the soul of Edinburgh between a rigid Calvinism which saw any deviation in doctrine or conduct as a moral threat to the community, and a new conviction of the privacy and variety of conscience."[37] Medical practitioners, like Dr. Pitcairne, and even their children, like Thomas Aikenhead, were in the middle of the fray, and so was Scottish medicine.

THE EDINBURGH MEDICAL OATH AS AN ALTERNATIVE TO THE *SPONSIO ACADEMICA*

The Edinburgh medical oath was a response to the Aikenhead incident and to centuries of censorship, repression, and intolerance. It was also an artifact of the Scottish Enlightenment,[38] a movement that, unlike its English and Continental counterparts, was *not* the child of free-thinkers like Aikenhead's intellectual mentor, the philosopher Thomas Hobbes (1588–1679); that is, it was not, as much of the Enlightenment was, "anti-Christian, anti-Church.... at the point of sliding into irreligion and proto-atheism."[39] It was rather a movement founded in the universities and intellectual circles with support from tradesmen and gentry to "preserve civilized society against any resurgence of religious enthusiasm and superstition.... of evangelical Protestantism and.... the barbarism of civil war."[40]

Reacting to centuries of intolerance, repression, and civil strife, the gentry and tradesmen of the towns allied themselves with moderate clergy and the intelligentsia in a quest for religious and political stability, investing in universities as independent centers of intellectual leadership and bulwarks against religious and political fanaticism.[41] It was just such an alliance that led to the 1720 appointment of Alexander Monro *primus* (1697–1767)—no relation to Edinburgh University Principal Andrew Monro—John Rutherford (1695–1779), and several others to the medical faculty of the university at Edinburgh.[42] Since Alexander Monro's son and grandson were also named Alexander, the eldest Monro referred to himself as *Primus*, to his son as *Secundus*, and to his grandson as *Tertius*.[43] In characteristic eighteenth-century nepotistic fashion, this father-son-grandson dynasty of anatomy professors—*Primus*, *Secundus*, *Tertius*—would hold sway at the Edinburgh medical college for 126 years.

In 1725, *Primus* received funding to open rooms in the university for teaching anatomy, an event that is often credited with founding the medical college.[44] As increasingly larger numbers of students received their medical doctorates,[45] the question arose of whether to require them to swear the university *sponsio*. The official text of the *sponsio* had been liberalized slightly in 1705, but graduates still had to swear to "maintain the Christian religion in truth and purity purged of all

Popish errors."[46] *Primus* and his colleagues evidently found this too oppressive, and, in the 1730s, a new medical *sponsio academica* was fashioned specifically for medical students.[47] The most recently published translation of this medical *sponsio* renders it as:

> I, A B, worthy of the title Doctor of Medicine, seriously and sacredly before God who sees into men's hearts, pledge that I will persevere in every duty of a worthy mind towards the University of Edinburgh until the last breath of my life. Furthermore indeed that I will exercise the Art of Medicine cautiously, purely and honorably, and, as far as I can, to take care faithfully that all [my actions] are conducive to [effecting] health in sick bodies. And finally that it behoves [me] to keep silent on all matters seen and heard during the course of healing, unless there is a pressing need to reveal these matters. Thus may the divine presence be favourable to me as I make this pledge.[48]

To appreciate the significance of this *sponsio,* one needs to recall the trial and hanging of Thomas Aikenhead, the censorship and indictment of Dr. Pitcairne, and the university purges that forced medical faculty to resign, flee, or perjure themselves because they gave a suspicious lecture or subscribed to unorthodox religious views. Words unspoken in this *sponsio* insulated medical students and faculty alike from these threats. Notably absent were such terms as "Christian," "Christ," and expressions like "Reformed Christian Religion," and "Popish errors."[49] Breaking with centuries of religious intolerance and political repression, this oath does *not* include a pledge of loyalty to the church, to crown, or even to Christianity. It envisions the physician as someone who could vow before "*Deo*," without invoking any particular religion. It was a vow that could be, and which was, pledged by Presbyterians, Episcopalians, and even by Catholics. Michael Ryan (1800–1841), a Catholic alumnus of the Edinburgh medical school,[50] translates the Latin "Deo" as, "the deity,"[51] a characterization that would make the oath acceptable to deists and even to Newtonians like Dr. Pitcairne.

Principal Andrew Mono had been forced from the university in part because of his abortive 1687 attempt to liberalize the *sponsio*. Four decades later, the new medical *sponsio* permanently opened Edinburgh's medical school to anyone holding any variant of any religious belief common in eighteenth- and nineteenth-century Britain or its colonies. Quakers were the one significant group of British religious dissenters who could not swear the medical *sponsio* as formulated.[52] It is indicative of the liberalizing intent of the new oath that, early in the eighteenth century, a version was drafted specifically for Quakers.[53] Generations of Quaker physicians would affirm this oath—a point of pride celebrated by Edinburgh alumni.[54] Importantly for American medicine, one Quaker alumnus, John Fothergill (1712–1781), supported the efforts of fellow Edinburgh alumni, the young

Americans John Morgan and William Jr., assisting them in founding a medical college in the British colony of Pennsylvania by sending them anatomical drawings, casts, and books.[55]

To reiterate, Edinburgh was the only eighteenth-century British medical college whose alumni network could include a Quaker like Fothergill, a Presbyterian like Shippen, and the son of a Baptist father and Quaker mother like Morgan (who later left both religions to become an Episcopalian). Religious tests and restrictive *sponsio academica* barred all of the above-named physicians from receiving medical degrees from other Scottish medical colleges and from the English colleges at Cambridge and Oxford. Edinburgh's medical *sponsio* opened the college to generations of students whose religious beliefs would otherwise have barred them from attending British medical schools, thus transforming Edinburgh into a beacon of tolerance in an era of intolerance.

THE TRANSFORMATIVE NATURE OF THE EDINBURGH OATH

What was said in the medical oath was as important as what was left unsaid. Like traditional oaths, the medical *sponsio* is a loyalty oath; however, instead of pledging loyalty to the state and its religion, loyalty and fidelity are pledged to the university and to the health of the sick—undermining the intent of the traditional *sponsio*, the purpose of which was to instill loyalty to crown and church above any other institution or person, including the sick. In a Scotland riven by factionalism, riots, and armed conflict, physicians and surgeons were inextricably faced with questions about whether to treat enemies or to inform on friends. The new medical oath answers unequivocally that, as a physician, one's actions should always be "conducive to [effecting] health in sick bodies" and, just as significantly, a physician should "keep silent on all matters seen and heard during the course of healing, unless there is a pressing need to reveal these matters."[56] As Irish Catholic alumnus Michael Ryan explained to his London medical students, the Edinburgh oath means that the secrets patients reveal to their physicians "ought not to be divulged even at the risk of liberty and life"[57] and that "[i]n time of war, medical men feel equally bound to aid friends and enemies."[58]

The impact of these commitments was transformative. The traditional *sponsio academica*, like the traditional midwife's oath, made physicians agents of the state, oath-bound to breach confidences and to spy on the sick. Just as the midwife was expressly bound by her oath to breach confidentiality since she "will not collude to keep secret the birth of a child.... and will not conceal the birth of bastards,"[59] the traditional medical *sponsio academica* obligated physicians not to collude with their patients in opposing church and sovereign. The Edinburgh oath, in contrast, stipulates that, by virtue of their occupation, medical doctors' primary fidelity is to their patients rather than to the crown or the church. The ethics of the oath, or to use the Latin term for an oath, the ethics of the *profession*, prioritizes fidelity to the sick and the duty to keep their confidences over loyalty to church or state.

Occupationally acquired professional duties of fidelity are a distinctive innovation in the eighteenth-century European context. In the modern and early modern period, European medical practitioners were regulated by religious edicts, contracts, guild and college regulations, and the law, but not by a self-imposed occupational ethics symbolized by an oath. Within Scotland and in the entire English-speaking world, the new Edinburgh medical oath was singular. No other Anglo-American medical institution required medical students to swear an oath stipulating their occupational ethics or pledging their fidelity to the sick:[60] not the Moral Statutes of the Royal College of Physicians of London, not the oath of the Royal College of Surgeons in London, not the graduation oaths of other Scottish medical schools at Aberdeen[61] and Glasgow,[62] and not the *sponsio* of Cambridge or Oxford. The Edinburgh medical oath is, in this sense, the *ur*-text, the mother text, so to speak, of physicians' conception of the foundational ethics of what came to be called "the physician–patient relationship."

A linguistic-conceptual note about "the physician–patient relationship." Both the Edinburgh oath and one of its likely authors, Alexander Monro *primus*, use the traditional expression "the sick," rather than the newer term, "patient." Linguistically and conceptually, the concepts of "the sick," "the sick poor," and "patients" were in transition in seventeenth- and eighteenth-century English usage. As early as the seventeenth century, some English-language medical writers began using the term "patient" (introduced into English from the French, possibly as early as the fourteenth century, from the Latin, *patiens*, "one who suffers") to differentiate between paying "patients" and nonpaying "sick poor;" however, "the sick" was used as a generic reference that encompassed both private patients and the sick poor.[63] *Primus*'s writings, the Edinburgh oath—even in the nineteenth-century descendent form used by the New York medical societies—use only the broad generic expression, "the sick." It is thus something of a misnomer to use the expression "physician–patient relationship" to refer to the relationship between seventeenth- and eighteenth-century physicians, surgeons, surgeon-apothecaries, and "the sick." The physician–patient relationship, as we understand it today, was first being constructed during this period. The concept of "the sick" was precursor terminology; not until the nineteenth century did American physicians begin to have a clear conception of the physician–patient relationship—and that conception differed from its twenty-first-century interpretation.

Just as the physician–sick person/physician–patient relationship was under construction during the eighteenth century, so too was the ethics of that relationship. As historian of eighteenth-century British medicine Mary Fissell has observed, before the Scottish Enlightenment "no ethics particular to their profession or vocation governed [medical practitioners] conduct. Rather, appropriate behavior was inculcated through the institution of apprenticeship, shaped by general norms of master/servant and client/patron interactions."[64] Fissell's observations challenge a "truism" accepted by many writers on medical ethics: that fidelity to the sick—the nub of the issue in the case of errant intern N and a central feature of the Edinburgh oath—"is the most ancient and universally acknowledged principle of medical ethics."[65] The truth inverts this truism: as the history of midwives' oaths and the *sponsio academica* attests, in every known medical oath sworn by practitioners in the Anglo-American cultural sphere prior to the Edinburgh oath, loyalty to crown/state and/or to the church preempted fidelity to the sick or to the laboring woman. Prior to the Edinburgh oath, medical professionals' oath-sworn loyalty was officially to parties other than the sick person—and, as we saw in the previous chapter, midwives generally conformed their morality and conduct to their oaths.

To put this point in perspective, it is helpful to recall that in the not too distant past oaths sworn by communist and Nazi doctors prioritized a commitment to their people and to their country over their obligations to their patients.[66] Medical oaths sworn in the Union of Soviet Socialist Republics (USSR) and allied communist countries during the 1970s and 1980s obligated physicians to be guided in all their actions, first and foremost, by "the principles of communist morality.... and.... [by their] responsibility to the Soviet state."[67] Substitute "religion" for "communist morality" and "King" for "Soviet state" and you again have the traditional *sponsio academica* sworn at Aberdeen, Cambridge, Glasgow, and Oxford. These oaths served the same purpose: to ensure the loyalty of the physician to parties other than the sick person/patient.

In the eighteenth century, the Anglo-American conception of physician/surgeon/apothecary-customer/patron/sick person/patient relationship was under construction, and it could well have evolved in a variety of ways that did *not* involve prioritizing fidelity to the sick person/patient.[68] When the Edinburgh medical oath was initiated, no single occupational ethics governed the practice of physic or surgery, and no formal statement of physicians' ethics obligated physicians to fidelity to the sick person. For example, except when expressly contracted to serve as plague doctors, British physicians routinely abandoned the sick during epidemics.[69] As one seventeenth-century observer remarked, "Never let any man aske me what became of our Phisitions in this Massacre [the epidemic], they hid their Synodicall heads as well as the prowdest.... not one of them durst peepe abroad."[70] In the eighteenth century, physicians did not censure fellow physicians for abandoning their patients during epidemics.[71] The notable absence of criticism arises because the concept of an occupation-specific role obligation of fidelity to the sick/patient was as alien to medical doctors as it would have been to butchers, bakers, and candlestick makers. There was no occupational ethics for physicians or surgeons prior to the Edinburgh oath; neither the sick person, nor the public, nor physicians themselves had expectations of physician fidelity beyond what custom dictated in customer-client-patron relationships.

To further illustrate the absence of specific occupational ethics governing the physician and surgeons relationship to the sick in eighteenth-century Britain, consider historian Mary Fissell's analysis of a pamphlet war conducted in the 1740s between the governors and staff of Bath General Hospital and an English surgeon, Archibald Cleland (circa 1700–1771), a surgeon who had served his apprenticeship in Edinburgh but who had not attended the university and so had not signed the Edinburgh oath. Cleland had performed vaginal examinations, "the touch," on two women hospital patients who interpreted these examinations as sexual rather than medical. The women complained to the hospital governors that Cleland had done them "business" (i.e., sexually molested them). After reviewing the charges, the governors dismissed Cleland.[72] "Nowhere in the accusations and counter-accusations," Fissell remarks, "do we see this incident in the light of Hippocratic injunctions which forbids sexual intercourse between doctor and patient."[73] Moreover, the language Cleland used in his own defense, that "no Man living would have thrust his Fingers into the *Common-shores* of a Couple of *Nasty pocky leperous Whores*, but out of a Laudable Zeal of being helpful"[74] is not "construct[ed] around a notions of medical behavior or medical institutions."[75] "The absence of such references," Fissell argues, "underlines the point that what is at issue is not medical ethics (as we would understand this subject today), but correct behavior (etiquette) between those of different social ranks."[76]

Similarly, in explaining their reasons for dismissing Cleland, the governors never invoked an occupational ethics of physicians; instead they invoked a conception of duty based on status and charity:

> The *Rich* and *Powerful* are capable of *repelling Insults* and *Punishing Injuries*; but the *Objects* of a HOSPITAL CHARITY are *Helpless* and liable to every kind of *ill Treatment*; if they are not protected by those, to whose Care they are entrusted.[77]

This passage is entirely about the powerlessness and helplessness of the objects of charity, and of relations between persons giving and receiving charity. No mention is made in this exchange about some special occupational ethic governing physicians' relationship to the sick. The reason: except for those who signed the Edinburgh medical oath, no such special occupational ethics for medical practitioners was recognized in the eighteenth century, not in oaths, and not, as this case illustrates, by hospital administrators. The oath was a transformational document: the first Anglo-American institutional attempt to formalize an occupational ethics for physicians.

A HIPPOCRATIC HERITAGE FOR THE EDINBURGH OATH

The Edinburgh oath may have had a Hippocratic precedent. Hippocratic works had been studied at the Edinburgh medical college since at least 1706, when Sir Robert Sibbald published a commentary on Hippocratic texts.[78] Perhaps more to the point, eighteenth-century Edinburgh alumni, such as John Morgan, characterized the Edinburgh medical oath as "Hippocratic," as did some early nineteenth-century commentators on the oath.[79] Twenty-first-century readers might be perplexed by this claim. The dissimilarities between the language of the Edinburgh medical oath and familiar renditions of the Hippocratic oath seem overwhelming. Yet to eighteenth- or early-nineteenth-century eyes, the Edinburgh medical oath would be read against the background of *sponsio academica* and, unlike the *sponsio* but like the classical Hippocratic oath, the Edinburgh oath contains a pledge of fidelity to the health of the sick person. For this reason alone, one twenty-first-century commentator remarked that "while [the Edinburgh medical oath] is not the Hippocratic Oath or even a loose modernized translation.... this oath could reasonably be called Hippocratic in character."[80]

Furthermore, eighteenth- and early-nineteenth-century commentators would appreciate that, unlike other medical oaths of the period, the Edinburgh oath was not designed to impose dictates of external state or religious authority on practitioners. Moreover, like the classical Hippocratic oath, the Edinburgh oath contains a pledge of loyalty to one's teachers, or at least to one's educational institution, and it is a fraternal vow in which an older generation of physicians initiates a new generation into the field. By contrast, *sponsio academica* and midwives' oaths are instruments of external authority. Nonmedical males drafted midwives' oaths to impose male social authority on the female practitioners and the culturally demarcated feminine world of childbirth. These oaths bristle with dictatorial impositions. The New York Midwives' Oath, for example, reiterates the expression, "she will not," seven times. In contrast, the Edinburgh oath emphasizes positive affirming adverbs—cautiously, chastely/purely, honorably, and faithfully.

Yet, to a twenty-first-century reader, the absence of familiar prohibitions, such as the prohibition against having sexual relations with patients, may seem to render the Edinburgh oath irremediably non-Hippocratic. From an eighteenth-century perspective, however, the adverbial admonitions to "exercise the Art of Medicine *cautiously, purely and honorably*," would appear to state these prohibitions. The duty not to engage in "sexual acts both upon women's bodies and upon men's"[81] is adverbially parsed as the virtue of acting "chastely" (Edinburgh oath) or "purely" (New York oath). Importantly, this reparsing shifts the focus of the prohibition from the action to the *motive* for acting.

The adverbial shift emphasizes what is important from an eighteenth-century perspective: not the prohibited action per se, but the *motive* underlying the constraint on the action—the virtue of acting cautiously. Similarly, the adverb, "faithfully," in the Edinburgh and New York oaths—"faithfully to procure all things conducive to the health of the bodies of the sick" (Edinburgh); "with fidelity and honour, do every thing in my power for the benefit of the sick committed to my care" (New York)—parses the duty of fidelity in a way that also emphasizes the physician's motives. Such systemic displacements of language signal a paradigm shift. By replacing the action-emphasizing verbs and gerunds of the classical Hippocratic oath with adverbs characterizing the motives underlying an action, the Edinburgh medical oath transforms an ethics of duty into a virtue ethics emphasizing motivation and character. As *Primus* wrote to his daughter, "Nothing, My Dear, shews a noble, generous, social well turn'd Mind [more] than Benevolence and Humanity."[82] As he observes elsewhere, "the Opinion of the World" is also "a considerable Inducement to do what is right and to shun what is generally reputed wrong."[83] Acts of benevolence and humanity should thus be internally motivated but, by demonstrating to the world one's noble, generous, well-turned-out mind, they raise one's status in the opinion of the world.

In an autobiography that *Primus* wrote to encourage his progeny and his "[s]tudents… towards obtaining such a Character as they ought to aspire at,"[84] he describes various actions that he performed as evidence of his own noble, generous, well-turned-out mind. He was a "general Benefactor to the Poor in Distress [who]….never refused Access to any Sick who desired to have his Advice; to many of them he gave medicines."[85] He was of "a tender Heart,"[86] and "[s]o little Doubt was make of this Gentleman's Veracity and Integrity that his Affirmation of any Fact from his own proper Knowledge was never suspected" and he had a "Love of Integrity."[87] *Primus*'s point in reciting these achievements was to establish that he acted from noble motives, displaying gentlemanly virtues; it was not to demonstrate that he was acting dutifully.

The ethics to which *Primus* subscribed, and to which he encouraged his children and his students to subscribe, viewed actions as testimonials to the motives and character of the actor. Theirs was not an ethics focused on dutifulness or avoiding prohibited actions—a deontological ethics, to use a technical term derived from the Greek *deon*, literally, "that which binds" (i.e., one's duties).[88] For eighteenth-century gentlemen and ladies, duties and prohibitions were less important than the motives and character of the actor in performing these duties and in avoiding prohibited acts. This conception of morality profoundly affected expectations of conduct. As one of *Primus*'s American students, Samuel Bard, wrote to his father, in 1765, "the two Monros [*Primus* and *Secundus*] with Dr. Cullen, were in all my private [doctoral] examinations….and to all of them I considered myself much indebted, for their behavior on this occasion, in which, although they kept up the strictness of professors, they never lost sight of the politeness of gentlemen."[89] Edinburgh students, like Bard, expected to be treated like gentlemen. To rehearse the traditional Hippocratic prohibitions—a deontological ethics—in the manner of the New York Midwives' oath would have insulted their honor. Any version of the Hippocratic oath intended for eighteenth-century medical students had to be appropriate to their status as gentlemen.

Since a list of the traditional Hippocratic prohibitions would have been unacceptable to graduates' gentlemanly sensibilities, the duties and prohibitions of the traditional oath were parsed to shift the oath's focus from prohibited actions to the gentlemanly virtues and motivations of the actor. A prohibition against sexual engagement is thus transformed into an admonition to cultivate the virtue of chastity or purity. These transformations may make the oath appear non-Hippocratic to a twenty-first-century reader, but to eighteenth- and nineteenth-century commentators, and to generations of Edinburgh medical students and alumni, the oath read as Hippocratic.

THE EDINBURGH OATH AS AN ETHICS OF GENTLEMANLY HONOR

The Edinburgh oath was drafted in a format consistent with the gentlemanly aspirations of the medical students who signed it. These aspirations were set out not only in *Primus*'s unpublished manuscripts but in such widely read publications as *The Compleat English Gentleman* (1729) by Daniel Defoe (1661?–1731)—better known as the author of *Robinson Crusoe* (1719). Defoe explains that to be a gentleman is to be "a man of honour, virtue, sense, integrity, honesty" and that without these a man is "nothing at all."[90] Another guide to the eighteenth-century concept of an honorable gentleman is the 1755 edition of Doctor Samuel Johnson's *A Dictionary of the English Language*. The noun "gentleman" is defined, dictionary style, as "A man of birth; a man of extraction, though not noble.... A man raised above the vulgar by his character or post...." The adjective "honourable" is defined as: "1, Illustrious, noble; ...Not to be disgraced; Without taint; without reproach; Honest, without intention of deceit; Equitable."[91] The Edinburgh medical oath thus specifies what it means to act honorably and without taint or reproach in one's role/post as physicians and does so in terms of Hippocratic duties reformulated as the virtues of acting cautiously, chastely/purely, honourably, and faithfully.

Being a gentleman, or at least being perceived as one, was a prerequisite for practicing medicine among the status-conscious middling and upper classes—which is to say, those who could afford to pay decent fees for a physician's services. Practicing successfully among the more affluent classes, however, meant confronting the dilemma of patronage. As sociologist N. D. Jewson observed in a classic essay, "By virtue of their economic and political predominance the gentry and aristocracy held ultimate control over the consultative relationship."[92] Affluent patrons could and did patronize their physicians in both a literal and metaphorical sense, treating physicians as mere hirelings. Physicians were often unable to direct a course of treatment for their fickle and often noncompliant patrons who would nonetheless "tax their Doctors with responsibility for poor health, even if they disobey their doctor's instructions."[93] Exacerbating matters further, physicians' reputations were effectively held hostage to their patrons' health, since the world at large naturally judged physicians' skill by their success in keeping their high-status patrons healthy. As one physician remarked, "If they happen to tumble while you pretend to keep them up with your own Shoulders, they'll bury you in their Ruins."[94]

Hence, the dilemma of patronage: patrons being *patrons*, felt entitled to patronize their physicians, but physicians, if they wished to succeed as *physicians*, could not allow themselves to be patronized: "A Physician's oblig'd to exert his Authority. . . . to rule his Betters" and to eschew "such Compliances as wou'd do very well elsewhere"—the dilemma was that one's Betters, by definition, held a social position that allowed them to dictate to their "lessers."[95] Nonetheless, eighteenth-century physicians contended that "more Men lose their Lives by their own Obstinacy, than by all the Distempers in a Bill of Mortality put together"; "the Patient. . . . must be governable, and resign to those that have the care of him, especially the Physician: And neither the Sick Man nor they that are about him, may presume to impose upon the Physician, or elude his Directions."[96]

One strategy that British physicians' employed to cope with this dilemma was to elevate their perceived status by adopting genteel deportment, genteel dress, and genteel forms of discourse. By acting gentlemanly and speaking like gentlemen, they sought to become accepted as gentlemen. The Edinburgh medical oath recognizes the gentlemanly aspirations of medical students by offering a vision of the physician as gentleman. Inverting the vintners' trick of making new wine more saleable by pouring it into old bottles, the Edinburgh oath made old ideals of Hippocratic ethics more palatable by pouring them into the new format of gentlemanly honor. Young medical gentleman could thus embrace, as a matter of gentlemanly honor, an ethics of fidelity to the sick, confidentiality, taking heed not to harm or to risk harming the sick, and abstaining from sexual relations with them. Having poured the old ethics into new bottles, it was adapted to the matriculation requirement of swearing a *sponsio*, and students had to quaff this brew to receive a medical doctorate from Edinburgh University. A modernized version of the oath, stilled referred to as a "*Medical Sponsio Academica*" is still sworn at the graduation ceremonies of the University of Edinburgh (see text in note).[97]

MEDICAL MORALITY AND GENTLEMANLY HONOR: THE CASE OF CONFIDENTIALITY

The Edinburgh medical oath formalizes an occupational ethics for physicians, stating the norms of character and conduct of the virtuous physician. Yet, as noted in Chapter 1, medical morality, the standards to which practitioners *actually* hold themselves and their peers accountable, often differs from the standards avowed in oaths and other formal statements of medical ethics. Progress in medical ethics is often the history of a long and tortuous transition of ethical ideals, initially only given lip service, from ethics into everyday medical morality—or from morality into ethics. The evidence indicates that although the norms of Hippocratic ethics conserved in the Edinburgh and New York oaths would ultimately become the morality of American medical practitioners and would be disseminated and enforced in the corridors of American clinics—as the case of intern N illustrates—they were not fully embraced by either British or American practitioners until the mid-nineteenth century. A different, nonmedical morality dominated intrapractitioner relationships, the morality of gentlemanly honor.

Consider the norm of patient confidentiality stated in the Edinburgh medical oath but, tellingly, left unstated in its New York descendant. The norm was flaunted openly in eighteenth-century Britain, and there is no evidence that any Anglo-American practitioner was censured for violating patient confidentiality until 1869, when the New York Academy of Medicine censured and expelled a surgeon for such a violation (see Chapter 5). Cleland, for example, published the names and medical conditions of his patients, Sarah Appleby, Mary Hooke, and Mary Hudson, whom he calls "*Nasty pocky leperous Whores*."[98] He declares his reasons for publicly castigating these patients in the opening lines of his pamphlet:

> The Reputation and Character, which every Honest Man wishes to maintain in the World, is so dear and tender in his own Eye, and of such Consequence to his Family and Friends, that when we find ourselves openly attack'd in our good Name, or privately vilified by Slander of evil Reports, and oblique Insinuations, we cannot too publicly, or too firmly repel the Injury.[99]

A gentleman's honorable reputation had to be defended at all costs—including publicly disparaging a patient's character and publicly revealing the patient's medical condition.

Cleland was not an Edinburgh medical college alumnus, and he had never signed the Edinburgh medical oath. Yet Edinburgh alumni routinely breached confidentiality in their flytes and pamphlet wars. Consider, for example, a flyte and pamphlet war between two physician alumni of Edinburgh University: William

Withering (1741–1799),[100] a classmate of Samuel Bard's who became famous for discovering digitalis, and Robert Darwin (1766–1848),[101] famous for being the son of a famous Cambridge and Edinburgh-educated physician, Erasmus Darwin (1731–1802), and the father of the even more famous biologist, Charles Darwin (1809–1882). The flyte erupted in 1789, after an apothecary involved in caring for one of Dr. Darwin's patients, Mrs. Houlston, recommended that Dr. Withering be called in to consult on the case. Withering visited Mrs. Houlston and changed the treatment plan without paying the young Dr. Darwin a courtesy call or consulting with him in any way—a breach of gentlemanly etiquette that was a common cause of physician flytes.[102] Dr. Darwin protested, and the flyte became public in a pamphlet war in which both physicians published details about their patient's medical condition, publicly declaring her name. At one point, for example, Darwin wrote

> I understand you told Mr. Houlston that [his wife] had no fever, when her pulse was 126 a minute; and she had an inflammation in her liver, when she had neither pain, nor soreness on the hepatic region nor any yellowness of the skin, or increased evacuation! What was your design in asserting what you knew to be untrue, if you know anything of the matter?[103]

Not content to reveal a patient's name and medical problems, Darwin proceeds to name several other patient whom, he charged, were mistreated by Withering: "Mrs. Willes of Newbold" and "Mr. Inge of Lichfield."[104] No attempt is made to protect patient confidentiality in this or most other eighteenth-century pamphlet wars. More important, no one condemned such public statements of patients' names and medical conditions as immoral, unethical, or even unseemly. Not a scintilla of censure attached to public broadcasts of patients' medical condition. No one acted, or pretended to act, as if public dissemination of medical information about patients was in any sense wrong.

As in the Cleland pamphlet war, the ethical concepts deployed were *not* specific to medicine or to the physician–patient/sick person relationship. The only ethics in evidence is the ethics of gentlemanly honor. Thus, Darwin objects to Withering's "ungenteel medical behavior toward me,"[105] and his unworthy "conduct as a gentleman" in changing a prescription without "desiring to meet me in consultation."[106] Using a standard flyting strategy, Darwin contends that Withering is acting from "paltry motives, which have always induced you to slander those of your own profession, among the other mean arts by which you attempt to support your business."[107] As Dr. Johnson observed, in eighteenth-century usage, a "gentleman" was supposed to be magnanimous, generous, and elevated above the common and thus to have no "paltry motives," no involvement in vulgar "business," and certainly to rise above the practice of "mean arts." This was thus a dispute about ungentlemanly conduct, about an insulting lack of consultation, about respect and disrespect. Nowhere in this or in other eighteenth-century pamphlet wars do we find a sense of moral conduct that corresponds to the ethics of the Edinburgh medical oath or to the norms it derived from its Hippocratic inspiration. The dominant ethos evident is the nonmedical morality of gentlemanly honor.

Flyting, pamphlet wars, and even duels are artifacts of the morality of gentlemanly honor. The virtue ethics of noble character exemplified by humane and beneficent acts taught by *Primus* and Defoe tends to be holistic. A virtuous person may on occasion fail to do what is virtuous—fail to tell the truth, for example—and still be considered honorable. Yet even a hint that a person indulges in a vice, like lying, if perceived as evidence of an ignoble character, of being a "liar," can become a revelatory tipping point. As Cleland might have remarked, like Humpty Dumpty of nursery rhyme fame, once one's reputation has been shattered, it may be impossible to put it back together again: innumerable acts of truth telling may fail to restore one's reputation for honesty. Consequently, gentlemen assiduously projected and protected their honor—which is why the history of eighteenth- and nineteenth-century Anglo-American medical gentlemen is suffused with tales of pamphlet wars, flytes, and the occasional duel.

Flytes and pamphlet wars were verbal duels, ways to publicly "disrespect" a rival in order to project and protect one's status and honor.[108] Much like actual duels, whatever the nominal subject of the dispute may be, the underlying issue is always status or respect.[109] As is evident in the Darwin-Withering pamphlet war, the rhetoric of a flyte is invariably *ad hominem*, challenging the character of the opponent, verbally disrespecting, or, to use American street culture jargon, "dissing" him, in an attempt to undermine his status. Since honor and its defense are about one's standing with others as much as with oneself, like actual duels, flytes and pamphlet wars are characteristically witnessed or conducted in public venues to spread the fame of the winner.[110] In this process, the ethos or morality of honor routinely overrode the medical ethics of patient confidentiality.[111]

When flytes and pamphlet wars failed to affirm honor in the face of some perceived challenge or insult, physicians sometimes faced each other with pistols rather than lose face and incur "the dreaded stigma of the censorious world."[112] American physicians were more inclined to resort to pistol duels than were their British counterparts.[113] Granville Sharp Pattison (1791–1851), a Glasgow-trained Scottish-born American anatomist, surgeon, medical educator, and founder of the departments of anatomy at three major medical schools—Jefferson Medical College in Philadelphia, the University of London, and New York University[114]—was a leading medical duelist. He was famous for his public challenge to no less a figure than Professor Nathaniel Chapman of the University of Pennsylvania (1780–1853), founding president of the American Medical Association (AMA). Pattison "posted" Chapman—literally nailing a statement to a post—in which he declared Chapman a "Liar, a Coward, and a Scoundrel."[115] On winning the resulting duel with Chapman's brother-in-law, General Thomas Cadwalader (1795–1873)—who was shot in the leg and walked with a limp and a cane for the rest of his life—Pattison mounted the dueling pistols over his fireplace and publicly bragged about the encounter to his students.[116]

To appreciate the pull of gentlemanly honor in Britain and colonial and post-colonial America, not only in medicine but in the culture generally, consider the near-death reflections of one of the most prominent figures in the era of the American Revolution and the early republic, Secretary of the Treasury Alexander Hamilton (1755–1804). On the night before his fatal duel with Vice President Aaron Burr (1756–1836), Hamilton wrote out five reasons why he should decline to duel: he risked everything and had little to gain from the duel; his differences with Burr were political, not personal; his finances were not in order; he had obligations to his wife and children; and he opposed "the practice of dueling" on religious principles. Nonetheless, Hamilton wrote, "all the considerations which constitute what men of the world denominate honor, impose on me a peculiar necessity not to decline the call."[117] On July 11, 1804, attended by his physician, David Hosack (1769–1835), Hamilton took a boat from Manhattan, where dueling was illegal, to face Burr on Weehawken Heights in New Jersey. According to Dr. Hosack, Hamilton's dying words were a caution and a declaration of nonlethal intent.

> "Take care of that pistol; it is undischarged, and still cocked; it may go off and do harm.... I did not intend to fire at him" [Hamilton said.] He then closed his eyes and remained calm, without any disposition to speak.... He asked me once or twice how I found his pulse; and he informed me that his lower extremities had lost all feeling, manifesting to me that he entertained no hopes that he should long survive.[118]

As Hamilton's death attests, asserting and protecting honor was a serious matter—a matter of life and death—in Britain and its colonial and postcolonial colonies.

PRIMUS'S HIDDEN CURRICULUM AND MORALLY DISRUPTIVE INNOVATIONS

In Edinburgh, as in all medical schools, a "hidden curriculum" imparts a sense of implicit morality that often conflicts with the ethics formalized in oaths and propounded in lectures. A prime example of teaching morality through the hidden curriculum involves Monro *primus*. *Primus* deeded to posterity two unpublished manuscripts: a family autobiography intended to be read only by his students and his progeny, and an *Essay on Female Conduct* that he wrote to educate his daughter. In the *Essay*, he extolled the virtues of beneficence and humanity, and, in his autobiography, he tried to show how he exemplified these virtues as a founder of the Edinburgh infirmary, a charitable institution that cared for the deserving poor. *Primus* also observed that although his intent was benevolent and humane in offering "private Care of the Poor," nonetheless,

> his tender Behavior to those in the Infirmary was of considerable Advantage to him. He became thereby such a Favorite of the Populace, that when the Mob was in great Fury endeavouring to destroy the Houses of the other Surgeons in Town on account of stealing and dissecting dead Bodies, their Ring leaders would not allow a Stone to be thrown at the House of a Surgeon, which was next to P[rofessor] M[onro]'s, lest by aiming wrong some of his Windows might be broken.[119]

Yet the crowds were not always this respectful. In 1725, violent protests against grave robbing and body snatching targeted the Surgeon's hall in which *Primus* performed dissections, forcing him to move his anatomy lectures and dissections to the University.[120] The hanging of Margret Dickson was probably the precipitating incident for this protest. Margret was a young woman discovered to have concealed the corpse of her newborn infant, in violation of the Scottish version of the Puritan Act to prevent the destroying and murdering of bastard children discussed in the previous chapter. She was convicted and hung in a public square. When her body was taken down from the scaffold and placed in a coffin, "there happened a scuffle between her friends and surgeons-apprentices" for possession of it. "One, with a hammer, broke down one of the sides.... of the chest [coffin]; which, having given some air, and, together with the jolting of the case, set the blood and vitals agoing." The effect was to resuscitate Margaret Dickson, who lived for another four decades and had several children. She was nicknamed "Half-hangit Maggie Dickson."[121] To this day, an Edinburgh pub in Grassmarket is named in her honor, reminding Edinburgh of the conflict between medical science and familial loyalty—and Maggie's marvelous resurrection.[122]

Such incidents were not uncommon: because of the limited supply of legally dissected bodies of executed criminals in eighteenth-century Britain "any [anatomy] teacher who wished to offer his students a practical foundation in anatomy.... was forced to break the law."[123] *Primus*, who offered the only course of anatomy lectures in Edinburgh, usually delivered 115 lectures from October to April to between 60 and 150 students.[124] He used only one or two cadavers at a time; supplementing cadaveric dissections with demonstrations by vivisecting live animals and dissecting dead ones.[125] This mix of human and animal dissections enabled *Primus* to offer an entire course with as few as two human corpses. Nonetheless, as the half-hangit

Maggie Dickson incident indicates, although the law permitted medical dissection of condemned criminals' corpses, medical assistants and medical students had to engage in public bodysnatching to acquire them. As one historian observed "the crowd [surrounding the gallows] disregarded legal permission and contested the right of surgeons to *any* felon's body. Dissection was a violently unpopular punishment."[126]

The half-hangit Maggie Dickson incident illustrates the Edinburgh populace's visceral objection to having their loved ones kidnapped from funeral processions by medical students in search of cadavers or having the bodies of their newly deceased relatives dug up for dissection without anyone's knowledge or consent. How did *Primus* react to such objections? What did he teach his students? One might expect that, as "a man of Tender Heart," *Primus* might sympathize with angst of the protesters.[127] Instead, he informed his students in his autobiography that the protest was a misguided "[p]rejudice of the People to dissections of human Bodies, [they] foolishly believed that [I, as Professor] stole living people to dissect them alive. These prejudices occasioned frequent violent mobs from whom the Professor was in great danger of his life."[128] Popular dissent was thus dismissed as "prejudices of the people," who "foolishly believe" untruths about medicine. *Primus* fails to appreciate, or perhaps cannot allow himself to appreciate, the morally disruptive nature of his innovative mode of medical education—dissecting cadavers to teach anatomy. Most Scottish anatomists shared *Primus*'s views, which they imparted to their students, who would carry these practices and these attitudes with them to their communities—some located in the American colonies.

ON MORALLY AND ETHICALLY DISRUPTIVE INNOVATIONS

The expressions "morally disruptive" and "ethically disruptive" are inspired by the work of Clayton Christensen, who coined the expressions "disruptive innovation" and "disruptive technology" to characterize innovations like the internet and the refrigerator that disrupt accepted forms of commerce and obviate the need for a network of support services supplied by on-ground delivery of records or digital disks in stores (in the first case) or ice and milk by milkmen and icemen (in the second case).[129] Christensen contrasts disruptive innovations with sustaining innovations, which, as their name implies, sustain rather than disrupt preexisting patterns. Antibiotics, for example, changed medicine, but the innovation was not disruptive because it sustained existing patterns of healthcare delivery, requiring no greater change than substituting one type of pill for another. Thus, insofar as revolutionary medical breakthroughs do not require physicians or patients or the public to act differently, they *sustain* rather than disrupt accepted modes of practice. The Salk-Sabine polio vaccine, in contrast, was a disruptive innovation because it obsolesced an entire medical industry, the Emerson iron lung industry, and closed hospitals wards that had once been filled with rows of iron lungs assisting the breathing of polio patients.

Technological or scientific innovations are morally or ethically sustaining or disruptive insofar as they sustain or undermine established moral norms or ethical codes. Thus, the Salk-Sabine polio vaccines, although technologically disruptive innovations, were sustaining with respect to medical ethics and morality because they were consistent with and did not undermine concepts or disrupt norms in existing codes of medical ethics or accepted understandings of medical morality. Perhaps the clearest example of a morally disruptive medical innovation is the ventilator—a mechanical pump to assist breathing—invented at Copenhagen's university hospital in 1952 by the Danish anesthesiologist, Bjorn Ibsen (1915–2007). Ibsen invented the ventilator during a polio epidemic because he was desperately trying to save the life of a twelve-year-old girl dying of polio. His invention—pumping oxygen directly into the lungs—saved her life and cut the mortality rate for polio victims in half.

By assisting respiratory functions with a machine, however, the ventilator kept some patient's hearts and lungs functioning even though they appeared to be in an irreversibly comatose state, with little or no brain function. This physiological phenomenon proved morally and ethically disruptive because medical ethics and morality mandated, to quote the New York oath, that physicians "do every thing in [their] power for the benefit of the sick committed to [their] charge," and this mandate was understood as preserving life. Since the presence of a pulse/heartbeat had traditionally served as the primary criteria demarcating the living from the dead,[130] a physiological correlative of this mandate seemed to be that a physician was obligated to keep a patient's heart beating as long as possible—even if the patient had no functional brain. Ibsen's innovation thus left physicians in an ethical and moral quandary: it was *morally disruptive* because neither physicians nor families now knew how to treat patients in this ambiguous state. If they were alive but in an irreversibly vegetative state, would it be moral to turn off the ventilator ("pull the plug") that was keeping them in this state? Would it be moral to declare them dead? And, if it was moral to turn ventilators off, who could authorize such an act? Judges? Physicians? Expert committees? Patients? Families? Surrogates? Proxies? The point to appreciate is that although most technological innovations are morally sustaining, a few are morally or ethically disruptive, and these may become important catalysts for changing medical morality and ethics.

A further point to appreciate is that morally disruptive technical innovations date to the birth of modern medicine. Monro *primus*, for example, founded his school and his career on a morally disruptive innovation. *Primus* belonged to the generation of anatomist that developed new formulas for effectively preserving human corpses and organs. He could thus introduce anatomical dissection as the central feature of his course on anatomy; however, this innovation required a steady supply of corpses. In theory, corpses could be obtained legally by using the bodies of condemned prisoners, like that of half-hangit Maggie Dickson. Yet procuring the corpses of the condemned challenged the accepted moral responsibilities that the living had toward the newly dead.

As noted earlier, eighteenth-century virtue ethics focuses on motives underlying actions. A virtuous person has a noble mind motivated by beneficence and humanity; the outside world, however, judges a person's internal motives by such external actions as providing a proper burial for one's dead family members. Failure to do so reflects poorly on the living.

> The reputation of survivors depended upon their burying their dead properly. Throughout this period, funerals which fell short of what observers thought appropriate to the status of the deceased attracted unfavorable comment..... The appearance of neighbors, kinsfolk, and members of the deceased's craft or profession at the funeral, their donning of mourning-garb or tokens, and their participation in funeral ritual, expressed their sharing in the bereaved sense of loss and their support for the surviving family.[131]

So, when medical students lawfully took a body from a funeral cortege for a condemned person, like Maggie Dickson, they disrupted more than the procession; they impeded fulfillment of familial and communal duties to the dead as displayed in the cortege. They insulted the honor of the living as well as the memory of the dead, and although the upper classes might protect their honor with flytes and duels, the general populace responded in a more visceral and less controlled manner—deemed a riot by the gentlemanly classes.

Moreover, since bodysnatching the corpses of the publicly executed criminals provided a limited and uneven supply of bodies for dissection, during the inevitable shortages, the required corpses were supplied by grave robbing—another ethically and morally disruptive act. In eighteenth-century Scotland, the living did their duty to the dead by properly protecting the corpse. "Once the breath was out of the body," it was prepared for burial by being wrapped in a "winding sheet of wool.... [with] woolen stockings for the corpse's feet.... [and] laid out on view for all who wished to see the 'corp[se]' in [a] room with chairs and other furniture covered with white linen. When means allowed it the chirurgeon [surgeon] half-embalmed the body and provided a cerecloth [shroud of waxed cloth] to envelope the corpse."[132] Grave robbing undid these preparations, violating the belief system and moral norms that underlay them. Unburying the dead was outrageous, and the population of Edinburgh expressed their outrage viscerally and violently.

Primus role modeled for his students the anatomist's response to public outrage over bodysnatching: dismissive rationalization and gentlemanly sang-froid.

This attitude was part of the hidden curriculum that *Primus, Secundus*, and other Scottish anatomists (including Granville Pattison and William and John Hunter) taught their American students: an elitist, gentlemanly obtuseness toward popular protest against morally disruptive medical innovations. Gentlemanly indifference to popular protest was as integral to the Edinburgh legacy as the oath—and, like the oath, Edinburgh alumni carried this legacy of disdainful indifference to the morally disruptive aspects of medical innovation with them when they returned to America.

4

THE LECTURERS: SAMUEL BARD AND BENJAMIN RUSH

In your Behavior to the Sick remember that your Patient is the Object of the tenderest Affection, to some one.... Let your Carriage be humane.

Samuel Bard, lecture to students, New York City, 1769[1]

[Of] those moral qualities peculiarly required in the character of a physician. The most obvious of these is humanity; that sensibility of the heart which makes us feel for the distresses of our fellow-creatures.

John Gregory, lecture to students, Edinburgh, Scotland, 1770[2]

Humanity has been a conspicuous virtue among physicians... they are called upon to exhibit their humanity by sympathy, with pain and distress in persons of all ranks.

Benjamin Rush, lecture to students, Philadelphia, 1801[3]

LECTURING ON MEDICAL ETHICS: AN EDINBURGH HERITAGE

For a little more than a half century, from 1769 to 1822, every major publication on "medical ethics" emanating from the colonial or postcolonial United States was authored or commissioned by physicians who had studied at the medical college of the University of Edinburgh. In fact, every important English-language publication in "medical ethics" written by a physician during this period was by someone who had either taught or studied at the Edinburgh Medical College. John Gregory published his first lectures on "medical ethics" in 1770. Samuel Bard, an American colonial who probably attended Gregory's lectures, beat his mentor to the printing press by publishing his Americanized version of Gregory's lectures in 1769.[4] Another of Gregory's American students, Bard's classmate, Benjamin Rush, took notes on Gregory's lectures on "medical ethics" and used them as the basis for his own lecture on the subject in 1789. Yet another of Bard's classmates, the English physician Thomas Percival (1740–1804), produced a draft code of medical ethics for physicians and surgeons in 1794, publishing a final version in 1803. Nicholas Romayne (1756–1817), who belonged to a later generation of Americans studying at Edinburgh, persuaded the medical societies of the state of New York to adopt an English-language version of Edinburgh's "medical ethics" oath in 1806 and 1807. Moving a few years forward, in 1829, another Edinburgh alumnus, Michael Ryan (1800–1841), began publishing lectures on medical ethics.

From 1769 to 1822, Edinburgh faculty and alumni held a monopoly on oaths, codes, lectures, and other English-language literature on "medical ethics."[5] Such exceptionalism cries out for explanation. Likely factors were the use of English rather than Latin as the language of instruction at the Edinburgh medical college, a graduation oath stating an occupational ethics for physicians, and faculty and students drawn largely from dissenters and minorities. This last suggestion, the notion that Edinburgh's environment was conducive to discussions of the relationship between medicine and morality because it was a magnet for dissenters, is prompted by the work of medical historian Winfred Schleiner who observed that, during the Renaissance, the subject that would later be called "medical ethics" was uniquely the province of refugee Jewish physicians seeking to legitimize themselves in the context of a potentially hostile Christian culture.[6] Something akin to this dynamic appears operative at the Edinburgh Medical College where deists like William Cullen[7] (professor at Edinburgh 1755–1790) and dissenters, like Percival, had to attest to the moral character of their medical practice to those who held different religious views. As a Unitarian, for example, Percival was barred from admission to Cambridge and Oxford, deprived of his civil rights, and subject to mob violence. In 1791, the year before he began work on the text that would be published as *Medical Ethics*, an Anglican mob burned the chapel at which he worshiped. Similarly, the first person to denominate himself a "professor of medical ethics," Michael Ryan was an Edinburgh alumnus struggling against anti-Irish, anti-Roman Catholic prejudice as he attempted to practice and teach obstetrics in Anglican London. Modeling his own lectures on those of his teachers, Ryan offered formal lectures on medical ethics and was the first person to claim a professorship in the subject. Religious outliers and dissenters, these Edinburgh faculty and alumni needed to invent a secular substitute for religious ethics, and this substitute came to be called "medical ethics."

This chapter deals with the two American colonials, both Edinburgh medical school alumni, who brought the preoccupation with medical ethics they imbibed at Edinburgh back to America: Samuel Bard and Benjamin Rush. The two differ fundamentally in temperament. Conservative in politics, in love, in life, and in medical practice, through his life and writings Bard adhered to the fundamental tenets of Edinburgh ethics, including the dictate of experimenting and practicing medicine cautiously. Revolutionary to the core, Rush rebelled against his Presbyterian religious heritage; against his mother country, Britain; against his military commander-in-chief, George Washington; against his Edinburgh teacher, Cullen; against the Edinburgh secularization of physician's ethics; and against the Edinburgh dictum of practicing medicine and medical research "cautiously"—but not against the Edinburgh practice of lecturing on "medical ethics."

SAMUEL BARD

"Discourse on the Duties of a Physician" (1769)

Lectures enter the pubic realm as oral performances. Their performative nature binds them to the occasion for which they were delivered and to their intended audience. Bard brought the Edinburgh practice of lecturing on medical ethics back with him to colonial New York and regularly lectured his students on the moral duties of physicians. Although we have student notes on many of these lectures, only one of Bard's lectures on ethics found its way into print, the "Discourse on the Duties of a Physician." This lecture, delivered on May 16, 1769, was young professor Bard's first public address. The occasion was another first, the first commencement exercise for the medical students at King's College (now Columbia). A handful of graduates, their families, the faculty, and patrons—including the Royal Governor of New York Colony, Sir Henry Moore (1713–1769, Governor from 1765–1769)—gathered in the intimate and charming confines of Trinity Church (chartered in 1697) for the occasion. It was a moment that, as the young twenty-seven-year-old Bard fully appreciated, could make or break his career.

Despite his youth, Samuel Bard had been involved with medicine since he began a surgical apprenticeship with his father, John Bard (1716–1789), at the age of 14—the age at which he enrolled as a student at King's College. Two years into this education, Bard's family yanked him out of King's to send him abroad to complete his studies at the Edinburgh Medical College. This abrupt change of plans was precipitated by John Bard's discovery that Samuel had become secretly engaged to his pretty but penniless cousin Mary Bard (1746–1821). As John explained to 16-year-old Samuel, "while I do not wish to extinguish in your breast the passion of love; marriage ever did and ever will put a sudden end to all the extravagant heights of love and then you will be convinced that nothing can insure your happiness in that state, but a calm judicious, and dispassionate choice, which results from reason, judgment and friendship."[8]

Samuel's journey to Edinburgh, like his love life and his education, was disrupted when French privateers captured his ship as it was headed toward London, holding the young Bard hostage until his father's friend, American diplomat Benjamin Franklin (1706–1790), arranged for his release. After a brief sojourn in London, Bard made his way to Edinburgh, commencing his studies under Cullen, Monro *Primus* and *Secundus*, and other distinguished faculty. He received his doctoral degree on December 28, 1765.[9] On returning to New York City in 1766, Samuel joined with five other physicians to found America's second medical school at King's College and was, on that day in May 1769, delivering the college's first commencement address.

Loyalty was one of Bard's defining characteristics: he was loyal to his family, to the Edinburgh Medical College, to its oath, and to Britain—supporting the British side during the American Revolution (1775–1783).[10] Later, loyal to an oath that placed patients above politics, Bard became physician to former rebel commander George Washington (1732–1799), successfully treating him for "a malignant carbuncle" (probably a large infected boil).[11] Bard was also loyal to his first love, his cousin Mary, and resumed that relationship on his return to America. They married in 1770, becoming inseparable through life and death—dying within days of each other in 1821.

Bard's marriage took place the year after he delivered his commencement address at Trinity Church. This sequence of events may explain an odd aspect of Bard's graduation speech: its focus on his father's pet project—founding a public hospital in New York City. One might speculate that in publicly taking up his father's pet project, in thanking his father's medical society for its role in establishing the medical college, and in securing the patronage of Governor Henry Moore to bring to fruition his father's dream of creating New York Hospital, Samuel Bard was making peace with his family and thereby setting the stage for his marriage to Mary Bard soon thereafter.

Whatever Bard's personal motives, publicly appealing to the patrons and the governor for funds to found a public hospital in the context of a graduation speech was a delicate matter. Bard handled it by skillfully transitioning from physicians' duties to provide medical care to the "unhappy victims, both of Poverty and Disease,"[12] to patrons' duties to provide a facility in which such care can be provided. Assuring his audience that they were above vulgar appeals to emotions and that he would not insult them by evoking the "Miseries of Sickness and Penury" or the "Despair of an affectionate Wife, and a tender Mother" since "*you*, I know, want no such Incitements to Duty and Benevolence."[13] Then, having cited these very cases even as he denied the need to do so, Bard observed that a public hospital would provide opportunities for medical research unavailable in private practice and would "afford the best and only means of properly instructing Pupils in the Practice of Medicine, breeding good and able Physicians."[14]

Bard's appeal was a memorable success. The governor pledged a £200 donation, other private parties pledged £600, and New York City would ultimately contribute £3,000 in funds (in 2010, a total equivalent to more than one million US dollars). Samuel Bard's plans, however, were again disrupted: the hospital building was destroyed by fire during construction, and the advent of the Revolutionary War further delayed the project. John Bard never lived to see the hospital completed. Ever loyal, Samuel ensured that, when the hospital finally opened its doors in 1791, the building was dedicated to the memory of his father, John Bard.[15]

Medical Knowledge: On Continuing Medical Education

Bard's lecture was more than an excuse for fundraising; by virtue of the occasion, it was also a graduation address. So, Bard spoke about graduates' duties as they assumed their lives as physicians. Foremost of these was dedication to lifelong learning: the "[p]rofession...that...you have embraced [has as its] Object the Life of a Man"; consequently, Bard charged the graduates, "you are accountable even for Errors of Ignorance, unless you have embraced every Opportunity of obtaining Knowledge."[16] To allow someone's death from ignorance, Bard's text shouts in capital letters, is to violate the "Sixth Commandment, 'THOU SHALT DO NO MURDER.'"[17]

Turning to graduates' duties to fellow physicians, Bard states that they are to be guided by the virtues of "Integrity, Candour and Delicacy."[18] Graduates, moreover, were not to "Raise [their] Fame on the Ruins of another's Reputation," undermining the work or the worth of fellow practitioners by a sly word, a smirk, or a lifted eyebrow. Their duties to their fellow practitioners also required them to share their medical knowledge, hence they should not try to profit from secret nostrums. The term "nostrum" derives from the Latin *nostor*, which means "ours," as opposed to everyone's. A "secret nostrum" is a medication or medical device whose composition or nature is kept secret from other physicians. In Western medical ethics tradition, physicians' duty to share medical information with each other dates to the Hippocratic oath, where the duty is formulated as an obligation to fellow practitioners "to teach...this *techne*, should they desire to learn [it], to [anyone who has] sworn a medical [oath] but no other."[19] The 1766 Instruments of Association of the New Jersey Medical Society, formulated just three years before Bard's speech, also characterizes the prohibition against secret nostrums as "inconsistent with the generous spirit of the profession, [we] will at all times be ready to disclose and communicate to any member of the Society, any discovery or improvement we have made in any manner respecting the healing art."[20] John Gregory, in his lectures of 1767–1768—which Bard probably attended—condemns secret nostrums as unscientific and often felonious,[21] remarking that the "the practice has an interested and illiberal appearance"[22] that reflects poorly on the character of the practitioner.[23]

Perpetuating the received wisdom, Bard informed the graduating class at King's College that they should

> not pretend to Secrets, Panacea's and Nostrums, they are illiberal, dishonest, and inconsistent with your Characters as Gentleman and as Physicians and with your Duty as Men—For if you are possessed of any valuable Remedy, it is undoubtedly your Duty to divulge it, that as many as possible may reap the Benefit of it; and if not (which is generally the case) you are propagating a Falsehood, and imposing upon Mankind.[24]

The Edinburgh Medicalization of Moral Sense Theory

Scottish moral philosophers Adam Smith and David Hume and the Scotch-Irish philosopher Francis Hutcheson (1694–1746) embraced a virtue ethics emphasizing a person's character, as evidenced in their sentiments of beneficence, humaneness, and sympathy. Alexander Monro *primus* also embraced this position, writing to his daughter that, "[n]othing, My Dear, shews a noble, generous, social well turn'd Mind [i.e., one's character, more] than Benevolence and Humanity."[25] Beneficence and humanity were thus among the virtues expected of honorable gentlemen; however, neither the Edinburgh oath nor any other text through the mid-eighteenth century specifies these virtues as essentially connected to the moral practice of medicine. As the quotations from Bard, Gregory, and Rush prefacing this chapter indicate, however, by the late 1760s, Edinburgh lecturers and their students were associating the virtues of beneficence and humanity that *Primus* expected of *any* honorable lady or gentleman as specific to the role of physician. They became "moral qualities *peculiarly* required in the character of a physician." Moral sense theory had thus become medicalized, in the sense that, in Edinburgh medical school culture, the virtues of beneficence and humanity were now specified as essential to the character of a physician.

Bard's Moral Sense Construal of the Physician's Role

Bard's 1769 commencement address disseminated the Edinburgh medicalization of moral sense theory to his American medical students:

> In your Behavior to the Sick remember that your Patient is the Object of the tenderest Affection, to some one, or perhaps to many about him; it is therefore your Duty not only to endeavour to preserve his Life, but to avoid wounding the Sensibility of a tender Parent, a distressed Wife, or an affectionate Child. Let your Carriage be humane and attentive, be interested in his Welfare.[26]

It is noteworthy that the medical virtues that Bard inculcates in this passage are not the virtues of caution, purity, honorableness, and fidelity to the bodily needs of the sick that he himself had pledged by signing the Edinburgh oath; they were instead the moral sense virtues of attentiveness and humaneness. Student notes on Bard's unpublished annual medical school lectures document his repeated emphasis on the psychodynamics of the physician–patient relationship, indicating his awareness of the limits of the purely physical medicine (i.e., the medicine of attention to patients' *bodies* of the sort presumed by the oath). Thus, he warns that

> the physician who confines his attention to the body, knows not the extent of his art: if he know not how to soothe the irritation of an enfeebled mind, to calm the fretfulness of impatience, to rouse the courage of the timid, and even to quiet the compunctions of an over tender-conscience... and this he cannot do without he gain the confidence, esteem, and even the love, of his patients.[27]

Writing in 1794, Bard's classmate, Percival, also emphasizes the psychodynamics of the physician–patient relationship. Thus, physicians are to "inspire in the minds of their patients gratitude, respect and confidence,"[28] and "every case, committed to the charge of a physician or a surgeon, should be treated with attention, steadiness and humanity."[29] For Bard, Gregory, Percival, and Rush, physicians' duties derive in large measure from their emotional connections to the sick. The fact that a patient is "the Object of the tenderest Affection, to some one, or perhaps to many about him" thus justifies humaneness and attentiveness not only to the patient, but also to family—"a tender Parent, a distressed Wife, or an affectionate Child."

American popular culture today expects physicians to be attentive and humane in their interactions with patients' families and friends, as well as with patients themselves. But no such expectation about the psychodynamics of the physician–patient–family relationship is evident in eighteenth-century Anglo-American culture before Bard and Gregory offered their lectures. Thus, the Edinburgh oath obligates physicians "to take care faithfully that all [my actions] are conducive to [effecting] health in sick bodies."[30] These obligations are specifically to promote health in the *bodies* of the sick. No mention is made of patients' feelings, much less the feelings of their families or friends. Words like "mind," "humane," "sensibility," "affection," and "tenderness" are notably absent. Similarly, a 1753 article by the trio of colonial American lawyers arguing for the regulation of medicine characterizes the physician as a godlike person whose "proper duties" are to relieve the sick, assuage pain, and prevent preventable deaths.[31] Again, notably missing from this list are the Edinburgh virtues of attentiveness, humaneness, and sympathy. The notion that physicians have *special* professional obligations to act attentively, humanely, and sympathetically to the sick person and to that person's family and friends is the Scottish Enlightenment's most notable contribution to American medical ethics—and Bard's Discourse of May 1769 is its first published statement.

An Anglo-American Divide on Delivering a Terminal Prognosis

Bard and Rush part company from their British counterparts Gregory and Percival in their understanding of the physician's duty to honestly inform dying patients of their terminal prognosis. The British ethicists hold that this is a familial responsibility, undertaken by physicians only as a last resort; the Americans, however, hold that patients themselves are to be directly and forthrightly informed of their terminal prognosis. Bard puts the point bluntly, "never buoy up a dying Man with groundless Expectations of Recovery, this is at best a good natured and humane Deception, but too often it arises from baser Motives of Lucre and Avarice: besides it is really cruel, as the stroke of Death is always most severely felt, when unexpected."[32]

In his clinical teaching, Bard reiterated the physician's duty to communicate directly and honestly with terminal patients:

> There is in the human mind a principle of acquiescence in the dispensations of Divine Providence, which, when treated with prudence, seldom fails to reconcile the most timid to their situation. Such information I have generally found rather to calm perturbation of mind, than to increase danger, or hasten the event of the disease. Whenever, therefore, the duties of piety, or even the temporal interests of friends have demanded it, I have never hesitated making, and seldom, or never, repented such communication.[33]

In a lecture on the "On the Vices and Virtues of Physicians" that Rush delivered two decades later, in 1801, he makes the same point:

> Falsehood: This vice discovers itself chiefly in the deceptions which are practiced by physicians with respect to the cause, nature, and probable issue of diseases.... [C]riminal is the practice among some physicians of encouraging patients to expect a recovery, in diseases which have arrived at their incurable stage. The mischief done by falsehood in this case, is the more to be deplored, as it often prevents the dying from settling their worldly affairs, and employing their last hours in preparing for their future state.[34]

Where the Americans Bard and Rush emphasize direct honest communication, Percival and Gregory suggest that compassion may dictate that, as Percival put it, the physician become "minister of hope and comfort to the sick [to]... smooth the bed of death... and counteract the depressing influence of... maladies" by informing only a patient's relatives of a terminal prognosis—so that these relatives may discretely break the news to the patient.[35] In nineteenth-century America, as Gregory and Percival became more influential than Bard and Rush, their ministry of hope and comfort superseded the Bard-Rush model of straightforwardly and directly communicating a terminal prognosis.

On Autopsies and Dissections

Bard advised graduates that "whenever you shall be so unhappy as to fail in your Endeavors to relieve; let it be your constant Aim to convert particular Misfortune into general Blessing, by carefully inspecting the Bodies of the Dead, inquiring into the Causes of their Diseases; and thence improving your own Knowledge, and making further and useful Discoveries in the healing Art."[36] Bard appreciates that this line of action will meet with "[o]bstacles... from the Prejudices of the People in general. And a false Tenderness and mistaken Delicacy in Relations."[37] Rush makes the same recommendation to his students: "Give me leave to recommend to you, to open all the dead bodies you can, without doing violence to the feelings of your patients, or the prejudices of the common people."[38]

It was a truism of Edinburgh medicine that a key to advancing medical knowledge lay in the use of autopsies and dissections. Although laypersons sometimes confuse these two procedures, they are quite different. The term "autopsy" derives from the Greek *auto* for "self" and *opsis* for "eye;" it literally means "to see for one's self." Bodies are autopsied to "see for one's self" the inner cause of death by establishing clinico-pathological correlations (i.e., correlations between externally observable clinical symptoms of disease recorded in the medical record and abnormalities in organs and other bodily parts). Autopsies leave a body intact and should not be confused with dissection—a term deriving from the Latin *secare*, "to cut," and "*dis*," asunder, and thus, "to cut up"—in which the body or its parts are disassembled and may not remain intact.

In encouraging autopsies, Bard and Rush's advice is similar to that of another Cullen student, William Hunter (1718–1783), who, in lectures published in 1784 observed that "if we look among the physicians of best character ... we shall find them constantly taking pains to procure leave to examine the bodies of their patients after death."[39] As Hunter acknowledges, the relatives of those who died under the care of a physician are presumed to have a right to refuse to turn bodies over to physicians for autopsy—thus, the physician must "procure leave to examine ... bodies." For Bard and Rush, the familial right to give leave to autopsy a body, or to decline to do so, is justified by relatives' feelings of "Tenderness." This justification contrasts with the position of twentieth-century bioethicists who defend the right of informed consent to autopsies (and organ donation) on the basis of rationality; according to eighteenth- and early-nineteenth-century moral sense theories of medical ethics, however, patient and family refusals of medical advice are properly justified on the grounds of sensibility and humaneness (i.e., people's "*feelings* and *emotions*"). As Percival put the point in a discussion of a patient's right to decline routine medical procedures like bloodletting, "even the *prejudices* of the sick are not to be contemned or opposed."[40]

Respecting a family's feelings and even their prejudices in declining to have a loved one's body autopsied, however, conflicts with the physician's duty to advance medicine by establishing clinico-pathological correlations. One interesting feature of the moral sense construction of a family's right to refuse access to a body is that it leaves the door open to an unusual possibility for resolving this conflict—subterfuge. Since the right to refuse rests on relations' "feelings," and since what relatives do not know cannot disturb their feelings, surreptitious autopsies might seem to offer an ethically acceptable way of fulfilling the physician's duty to advance medical science. It thus might appear to morally adventurous physicians that they could fulfill their duties to science by using effectively stealthy grave robbers to secure bodies for autopsies and dissections.

Bard countenanced no such behavior. According to one biographer, during the New York Doctor's Riot

> in the year 1788, against the physicians of the city, from suspicion of their robbing the grave yards.... Dr. Bard.... Conscious of his innocence of the alleged charge ... resisted the most urgent solicitations of his friends to flee or to conceal himself; but as the infuriated mob approached his house, ordered the doors and windows to be thrown open ... in full view of them, as they drew near. His calmness, or his character, saved him: they approached with

horrible imprecations; gazed a while in silence, and then passed on, with acclamations of his innocence.[41]

BENJAMIN RUSH

Lectures on the Duties, Virtues, and Vices of Physicians

On February 7, 1789, America's most famous physician, Benjamin Rush, delivered his closing lecture as professor of chemistry at his alma mater, the Medical College of Philadelphia (now part of the University of Pennsylvania). Anticipating promotion to professor of the theory and practice of medicine, Rush chose a topic in medicine, rather than in chemistry. This was more challenging than it might appear because Rush had achieved his fame from writing about temperance and abolitionism,[42] from his support of the American Revolution as a member of the Continental Congress, from his role as surgeon general to the Continental Army, and—more than anything else—as a signer of the Declaration of Independence. Rush was, in sum, America's most famous physician, but he had never distinguished himself as a practitioner, researcher, or teacher of medicine.[43] So, he chose as his topic a subject that did not demand expert medical knowledge, "Observations on the Duties of a Physician." As professors often do when venturing into new areas, Rush based this lecture on notes he had taken at the lectures delivered by one of his teachers at Edinburgh, John Gregory. Rush even borrowed Gregory's title, "Observations on the Duties of A Physician" but changed the subtitle to "Accommodated, to the Present State of Society and Manners in the United States."[44]

Much of Rush's lecture simply rehearses Gregory's favorite themes: avoiding "singularities of every kind in your manners, dress and general conduct... [which] we find... chiefly in little minds."[45] Rush also follows Gregory in encouraging temperance by avoiding "strong drink."[46] Additionally, Rush follows Gregory in advising physicians to "never... abandon a dying patient,"[47] and he urges his students to adopt a sliding fee scale, charging more to the rich but providing free services to the poor.[48] Channeling Gregory's thoughts, Rush also emphasizes the psychodynamics of the physician–patient relationship: "Let us avail ourselves of the aid of which these powers of the mind present to us in the strife between life and death."[49] Rush's believed in using placebos; that is, "remedies of doubtful efficacy... work[ing] up in my patients confidence, bordering on certainty, of their probably good effects... the success of this measure has, much oftener answered, than disappointed my expectation; and while my patients have commended the vomit, the purge, or the blister which was prescribed, I have been disposed to attribute their recovery the concurrence of the *will* in the action of the medicine."[50]

Rush's Rejection of Secularism and of "Caution" in the Conduct of Research

Rush differs from Gregory in rejecting the separation of religious ethics from medical ethics. A "New Sider" Great Awakening Presbyterian, Rush embraced highly emotional "Awakened" services that created a visceral connection between worshipers and the deity.[51] He held that belief in the "true" Christian God is a virtue in a physician and that neglect of religion is a preeminent vice of the medical profession.[52] By the end of his career, Rush would model the physician–patient relationship on the God-worshiper relationship and teach his students that the virtuous physician was a Christian whose primary duty was piety toward the Christian God.[53]

Rush not only rejected the Edinburgh heritage of building a wall of separation between religion and medicine, he also rejected the Edinburgh view that caution is a preeminent virtue of physicians. In Edinburgh parlance, the duty of caution and the correlative virtue of practicing physic cautiously refers both to the mode in which physic is practiced and to the responsible conduct of medical research. In his lectures to his medical students on the duty of practicing medicine "cautiously," as stipulated in the Edinburgh oath, Michael Ryan invoked the morality of the Golden Rule:

> The duty of *caution* in practice means, "care not to expose the sick to any unnecessary danger." The best rule of conduct on this important point is the simple and comprehensive, religious and moral precept "do unto others as you would they should do unto you."[54] Whatever the practitioner does or advises to be done, for the good of his patient, and what he would do in his own case, or in the case of those dearest to him—if he or they were in the same situation—is not only justifiable on his part, but it is his indispensible duty to do.... But if [the practitioner] administered a dangerous medicine, merely to gratify his own curiosity or zeal for science, to ascertain the comparative advantage or disadvantage of some new remedy, either proposed by himself or suggested by others; he is guilty of a breach of ethics and of a high misdemeanor, and a great breach of trust towards his patient; and if the patient died, I apprehend, he might be severely punished.
>
> Medical men have tried the most dangerous experiments upon themselves, from their zeal for science; and even sacrificed their lives, but patients in general have no such zeal for science, no ambition for such a crown of martyrdom, and generally employ and pay their medical attendants for the very opposite purpose..... [Yet] it is admitted by the best practitioners, that many remedies are still wanted for the cure of disease, and that this want leads us most justifiably to and most inevitably to try new remedies on many occasions; and such experiments are not blamable, for they are necessary....[55]

> From [such experiments] there results much inevitable danger in the practice of physic. From this acknowledged danger, results the important duty of caution in a physician, or care to make the danger as little as possible. Whatever is best for the sick, it is the indispensible duty of a medical man to do for them. It is [in the words of the Edinburgh oath] his duty and obligation, "faithfully to do all things conducive to the health of his patients;" and this is so complete and indefeasible, that it cannot be set aside by any cause whatever.[56]

Ryan recognizes the necessity of *therapeutic* experiments (i.e., experimenting with treatments that might benefit patients whose illnesses were unresponsive to traditional treatments); however, the intent of such experiments should be "for the good of [the] patient," and the experimental treatment should be subject to the Golden Rule, "what [a physician] would do in his own case, or in the case of those dearest to him." *Nontherapeutic experiments*, those conducted to "gratify [a physician's] own curiosity or zeal for science, [or] to ascertain the comparative advantage or disadvantage of some new remedy," are condemned as "a breach of ethics...a high misdemeanor, and a great breach of trust towards his patient." Ryan is also concerned that even seemingly justifiable therapeutic experiments endanger physic—the field of medicine itself—by tempting physicians to place their interests as researchers above the interests of their patients. To help physicians determine whether they are motivated by their own interests or by the patient's interests, Ryan recommends testing their desire to introduce an experimental treatment by using the Golden Rule, explicitly invoked as a moral principle. In later commentary, Ryan remarks that "the rule laid down by the profession [is] that dangerous experiments should not be made on the sick without their consent."[57]

Like Ryan, Gregory also appealed to the Golden Rule and to principles of "Justice & Humanity" to condemn students' nontherapeutic experiments on patients[58]:

> I know very well that it is a common opinion with many young Gentlemen, that the Physician who attends an Hospital should always try Experiments on the Patients; this I think contrary both to Justice & Humanity: I shall therefore give you my common Practice & not sport with the lives of poor people: I would not give a Person a Medicine that I would scruple [i.e., hesitate] to take myself. I shall always have in my Eye that moral precept, "Do as you would be done by."[59]

Gregory accepted that some therapeutic experiments were permissible "when the Medicines that I commonly use fail." As he elaborated in a different lecture, "Desperate measures should be used in some cases, where every other method has been proved ineffectual. In such circumstance we should have recourse to medicine which under more favourable circumstances might be thought dangerous."[60] In another lecture, Gregory discussed inoculation experiments, holding that such experiments were permissible only if they met the Golden Rule test: "Some I know have tried dangerous Experiments, such as inoculating people [with] Small pox . . . yet I would ask that man if he would have done so to his own child: if he would not do it to his own Child, why should he endanger the lives of other people?"[61] Since virtuous character and intent were primary for Gregory, the Golden Rule was invoked to validate the purity of one's intent. Gregory thus held that one could experiment with new therapies in desperate circumstances if conventional remedies have failed, but only if one would submit one's self or one's child to the same experiment. Gregory's student Samuel Bard abided by the Golden Rule ethics of experimentation by conducting nontherapeutic experiments for his thesis research on opium—then, as now, a major analgesic essential to effective palliative care—using as his subjects himself and his roommate. In an act of reciprocity, Bard submitted to his roommate's experiments on the medical uses of ammonia.[62]

Bard also taught his medical students the virtue of caution in research, explicitly warning against overtheorizing from inadequate data, especially when proposing new remedies:

> It is the error of ingenious men, and, therefore, should be guarded against by the young; who, in the warmth of their imagination, and pursuit of knowledge, are too ready to adopt such plausible theories as promise to shorten their labour, and advance their views; to remove all their doubts and difficulties, and enable them to give a reason for everything. Be *cautious*, therefore, how you admit new names, new theories, and new remedies. This rage for novelty pervades our profession, especially in this country. Hence our extended catalogue of new fevers, and hasty adoption of new remedies; hence the unlimited and unwarranted application of mercury with weight . . . and the lancet without discrimination; and hence, I am afraid, I may say, the sacrifice of many lives which might have been preserved, had they been left to water gruel, and good nursing.[63]

For Bard, "caution" meant skeptical scrutiny of "new names, new theories, and new remedies." In Bard's medical writings, caution is an operant virtue; he generally recommended less rather than more medical intervention.[64] Bard expressly condemns the "unlimited and unwarranted application of mercury with weight"—massive doses of mercury chloride, a poison used as a powerful and violent laxative or "purge," which was known as *calomel* in the eighteenth century. He also condemned the indiscriminate use of the lancet for surgical bloodletting or bleeding.

Bard's language is striking similar to that of his teacher, Cullen (also Rush's "master" or mentor). Cullen scorned systems built on "false facts," emphasizing cautious observation and the need to test new treatments through "cautious safe trial." According to the notes taken by Philadelphia medical students who studied with Cullen around the same time that Bard, Percival, and Rush attended his lectures, Cullen taught:

> We must be *cautious* of the difficulty of observation, we must trust to none that we have not had an opportunity of observing in all Circumstances and of repeating several times as we are liable to your same Credulity to the same bias in favor of System, and to the same partiality for remedies whose good effects we have once experienced or which we perhaps have recommended, and no man can be sufficiently guarded against these biases which may deceive his eyes....[65]
>
> I need hardly add, that particularly with regard to... Remedies there may be a vanity in believing too little or in believing too much. I hold that some degree of diffidence is the safe side but this must be always under the correction of a *cautious* safe trial and of a repeated observation by repeated Experiment as free from prejudices we have mentioned as we can.[66]

On occasion, Cullen expressed himself on these matters with startling frankness:

> Physicians fond of Theory have given us many false facts, perhaps with honesty adopting facts not well observed. Others, who thought they had made improvements in the cure of disease, have told downright lies especially those who have pretended to discover cures of new remedies, this is not confined to Quacks: the love of fame will produce it in many. The best things in the world are liable to abuse, one of the highest improvements of Physic is the agreement among Physicians of the necessity of increasing the Stock of facts. Many however seeking fame publish Experiments and observations, which are often inaccurately made and unfaithfully recorded. Their cases are often the Produce of their Closets [i.e., crap].[67]

As these passages from Bard, Cullen, Gregory, and Ryan (and comparable passages in Percival[68]) attest, within the Edinburgh school there was a widely shared conception of the duty to practice medicine cautiously and to be especially careful to avoid what Bard characterized as the "error of ingenious men," hurriedly introducing new diseases, new theories, and new treatments. The practice, the virtue, and the duty of caution was multifaceted: it involved caution in observation of experiments (repeated unbiased observation), cautious safe trials of new remedies, caution in using the least dangerous medicines or amounts, and caution in experimenting to find new remedies and in using new treatments only when traditional measures failed—and then only therapeutically, with the patient's benefit as the primary purpose. Physicians were to assure themselves of the beneficent intent of their experiments by using the Golden Rule: would they conduct this experiment on their own child? Nontherapeutic experimentation was ethical only if it was voluntary and—again following the Golden Rule—only if the researcher actually submitted himself or someone from his family to this or a comparable experiment. Ryan also added the condition that all experiments require the consent of the capacitated participant.

In striking contrast to his Edinburgh professors and fellow Edinburgh alumni, Rush snubbed the virtue of caution in treatment and research, expressly rejecting the standards for the responsible conduct of medical research taught by his contemporaries. As early as 1789, Rush derided cautious physicians as "pusillanimous." The word is derived from the Latin for "puerile" and "animus," lacking animation, or unmanly—a euphemism for cowardly or impotent. Instead, Rush urges his students to practice physic with Christian boldness:

> XIV... we should at all times risk, and even sacrifice reputation, to preserve the life of a fellow-creature. The pusillanimous, or as he is commonly called, the *safe* physician, who, absorbed only in the care of his own reputation, views without exertion the last conflict between life and death in a patient, in my opinion will be found hereafter to have been guilty of a breach of the Sixth Commandment [thou shalt not murder]; while the conscientious, or, as he is commonly called, the *bold* physician, who loses sight of his character, and even of the means of his subsistence, and by the use of a remedy of doubtful efficacy turns the scale in favor of life, performs an act that borders on divine benevolence. A physician who has only once in his life enjoyed the godlike pleasure that is connected with such an act of philanthropy, will never require any other consideration to reconcile his life to the toils and duties of his profession.[69]

Lampooning the virtue of caution as "pusillanimity" motivated by a self-serving concern for reputation, Rush extols the ideal of the bold physician who will respond to his Christian calling by trying any "remedy of doubtful efficacy" to save a patient's life, and who, if successful in this act, which borders on "divine benevolence," will experience the rapture of "godlike pleasure." Seldom have a few words of advice to a lecture hall of students proved as prescient, and rarely has following one's own advice proved so devastating. Within a few years of uttering these words, Rush would "enjoy the godlike pleasure" of defying conventional opinion to save patients' lives, becoming "the bold physician" experimenter he envisioned. In consequence, he would be expelled from the College of Physicians, caricatured in the press, and pilloried in the court of public opinion.

RUSH AND THE YELLOW FEVER EPIDEMIC OF 1793

Rush's repudiation of the duty of cautious conduct during the yellow fever epidemic of 1793 is pivotal to understanding his medical career and the fluctuating nature of his later reputation.[70] For, in the midst of that epidemic, Rush became the bold "heroic physician" he extolled to his students—providing a role model that would influence later American medical practice.[71] The turning point was his inaugural lecture as full professor of medicine in 1789. Had Rush been content to elaborate on "the System of medicine [he] had learned from the lectures and publications of Dr. Cullen,"[72] as he had done earlier that year in adopting Gregory's lectures, he could have composed the lecture with few problems. This time, however, Rush, was determined to be original.

As Rush remarked in an autobiography that he wrote for his descendants,[73] "After much study and inquietude," a new "[s]ystem . . . obtruded upon me suddenly while I was walking the floor of my study. It was like a ferment introduced into my mind. It produced in it a constant and endless succession of decompositions and new arrangements of facts and ideas upon medical subjects."[74] Rush's new theory of medicine thus came to him as a revelation, and, in accepting this revelation as a self-evident scientific truth, Rush abandoned Cullen's concept of cautious empirical investigation in favor of a New Side Great Awakening Presbyterian standard of truth. A vision revealed to Rush that "there was but one fever in the world"—a theory that would soon evolve into the more radical view that "there is but one disease in the world."[75] These visions of a new "[s]ystem . . . led to important changes in [Rush's] practice of medicine"[76] and he began "depleting" fever-generating overactive systems or organs by purging the body with massive doses of calomel (mercury chloride), supplemented by extensive bloodletting.

Neither purging nor bloodletting were new treatments. In 1789, Europe and its colonies were still captivated by the heritage of Greco-Roman medicine, according to which disease was a symptom of an imbalance in humors that could be righted by bleeding or purging. What distinguished Rush's practice from this tradition was his "heroic" use of massive, violent purges with calomel and frequent withdrawals of large quantities of blood. Rush would eventually reject as useless most standard medicines except for bark (quinine), diet, opium, bloodletting, calomel, and other purges, making "medicine . . . a science so simple that two years study, instead of five or more, were sufficient to understand all that was true and practical in it."[77]

"In the innovations which I attempted," Rush reassured his descendants, he "was not actuated by ambition, or a desire of being Founder of a new sect" like his "master, Dr. Cullen"—who had been the object of "too much veneration." It is rather that "[h]umble and unworthy instruments," like Rush himself, "are often employed in promoting the physical as well as the moral happiness on mankind."[78] Rush, protests too much: he was clearly rebelling against his master Cullen, rejecting and inverting Cullen's systematic classification of fevers.[79] Where Cullen found many diseases and causes, Rush found but one disease and one single cause, "overexcitement," and this could be cured by just one treatment: depletion through bleeding and purging. Rush would later claim that Cullen's nosology (i.e., his classification of diseases) and his search for clinical-pathological correlations "retarded the progress of medicine" because "the division of diseases into genera and species... has led physicians to prescribe exclusively for the names of diseases.... This practice has done the most extensive mischief, [in] epidemics.... It multiplies unnecessarily the articles of the material medica, by employing nearly as many medicines, as... forms of disease."[80] The College of Physicians of Philadelphia, however, rejected Rush's revelations and consequently Rush's "business"—the word Rush himself chose to describe his medical practice—declined as fellow Philadelphia physicians "precluded [him] from consultations."[81]

As fate would have it, the summer of 1793 provided Rush with a new opportunity to persuade his colleagues and to increase his "business." Philadelphia, at that time the national capital and America's largest metropolitan area (with a population of about 40,000) was stricken by a yellow fever epidemic. Throughout the summer of 1793, the city lost a quarter of its population: an estimated 4,000 (1 in 10) died of yellow fever; another 6,000 fled. The city became a charnel house as bodies piled up unburied. Many physicians fled city with their affluent clientele but, to his credit, Rush refused to flee. Adhering to Christian precepts, he treated everyone who sought his services, poor and rich alike, irrespective of payment.

In the second month of the epidemic, Rush discovered an unpublished manuscript in which it was reported that extreme purges had cured "yellow fever" during an outbreak in Virginia a half century earlier.[82] Chance favoring the prepared heart, Rush "paused,"[83] as he realized that the treatment described in the manuscript fit the theory of treating fever that he had announced in 1789. The manuscript "dissipated [his] ignorance" and, using the New Sider Presbyterian revelatory standards of truth, Rush "adopted his theory, and practice, and resolved to follow them. It remained now only to fix upon a suitable purge to answer the purpose of discharging the contents of the bowels."[84]

After deciding on a truly violent purge, a combination of calomel and jalap (a powerful root laxative), Rush reported, "It perfectly cured four out the first five patients."[85] So, on the basis of an old manuscript, an epiphany, and the unrepeated observation that four out of five patients remained alive after one or two days of treatment, on September 9, Rush informed the College of Physicians of Philadelphia that he had discovered a new "cure" for yellow fever. Responding on the next day, Adam Kuhn (1741–1817), a fellow Edinburgh alumnus and another Cullen student, replied in an open letter published in a local newspaper that yellow fever could be treated successfully using mild medicines. "I do not administer any emetic," Kuhn wrote, "neither do I give a laxative, unless indicated by costiveness [constipation]."[86] Kuhn also warned that, in the West Indies, where yellow fever is common, "laxatives are never employed."[87]

"Hereafter my name should be Shadrach, Meshach or Abednego,"[88] Rush wrote to his wife later that day.

> For I am sure that the preservation of those men from death by fire was not a greater miracle than my preservation from the infection of the prevailing disorder. I have lived yet to see the close of another day, more awful than any I have yet seen. Forty persons, it is said, have been buried this day, and I have visited and prescribed for more than 100 patients.... Amidst my numerous calls to the wealthy and powerful, I do not forget the poor.... Drs.[names] have all adopted my method of treating the disorder, and are all successful with me. Dr. Kuhn has set his face against it, and many follow him, and hence the continuance and mortality of the disorder.[89]

Identifying with Shadrach, Meshach, and Abednego, heroes of the Hebrew Bible who survived near-martyrdom by adhering to their beliefs, Rush claims that, like them, he too will survive the fiery ordeals of disease and skeptics through his unwavering belief in his newly revealed system of treating yellow fever.

To obviate the effects of Kuhn's letter on the minds of citizens, the following day Rush, "published an account of the ill success which had attended the use of the remedies recommended by Dr. Kuhn."[90] He also accused Kuhn of misdiagnosing, "Prescribing for the *name* of a disease, without regard to the above circumstances, has slain more than the sword."[91] On September 11, Rush wrote to his wife, "Thank God! Out of one hundred patients, whom I have visited, or prescribed for, this day I have lost none."[92] The next day, September 12, Rush published two letters in a newspaper: one addressed to the public announced—apparently because none of his patients had died on the previous day—that "the almost universal success with which it has pleased God to bless the remedy of strong mercurial purges and bleeding."[93] Rush then advised the citizens of Philadelphia not "to leave the city... because the disease is now under the power of medicine [and] because the citizens who now wish to fly into the country cannot avoid carrying the infection with them."[94] Published alongside this letter were advertisements for "Doctor Rush's Mercurial Sweating Powder for Yellow Fever."[95] The second letter "To the College of Physicians: The Use of the Lancet in Yellow Fever," announced that

Rush "consider[ed] intrepidity [i.e., resolute fearlessness] in the use of the lancet at present to be as necessary as mercury and jalap in this insidious and ferocious disease." Rush also reiterated his accusation that his colleagues had misdiagnosed the disease.[96]

Rush noted with satisfaction in his autobiography that these letters "brought me an immense amount of business."[97] This may have been the intended effect. As Rush would later remark in a revealing lecture to his students, "[]opposing the principles, and traducing the practice and characters, of brother physicians.... Performing great and sudden cures" are effective if "dishonorable method[s] of acquiring business."[98] Rush's faith in his cure seemed to render honorable these otherwise disreputable acts.

On October 3, Rush confidently proclaimed, "I think I was the unworthy instrument in the hands of kind Providence of recovering *more* than ninety-nine out of an hundred of my patients before my late indisposition. A number died...for want of well timed bleeding and purging.... [S]ome have died under my care from my inability...to be early and punctual in my attendance on them; for recovery often depends upon the application of the remedies, not only on a *certain* day, but frequently at a *certain* hour."[99] Reflecting on these claims years later, Rush reiterated that he lost patients during the 1793 epidemic *only* because of mistimed treatment: "In one of my publications in the year 1793, I asserted that the yellow fever was as much under the power of medicine as the influenza, or an intermitting fever. This was strictly true in the beginning of the epidemic of that year, and continued to be so [except for] delays in sending for physicians."[100]

By making the success of his treatment time dependent, Rush rendered it unfalsifiable, since any reported death was automatically explained away as a mistimed application of his treatment methods. Thus, Rush could and did deny that the yellow fever deaths of his sister and of four out of five his apprentices—all of whom had received the full Rush purge and bleed treatment—counted against his claim of a 1 percent mortality rate. Like Shadrach, Meshach, and Abednego, Rush had unshakable faith in his cures, and any mortality greater than 1 percent had to be explained away by other factors.

Cullen had warned his students that progenitors of a priori systems pollute the medical literature with "false facts" produced "from the design of supporting favorite theories—from the design of supporting particular remedies...from the vanity of giving false observations; in short, as I have often said there are more false facts than false opinions in physic."[101] Yet Rush, jealous of Cullen's fame, desperate to be original and to avoid parroting his "master," and influenced by New Sider Great Awakening standards of revealed truth, rejected Cullen's standard of cautiously repeatable empirical observations, embracing instead a revealed theory of medical truth that transubstantiated medical science into medical theology.

Cullen, the skeptical deist, characterized such theories as "crap" and predicted that the authors of crap theories would manufacture "false" facts to prove them. Rush's actions seem to substantiate Cullen's prediction.

THE CONTEMPORARY CRITIQUE OF RUSH'S THEORY AND PRACTICE

Rush had violated the basic precepts of scientific experimentation, as understood in his own time: cautious safe trial, cautious repeated observation, and caution in announcing success in advance of the "facts." He was, moreover, so confident of his revealed cure that he endangered the lives of thousands of Philadelphians by publicly advising them not to flee their plague-ridden city. Rush also violated ethics of gentlemanly honor by puffery in overstating his cure rate in the public press, by advertising secret nostrums, and by accusing his colleagues of mass murder. His fellow physicians criticized him publicly, ostracized him, and forced his resignation from the medical society. They carried the grudge to extent of remarking his faults in his obituary:

> Dr. Benjamin Rush, one of the... founders of the College, died April 19, 1813. He resigned in 1793[102].... He was dogmatic, impatient of contradiction, and often unreasonably resentful.... His attitude was unfriendly and resentful to those medical friends whose opinions in connection with the yellow fever were in conflict with his own. His relations with many of the medical men of Philadelphia became so unpleasant to his sensitive nature that, in 1797, he expressed readiness to remove to New York, provided he were appointed to a medical professorship in Columbia College [which was denied him].[103]

Rush's leading contemporary critic was not a physician but a muckraking journalist, William Cobbett (1763–1835), whose attacks on Rush were politically motivated. Cobbett characterized Rush's bleeding and purging treatment for yellow fever as "one of those great discoveries which have contributed to the depopulation of the earth."[104] Cobbett knew enough about eighteenth-century medical research standards to call Rush's claim of saving better than 99 in 100 patients an "intentional falsehood."

> Rush... modestly observed that he had been "the unworthy instrument in the hand of a kind Providence of recovering *more* than *ninety-nine out of a hundred of his patients;*" and he had... publicly proclaimed in Philadelphia, that, with the aid of *his* remedies, the Fever, was, "In point of danger and mortality, reduced to a level with the *measles,* the *influenza*, or a *common cold*." [Even] after he had time to reflect, and to retract these assertions, he

repeats them with additional effrontery, and thus deprives himself of all claim to an exemption from the charge of *intentional falsehood.*

[Rush however] gives no *list* of his patients; an omission not to be accounted for otherwise than by his assurance that such a list would give the lie to his assertions.... "I regret," says he, "that is not in my power to furnish a list of them, for a *majority* of them were poor people, whose names are still *unknown* to me." Can you imagine that this man, who was labouring...to establish his reputation on the success of a discovery, to which he prefixed his name, would omit to note down the names of those he cured? Recollect, too, that his system was opposed by other physicians[105]; that the public had been cautioned against his practice, as against "*certain death.*" Under such circumstances...had [Rush] cured but ninety-nine out of a *thousand,* can you believe that he would have omitted to note down the *survivors*? He says a *majority* of his patients were poor people. But...poverty does not deprive men of their *names*; nor are the names of the poor...more difficult to write down, than those of the rich....

Never did a healing discovery fail of success for want of certificates of its efficacy; on the contrary, wonder-working nostrums are always indebted for a great portion of celebrity, to the importance which each lucky patient attaches to its existence, and to the vanity which almost every one has, of appearing in print....

Fortunately, however, for Philadelphia, and unfortunately for Rush and his discovery, a bill of *mortality* was kept by the officers of the city.... The Yellow Fever of 1793 broke out on the first of August, and for that day to the eighth of September the number of deaths has been various, once as low as three and once as high as forty-two.... On September the twelfth Rush began to recommend his powders by public advertisement;...from the day on which Rush declared that his discovery has reduced the Fever to a level with a *common cold*; from the day on which he promulgated the infallibility of his nostrum; from that day did the bill of mortality begin to increase in a fearful degree, as will be seen by the following abstract.

Thus, you see, that...the deaths did actually increase; and, incredible as it may seem, this increase grew with that of the very practice which saved more than ninety-nine patients out of a hundred![106]

Cobbett's epidemiological methodology may have been crude, but the thrust of his observations was correct. The mortality rate for Rush's patients could not have been the 1 percent that he claimed. Historians currently estimate that the mortality rate for Rush's patients was about 46 percent, which is significantly higher than the 33 percent mortality rate that Thomas Jefferson estimated for the 1793 Philadelphia outbreak.[107] As Rush's contemporaries pointed out, there was then—and there

TABLE 4.1 William Cobbett's Table of Yellow Fever Deaths, September and October 1793

September	Deaths	October	Deaths
11th	**23**	1st	**74**
12th	**33**	2nd	**66**
13th	**37**	3rd	**78**
14th	**48**	4th	**58**
15th	**56**	5th	**71**
16th	**67**	6th	**76**
17th	**81**	7th	**82**
18th	**69**	8th	**90**
19th	**61**	9th	**102**
20th	**67**	10th	**93**
21st	**57**	11th	**119**
22nd	**76**		
23rd	**68**		
24th	**96**		
25th	**87**		
26th	**52**		
27th	**60**		
28th	**51**		
29th	**57**		
29th	**57**		
30th	63		

is now—no evidence that Rush's radical bleeding and purging treatment would do anything but weaken a yellow fever patient, increasing mortality by exacerbating the impact of the disease. Moreover, the discrepancy between the 1 percent morality rate that Rush claimed and the estimates of 33–46 percent found by others is so great that some combination of self-deception, radical hyperbole, and perhaps even intentional falsehood seems implicated.

Assessing Rush by Eighteenth-Century Standards of Medical Conduct

Cobbett accused Rush of various forms of ethical misconduct: (1) intentional falsehood in asserting exaggerated claims of cure in the face of overwhelming evidence to the contrary; (2) endangering the lives and health of Philadelphians in pursuit of (3) a messianic desire to be regarded as a "Saving Angel," sent by "a kind Province" to rescue the people of Philadelphia; (4) quackery in advertising his cure for yellow fever; and (5) failure to follow the accepted practice of "all other great discoverers, of registering the names of those patients who had received his treatment."

Perhaps Cobbett's most cutting charge is that of "quackery." Quoting the definition of "quack" used by Joseph Addison (1672–1719) as "a boastful pretender to physic; one who proclaims his own medical abilities and nostrums in public places," Cobbett argues that Rush's "conduct brings him up to this definition."[108] Following up on this charge, Cobbett compares Rush's newspaper letter of September 12, urging "fellow-citizens... to take *his mercurial purges*; which [enjoy] *almost universal success*,"[109] to advertisements of known quacks and notes that the language is virtually identical.[110] Rush is thus found guilty of conducting a quackish campaign to promote his own fame and fortune. The issue of record keeping (i.e., *lists*) probes more deeply into the distinction between innovation and quackery. Quacks are businessmen who sell a product to make a profit, irrespective of its actual efficacy. Proper physicians, in contrast, should be motivated by the virtue of beneficence rather than by profit and should prescribe only safe and effective remedies to their patients. New treatments should be based on cautious safe trial, cautious repeated observation, and meticulous record keeping. Rush violated all of these standards. He had not subjected his cure to repeated observations before offering it publicly and before assuring the public at large that they need not flee the epidemic.[111]

Although a layperson, Cobbett fully appreciated that meticulous record keeping, "lists," are integral to any form of prospective study, including those recognized as responsible science in the eighteenth century. Rush, however, had claimed a 1 percent mortality rate for his treatment and yet either kept no records or refused to publish his records. Then, as now, standard business practice required keeping a registry of patients' names, if for no other reason than to bill them.[112] Moreover, as Cobbett observes, the practice of "other great discoverers" involved a registry of subjects' names. It is difficult to imagine that Rush kept no such registry, especially since he reports recording in a "note book all the observations I had collected during the day, and which I marked with a pencil in my pocket book in sick rooms, or in my carriage."[113]

Lists and the Precedent of the Royal Experiment

The issue of "lists," or a registry of patients name, lies at the core of Cobbett's indictment of Rush. Bard, Kuhn, and Percival—all Cullen's students—emphasize the importance of record keeping. Medical texts of the period are filled with details of specific cases drawn from meticulously kept records. The standard for record keeping during epidemics had been set during a debate over smallpox inoculation that raged in the early eighteenth century. Physicians and laypersons were experimenting with a new method for preventing smallpox: inoculating healthy people with pus from smallpox to infect them with a milder form of the disease that then immunized them against more virulent attacks. Inoculation was common in Africa, Asia, and the Middle East but not well known in early eighteenth-century

Europe and its North American colonies—although accounts of the procedure had been reported in 1669 to the Royal Society and were published in 1714 and 1716 in a leading scientific journal, *Transactions of the Royal Society*.[114] In 1718, Lady Mary Wortley Montagu (1689–1762), wife of the British consul in Constantinople—a beautiful woman whose face had been ravaged by smallpox—introduced the practice of inoculation to Britain after complying with the Golden Rule (as understood at that time) by subjecting her own son and daughter, aged 5 and 4, to the Turkish practice of inoculation.

Lady Mary shared Gregory's understanding of the Golden Rule: "I would ask that man if he would have done [this experiment] to his own child."[115] As she wrote to a friend, "you may believe I am well satisfied of the safety of this experiment, since I intend to try it on my dear little son. I am patriot enough to take the pains to bring this useful invention into fashion in England, and I should not fail to write to some of our Doctors very particularly about it."[116] Having safely inoculated her son, on returning to England, Lady Mary engaged the Scottish physician Charles Maitland (c. 1704–1751) to inoculate her 4-year-old daughter in front of witnesses.[117] Her daughter survived unharmed. On August 9 1721, acting on a Royal Command, Maitland again demonstrated the safety and efficacy of smallpox inoculation by testing it on seven prisoners condemned to execution. The prisoners survived and then demonstrated their immunity by being exposed to smallpox without becoming infected.[118] Once the safety and efficacy of inoculation was established, the British Royal Family was inoculated, thereby setting a precedent for the practice in Britain and its colonies.[119]

The dramatic story of "The Royal Experiment" was well known, and Rush, who had published his own theory of inoculation in 1781,[120] was undoubtedly familiar with it. He must also have been aware that Dr. Maitland, following good eighteenth-century scientific practice, kept a register of his research subjects from John Alcock, age 20, to Anne Tompion, age 25. These records list the hour and day on which subjects were inoculated and offer evidence that, as Maitland observed, the time of inoculation did not affect efficacy. As is standard for the period, Maitland's records document all of his claims.[121]

The Boylston-Mather Lists

Rush must also have been familiar with the use of a register, a simple list of patients, to settle controversies surrounding the practice of inoculation during the Boston smallpox epidemic of the 1720s. The influential Puritan minister Cotton Mather (1663–1728) had read about the practice of inoculation that Lady Mary introduced to London in the *Transactions of the Royal Society* and had learned more about the practice from his slave, Onesimus, and other African Americans working in

Boston. One physician, Zadbdiel Boylston (1679–1766) was sufficiently persuaded by Mather's information to apply the Golden Rule for experimentation by testing the safety of the procedure on his own family members (his son and two house slaves).[122] They survived. Having established the safety of the procedure, Boylston inoculated more than 200 people. Initially, Mather and Boylston were publicly castigated for intruding on God's prerogative by "sporting" or gambling with human life. At the height of the debate, a bomb was thrown through Mather's window with a note, "Cotton Mather, you dog, dam you! I'll inoculate you with this; with a pox to you!"[123] However, when Boylston and Mather published lists of names showing that those inoculated were significantly less likely to contract smallpox than those not inoculated, condemnation gave way to praise. Only six of the 244 people on the list of those who had received inoculations died (2.5 percent), compared with 844 deaths in the 5,980 persons who were not inoculated (14 percent).[124]

These comparative data—these lists—convinced former critics like Benjamin Franklin and the Edinburgh-educated physician William Douglass (c. 1691–1752) to change their minds and become champions of inoculation.[125] As Cullen had taught Rush and generations of other Edinburgh students, medical science could resolve controversies and reconcile conflicting opinions because it rested on "facts." In the case in point, the facts were documented by a list of the names of those who had received the inoculation. Anyone could read the list and count who had survived and who had not.

These well-publicized cases involving the King and Queen of Britain in a "Royal Experiment" and an intense medical debate in the American colonies were well known to a layperson like Cobbett. They should have been well known to an Edinburgh-educated physician like Rush, who, to reiterate, had published on inoculation. Patient registers—*lists*—were the established means of attesting to the efficacy of experimental therapies during epidemics. Yet Rush proclaimed a "cure" or recovery rate of 99 percent, even though he claimed to have kept no register of those whom he and/or his apprentices had treated—thereby violating the basic rudiments for the responsible conduct of scientific research as understood in the eighteenth century. Rush's puffery, his uncorroborated claims of an exaggerated cure rate was, as Cobbett perceptively observed, more like quackery than science. Yet, when Cobbett and the College of Physicians challenged Rush's claims—the latter expelling Rush—he found ways to silence them.

RUSH'S ROAD TO REPUTATIONAL REHABILITATION

By 1797, Rush had been expelled from the College of Physicians of Philadelphia, ostracized by this fellow physicians, and caricatured and pilloried in the press. Yet he still proclaimed his theory, even as sought to avoid bankruptcy by fleeing from Philadelphia to New York. When the New Yorkers at Columbia rejected him, Rush was saved through the generosity of a political opponent—an old comrade-in-arms from the revolutionary period, President John Adams (1735–1826; Vice President 1789–1797; President, 1797–1801). Ignoring their political differences, Adams appointed Rush to the office of Treasurer of the Mint.[126] As Rush wrote a decade later, in a letter thanking former President Adams,

> Had it not been for the emoluments of the office you gave me I must have retired from the city and ended my days upon a farm upon the little capital I had saved from the labors of former years.... [Yet] in no period of my depression did I regret the conduct that occasioned it. My opinions and practice I was sure were correct, and I believe they would prevail. I acted uprightly and consulted the health of my fellow citizens and the benefits of society more than I did my own interest or fame. Most of my fellow citizens (the physicians excepted) have forgiven me, and *they* dare not openly, as they once did, assail my character.[127]

Rush's last comment, "they dare not openly, as they once did, assail my character," is a reference to his victory in a libel suit against Cobbett, *Rush v. Cobbett*, that he had won in 1800, shutting down Cobbett's Federalist newspaper, *Peter Porcupine's Gazette* (1797–1800) and silencing his medical critics.

As Rush would later remark to his students, "[w]riting and publishing a popular and useful book"[128] is an effective way to increase one's business. So even before Cobbett and his medical critics were silenced, Rush published a self-portrait, painting his conduct during the 1793 epidemic in heroic colors.[129] He was a modern Shadrach, Meshach, or Abednego: a near martyr who, unlike the cowardly physicians who had fled the city with their affluent clients, stayed to brave the fiery furnace of the yellow fever epidemic, treating the epidemic-stricken poor as well as the fee-paying rich. And yet, as Rush tells the tale, instead of being rewarded for boldly discovering a new cure, he was nearly hounded out of the profession by jealous, ungrateful, carping critics.

Rush also published a series of lectures exonerating his conduct and undermining his critics, often by invoking claims of medical ethics and donning the mantle of martyr:

> A physician is exposed to vexation from the false judgment which the bulk of mankind often entertain of the nature of certain medicines which he employs in his practice...few persons are ignorant of the unfounded and illiberal clamors, which exist, at this day, in every part of the world against the use of mercury and the lancet.... That bold humanity which dictates the

> use of painful remedies, in violent diseases, is branded with the epithet of cruelty...and a want of principles in medicine.[130]

Offsetting these vexations, Rush modestly informed his students, is the gratification of "becoming the instrument in the hands of Providence of discovering a remedy for a mortal epidemic, and thereby saving a whole city or country from destruction."[131] As to the pesky statistics that Cobbett challenged him with, Rush classified them and other forms of mathematics as among "the causes which have retarded the progress of [medical] science....What affinity have the abstruse branches of mathematics with medicine?"[132]

Rush, who offered a cheaper, shorter course of lectures for a medical degree than did his competitors, flooded the field with his students—especially in the states south of Pennsylvania. He was a popular medical lecturer, in part because the simplified system of medicine he taught was easier to learn than the complex nosologies and larger *materia medica* taught by other lecturers. His students worshipped him. The future Philadelphia physician Charles Meigs (1792–1869) wrote to his grandfather that

> Dr. Rush looks like an angel of light, his words bear in them, and his looks too, irresistible persuasion and conviction: in fact, to me he seems more than mortal. If ever a human being deserved Deification, it is Dr. Rush.[133]

Doctors as Demigods; Patients as Worshipers

In his lectures on "medical ethics," Rush lays out his notion of the Christian physician, duty bound to believe in "Divine and Superintending Power,"[134] who ought to "Thank God" rather than medicine for cures,[135] and who, like the Presbyterian God, stands in a benignly dictatorial but sympathetic and covenantal relationship to his patients. Just as these physicians' first duty is to choose the right religion, Christianity, "[t]he first duty...of patients is to choose no man for a physician who has not had a regular education."[136] Moreover, just as a good Presbyterian promptly, strictly, and universally obeys the dictates of his God, "[t]he obedience of a patient, to the prescriptions of his physician should be prompt, strict, and universal."[137] Rush's advocacy of deified medical paternalism contrasts strikingly with the views of other Edinburgh "medical ethicists" who urged physicians to respect the feelings and wishes of private and hospitalized patients, even in cases in which they believed the patient to be in error.[138]

Rush also held that patients should choose a physician "whose habits of life are perfectly regular,"[139] like the habits of life of the good Presbyterian. The properly deified physician should regard "the theatre, the turf, the chase, and even a convivial table in a sickly season [as] improper places of relaxation"[140] because, on Rush's covenantal Presbyterian vision of the physician as demigod, these are precluded by the duty of fidelity to the patient. The patient is entitled to "a monopoly of [the physician's] time and talents; and it is a breach of contract with them to apply them to any other purpose. [The physician's] mind [should be] concentrated on his duties to the sick."[141] Patients, in return, are to be monotheistic with respect to their physicians, confining their care "exclusively and constantly to one physician," to whom they should also apply for advice and communicate all of their concerns, "even in trifling matters."[142] Patients should also praise their physicians much as a Presbyterian praises his God, "do[ing] justice to his humanity and punctuality in attendance upon him as well as to his skill,"[143] and they must render to the physician his due: payments either partially during his attendance or after a cure, or "if this is impracticable, at the end of every year."[144]

For Rush, the physician–patient covenant "imposes an obligation of secrecy upon [the physician] and thus prevents his making public what he cannot avoid seeing or hearing accidently in his intercourse with the [patient's] family."[145] The covenant requires a sliding fee scale for poorer patients. Moreover, "[t]o undertake the charge of sick people, and to neglect them afterwards, is a vice of a malignant dye in a physician,"[146] since "[t]he most important contract that can be made, is that which takes place between a sick man and his doctor. The subject of it is human life. The breach of this contract by willful negligence, when followed by death, is murder."[147] Rush attributes physicians' breach of this contract to the vice of "avarice," which also "discovers itself, in, among other things denial of service to the poor."[148] Another major vice is "[i]nhumanity... which sometimes... discovers itself in the want of prompt and punctual attendance upon the sick, and in a careless or unfeeling manner in sick rooms... [an] insensibility to human suffering."[149] As in New Sider Presbyterian theology, emotions connect worshipers to a responsive deity: so the deified physician should respond humanely and sensitively to the suffering of the sick.

Rush projected an evangelical New Side Presbyterian conception of a benign, loving, but dictatorial deity onto the physician–patient relationship. In his view, the physician, as a Christian demigod, must be ever faithful to keeping his end of the covenant and so must be dedicated to serving the poor, must always be attentive to the patient's needs, and must never be neglectful. This demigod model of the physician–patient relationship is more than a historical curiosity. In 1832, it was integrated into the System of Medical Ethics of the Medico-Chirurgical Society of Baltimore (1832–1838), which, in turn, was integrated into the code of ethics adopted by the American Medical Association (AMA) in 1847. Rush's demigod-like conception of the physician–patient relationship thus became the dominant conception in American medicine from the mid-nineteenth through the mid-twentieth century. It was this conception that bioethicists would reject, embracing in its stead, ironically, something akin to the relationship envisioned by Gregory and Percival.

INFLUENCE AND REPUTATION: BARD AND RUSH

Two physician-educators, Samuel Bard and Benjamin Rush, are equally the protagonists in this chapter, yet Rush received about twice as much space as Bard. This is roughly proportionate to their influence. Like Rush, Bard never fled when the yellow fever epidemic of the 1795 hit his hometown of New York City, and, like Rush, Bard treated poor and rich alike. Also, like Rush, Bard helped to organize public health measures to stem the epidemic: however, unlike Rush, instead of picking a quarrel with his fellow physicians and announcing a self-promoting "cure" for the fever, Bard worked with a committee to correct unsanitary conditions (the breeding grounds of the mosquitoes causing the fever) and to publicize the dangers of numerous "cures" for the fever sold by quacks and by some physicians acting like quacks. Bard also published on yellow fever and other subjects, but, instead of announcing radical new "cures," he evaluated a range of treatments. Bard's magnum opus, *A Compendium of the Theory and Practice of Midwifery*, became the authoritative American text on midwifery through the first part of the nineteenth century, going through five editions from 1807 to 1819.[150] Unlike Rush, Bard was self-effacing: "I have attempted, to be useful rather than to appear learned; to say nothing but what is absolutely necessary, and easily understood; and to detail such facts and observations, and recommend such practices, as have been long known, and have received the stamp of time and experience, rather than to offer new opinions."[151]

Bard also opposed the interventionist medicine (later branded "heroic") championed by Rush, repeatedly warning against iatrogenic harm (i.e., the danger that medical interventions will cause patients more harm than benefit). He was "convinced that the use of instruments, and the introduction of the hand into the womb, as too frequently practiced by unskillful and presumptuous men, are more dangerous than the most desperate case of midwifery left to nature." Bard's "intention" was thus "to recommend *caution* and repress temerity."[152] He taught his students that nature was benign and that the job of the physician was to cautiously assist her, but only when necessary. He also taught them to skeptically appraise medical interventions that could endanger their patients.

Yet Rush was the more influential teacher. In an era in which an M.D. was a rarity that automatically conferred status, Rush taught nearly three thousand future "MDs between 1779 and 1812."[153] He is credited with "exert[ing] more influence on the medical profession than any other person during the quarter century following the War for Independence. His students practiced throughout the country, from Massachusetts to Georgia [the northern- and southernmost states] and kept in touch with his ideas through correspondence and through his published writings."[154] Where Bard taught his students that nature was benign, Rush taught his students that she was perfidious: "The natural, moral, and political world exhibit every where marks of disorder, and the instruments of this disorder are the operations of nature. Her influence is most obvious in the production of diseases, and in her hurtful or ineffectual efforts to remove them."[155] Medicine's goal, Rush explained, was to impose order on disorderly nature, to place it under the rule of the physician.

In 1884, the AMA campaigned successfully to erect a statue of Rush on the national mall in Washington D.C.[156] Still the only statue of a physician on the national mall, Rush's monument was erected in 1901 and dedicated in 1902.[157] On June 11, 1904, Philadelphia physician James C. Wilson (1847–1934) delivered an address at the official unveiling of the statue that bowdlerized the historical record to valorize Rush.[158] Wilson cast the College of Physicians of Philadelphia as the villain in its conflict with Rush. "In truth,"—two words that when conjoined often serve to preface a falsehood—"it was Dr. Rush's plan to shun rather than to seek controversy.... [H]e resigned from the College of Physicians...because...of the abuse and persecution he had sustained from that body on account of his treatment of the epidemic disease by blood-letting and calomel."[159] Wilson also explained away an embarrassing incident that called into question Rush's patriotism. Rush has been forced to resign as Physician-General to the Army in February 1778, probably as a consequence of a failed attempt to have George Washington removed as commander.[160] Washington never forgave Rush's treachery, reportedly remarking that, "[h]e had been a good deal in the world and seen many bad Men, but Dr. Rush was the most black hearted scoundrel he had ever known."[161]

Wilson tries to justify Rush's practice of radical bloodletting and violent purging by invoking a misplaced sense of historical relativism:

> We cannot measure his practice by ours, for old things have passed away and things have become new. But we must grant him the courage of his convictions. If his premises had been true—alas! The if,—his conclusions would have been inevitable and his practice logically correct. The Defense of Bloodletting makes us shudder. To him the facts amounted to a demonstration of the curative power of that sanguinary measure: to us they only show the enormous resistance of certain organisms to depletion.... Groping in the dark, he struggled towards the light. The traditions mislead him, but his own powers of observation set his feet upon the right way. He was father of Experimental Medicine in America.[162]

In this paragraph, Wilson outlines what was to become a standard portrayal of Rush as the martyred physician-hero, misled by tradition into adopting medical practices abhorrent to later generations but acceptable in his era. To be sure, every student of history has shared with Leslie Hartley (1895–1972) the thought "that the past is a foreign country: they do things differently there."[163] Wilson's eloquent defense of Rush draws on this sentiment, but Wilson does not really believe that Rush's bleeding and purging "cure" for yellow fever reduced the mortality rate of those affected to just 1 percent: Wilson states that Rush's "Defense of Bloodletting makes us shudder." Like other apologists, Wilson suggests that Rush was misled by tradition. Again, the facts belie this claim, for had Rush followed Edinburgh tradition, he would have tested his theories by repeated empirical observation and kept a register of treated patients. Rush rejected tradition. As we know from Rush's own hand, he embraced his radical bleeding and purging theories and practices not because he was practicing the medicine that he had been taught, but because he was searching for a new theory that would repudiate the views taught by his "master," Cullen, and that would establish Rush's own reputation. The profession of Rush's day condemned him, expelling Rush from the College of Physicians not because he was following tradition, but because he was breaking with tradition, with the accepted standards of conduct accepted in his day.

Wilson's comment, "Groping in the dark, [Rush] struggled towards the light," is also inadvertently ironic: Rush ridiculed the slow, empirical, collaborative, and cumulative understanding of science as a search of facts championed by Cullen and practiced by Bard, opting instead for a "bold," emotive, revelatory approach to medicine. In consequence, American physicians who followed him groped into a darkness in which the medical theology of radical bleeding and purging eclipsed whatever illumination the science of that era had to offer. It is thus the blackest of ironies that the words inscribed on the statute of Rush that Wilson dedicated are "Father of Experimental Medicine in America." Rush's belief in research as revelation, his callous treatment of data, and his embrace of heroic medicine were as poisonous to American standards of responsible conduct of research as his mercury treatment was to his patients. Rush's theology of heroic medicine set back experimental medical science in America for much of the nineteenth century, and, as we will see in Chapter 6, it also undermined scientific challenges to the alternative medical theologies of Samuel Hahnemann (1755–1843) and Samuel Thomson (1769–1843).

5

OATHS AND CODES OF MEDICAL POLICE AND ETHICS, 1806–1846

XXI. The use of Quack medicines should be discouraged by the faculty, as disgraceful to the profession, injurious to health, and often destructive even of life....

XXII. No physician or surgeon should dispense a secret *nostrum*.[1]

"The Use of Quack Medicines," Thomas Percival, *Medical Ethics*, 1803

Any physician or surgeon who divides his responsibility with a known quack, and associates with him in medical consultations, receiving a fee or the usual charges for such services, or practices with nostrums, secret medicines, or patent remedies, is guilty of quackery.[2]

"Quackery," Medical Society of the State of New York, *System of Ethics*, 1823

AMERICAN MEDICAL SOCIETIES: CENSORS, BYLAWS, AND CODES

American medical societies were modeled after the colleges of physicians of London (founded in 1518) and Edinburgh (founded by 1681). These were not academic institutions, even though they were called "colleges," but rather licensing organizations administered by presidents, vice presidents, treasurers, secretaries—and censors. This term, "censor," originates with the Romans who created the office to maintain an official list of citizens (a census) to supervise elections, the collection of taxes, and to oversee public morals. This last role evolved from the censor's power to exclude or strike names from the list of those enjoying the privileges of Roman citizenship. Medical college censors played similar roles: a subcommittee of censors known as the *comita minora* kept membership lists, collected dues, assessed applicants qualifications for a license to practice, and guarded the morals of members by investigating complaints, adjudicating disputes, and recommending punishments for misbehaving members. Sometimes, following the precedent of their Roman precursors, the *comita minora* recommended that a college strike the name of a miscreant from the membership list—an action that meant expulsion, potential ostracism, and, in some jurisdictions, loss of a license to practice.

On admission to a medical society, American physicians and surgeons signed an oath or pledge promising to abide by the society's bylaws and by its code of medical police or medical ethics.[3] "Bylaws" are rules regulating members' conduct, and these rules apply only to the members of the society. Thus, a typical bylaw might open with the phrase, "No member of this Association shall. . . . "[4] Codes of medical ethics, in contrast, address the conduct of anyone acting in the role of physician or surgeon, irrespective of their membership in a particular society. Thus, a typical provision in a code of medical police or ethics might open with a phrase such as, "*No Physician or Surgeon* shall. . . . " Nathan Smith Davis (1817–1904), later deemed the "father of the American Medical Association (AMA)," explained the difference between codes of ethics and bylaws as follows: "A Code of Ethics for our profession must partake . . . of the nature of a moral essay, developing principles or guidance equally applicable to all places and times, instead of a few simple rules applicable to the members of some particular society."[5] Davis then continues, "principles and rules of conduct enumerated [in a code of ethics] are equally applicable for the guidance of all who attempt to practice the healing art, whether they are members of any medical organization or not."[6]

Since codes of ethics were supposed to apply universally to all physicians or surgeons, irrespective of their membership in a particular medical society, they were published and circulated to all the respectable physicians and surgeons of a community. Nonmembers had good reason for taking an interest in the medical society's code because they could be censured for violating it, even though they were not members of the society and had never pledged to abide by its code of ethics or police. Nonmembers, in turn, had the right to press charges against members who violated a society's code of medical ethics. An investigative committee of the censors of a New York City society, for example, indicted a society member charged with wrongdoing by a nonmember. According to the society's records:

> During the prevalence of the Cholera in this City Dr. M. was called to visit a young man by the name of Tucker laboring under that disease; after he was prescribed Dr. W., who had previously seen the case, came in claiming the patient—Dr. W. however found that his attendance was no longer required and he attempted to prove that [this was because] Dr. M. represented him as having a murderous lack of success in the hospital. He retired from the case and in a state of consequent excitement wrote a letter to the mother of Mr. Tucker in which he urged the dismissal of Dr. M. from the case on the grounds of him being utterly incompetent and unsafe.
>
> [Faced with these charges] Dr. W. acknowledged to the *Comita* that he has acted indiscreetly and improperly and protests that he did not believe at the time that this society could have any cognizance in the premises in as much as he supposed that Dr. M. was not a member of this Society and could not therefore be amenable to them for his act.[7]

The wrongdoing Dr. W. was right about one thing: Dr. M. was not a member of the local county medical society; he belonged to a medical society in another county. Nonetheless, the *comita* recognized Dr. M.'s right to bring charges of interference, slander, and illiberal conduct and ruled in his favor—forcing Dr. W. to apologize for misconduct.[8] The point to appreciate is that medical society codes of medical police or ethics were held to apply to anyone assuming the role of physician, irrespective of their membership in a particular society.

It was common for medical guilds, colleges, and societies in Britain and continental Europe to issue bylaws or rules for their own members. Yet, only in America, as the expression goes, did nineteenth-century medical societies typically issue written codes of medical police or medical ethics, in addition to bylaws.[9] When, for example, the medical society later called the British Medical Association (BMA, from 1856) was originally founded as the Provincial Medical and Surgical Association in 1832, its founder, Charles Hastings (1794–1866) favored a written code of medical conduct.[10] His colleagues rejected the proposal at the point of the society's founding and in almost every subsequent decade from the 1840s to the 1960s. The proposal failed quite prominently in 1882, even after one if its members, Jukes Styrap (1815–1899), offered the BMA a comprehensive code of medical ethics.[11] The BMA would have no official written code of practitioner conduct until almost the end of the twentieth century.

The situation was similar in continental Europe, where French[12] and German[13] medical societies would adopt official written codes of conduct, or medical deontologies, as the French called them, only in the later decades of the nineteenth century.

Europeans rejected the notion of codes of medical ethics because such codes affronted ideals of gentlemanly honor. As discussed in Chapter 3, notions of gentlemanly honor lie at the root of all Western concepts of professionalism.[14] Written codes of conduct were deemed incompatible with these ideals because a gentleman's sense of honor was held to emanate from his very nature: one either had the inborn character and virtues of an honorable gentleman, or one did not. As Sir Benjamin Collins Brodie (1783–1862), surgeon to Prince Albert and later President of the Royal Society, observed in an address to medical students in 1843, in practicing medicine they should "feel and act as gentlemen"[15]—Sir Benjamin presumes, in this remark, that the students he is addressing would know intuitively what a gentleman feels and acts like.

The Medical Act of 1858 institutionalized this notion of "feeling and acting as a gentleman" by creating a quasi-autonomous nongovernmental institution (a quango) the General Medical Council (GMC), which was given the censor's power of "registering" (i.e., licensing) practitioners or "striking" their names from the official register—thereby delicensing them. The official explanation for striking a practitioner's name from the register was always the same: the council had "judged him to have been guilty of infamous conduct in a professional respect."[16] As professionals, practitioners would naturally be gentlemen who would know how to feel and act and would need no further explanation—and, if they needed an explanation, they were not proper gentlemen and so were not properly professionals.[17]

In 1883, the GMC began issuing notices explaining why specific cases were considered "infamous conduct in a professional respect." This list gradually expanded into a system of "Warning Notices" published in medical journals and collected as a pamphlet. As late as 1903, when the GMC received a petition from 133 Scottish practitioners requesting official written guidance that would allow them to anticipate *in advance* which actions would constitute "infamous conduct," the GMC declined to do so. Their reason: insofar as professional conduct is a function of gentlemanly character, written codes of conduct are useful only to persons who, lacking the ingrained virtues of an honorable gentleman, nonetheless wish to pretend to have them. It was, according to the GMC, "not *desirable* to pass a resolution condemning any practice in general terms."[18] Honor codes for gentlemen needed no written codification. Indeed, no official written British guide to ethical medical practice would be published until the 1980s,[19]—American colonials, in contrast, began to write out codes of conduct in the early nineteenth century.

NEW YORK MEDICAL SOCIETIES AND THEIR OATHS

The Weekly Society of Practitioners: New York's Earliest Medical Society

One of the first medical societies established in the American colonies was the Weekly Society of Practitioners. The society seems to have met as early as 1749,[20] when Samuel Bard's father, John Bard, hosted informal gatherings of perhaps a dozen physicians and surgeons at his house to discuss medicine and articles in medical journals. The practitioners shared the costs of subscribing to journals and thereby created a shared medical library. In 1788, the society renamed itself the New York Medical Society, electing John Bard and a former English military surgeon practicing in New York City, John Charlton (1731?–1801) as presidents.[21] Perhaps due to Charlton's influence, the society was reorganized along the lines of British colleges of physicians, assuming the grandiose name of the Medical Society of the State of New York (1794–1806).[22]

Despite this more formal organizational structure, the society remained a convivial reading group until the outbreak of a major yellow fever epidemic in New York City in 1795. The society then oversaw efforts to fight the epidemic and recommended policies to the governor for preventing recurrences. It pinpointed likely sources of the epidemic as "1st the [ac]cumulation of filth in the streets"; "2nd obstructed water drains, occasioning stagnant water"; "3rd putrefaction in certain houses"; and "4th intolerable stench" at low tide—and proposed governmental action to remedy these problems.[23] After the epidemic abated, the society might well have abandoned these proto-professional activities—information sharing, collaborative investigations, standard setting, lobbying—and returned to the life of a quiet reading group had not President Charlton called an emergency meeting on February 14, 1797. The reason: "a law now before the [New York State] Legislature to regulate the practice of physic."[24] Medical societies from Saratoga and other upstate counties[25] had lobbied the state legislature for the power to license medical practitioners. Objecting to this proposal, the New York City physicians appointed a committee "to draft a memorial to the Legislature on the Practice of Physic."[26] Nevertheless, the upstate societies prevailed, and the legislature created a statewide medical society that would have the power to license physicians and set the standards used by county medical societies to examine the qualifications of physicians. The same legislation also required county medical societies to register with the state, thereby empowering state bureaucrats to deregister and thus to regulate county medical societies.

The Manhattan-based New York City society found this "highly objectionable,"[27] especially since the new statewide society appropriated its name—the Medical Society of the State of New York (MSSNY)—thus forcing the New York City society to retitle itself the Medical Society of the County of New York (MSCNY—its current name). Worse yet, since membership in a county society was now required for licensure, the MSCNY's numbers swelled from a handful of gentlemen to 102 members. Very much against its will the MSCNY was transformed from a convivial reading group meeting in private homes into a professional society meeting in public places.

Transplanting Edinburgh Oath to New York

In 1806, the members of the new MSCNY elected Nicholas Romayne their president. It was a surprising choice. About a decade earlier, in 1797, Romayne had been arrested and imprisoned on the orders of President John Adams (1735–1826, President 1797–1801) and forced to testify at the impeachment trial of Senator William Blount (1749–1800)—the first impeachment trial in U.S. history. At issue was a violation of official oaths: Senator Blount was charged with violating his oaths of office in a conspiracy with Romayne and others to create an incident that would wrest the Louisiana Territory from the French and turn it over to Britain and the United States.[28] When this affair ended, Romayne took refuge in Britain.

In choosing Romayne as their president, the Manhattanites may have been expressing their resentment of the 1806 act that had placed power to regulate medicine in the hands of state officials and that had infringed on the autonomy of the New York City society, forcing it to abandon its name. As Romayne would later put it, the 1806 act

> affords the first instance in the modern history of Physic, of professional regulation being placed under the direction of men in power [bureaucrats], after being vested in the members of that profession. It may be doubted whether any advantages to the community are likely to arise from this regulation.[29]

For Romayne and for the forcibly renamed MSCNY, the law empowering the MSSNY to license physicians and surgeons was something of a devil's bargain: in gaining the authority to license, medical societies had compromised their autonomy by placing regulatory power in the hands of the state.

Romayne's ambivalence about the 1806 law provides the context in which he lobbied to have all physicians receiving a license in New York swear a version of the Edinburgh oath, thereby symbolically reasserting a measure of professional autonomy against a perceived threat "of men in power." To implement this initiative, the oath was translated from Latin to English (probably by Romayne), the unrealistic and unenforceable confidentiality clause was deleted, and a pledge of fidelity to the medical society and to one's peers was substituted for an invocation of the deity and a pledge of fidelity to the University of Edinburgh. The MSCNY version of the oath read:

> I, A. B., do solemnly declare, that I will at all times hereafter pay due consideration and respect to this Society from which I derive this privilege to exercise the profession of a Physician or Surgeon; that I will chastely, virtuously and honestly, conduct myself in the practice of physic and surgery, that I will, with fidelity and honor, do every thing in my power for the benefit of the Sick committed to my charge, and recommend to them if necessary the best medical advice and I do further declare that I will consider all persons who are licensed to practice Physic or Surgery by this Society or any other incorporated Society of this State as Brethren of the same profession with which I am now invested and I will on no occasions wantonly attempt to injure their Medical Reputation.[30]

In 1807, after Romayne was elected president of the state society, the MSSNY, he adopted the following stripped-down version of the MSCNY oath as an official oath for use in all county medical societies as part of their induction ceremonies:

> [A]ll students of medicine who shall have presented to the majority of the censors of this said Society, satisfactory testimony that they have studied physic and surgery, as is directed by the statute for incorporating this Society, and who shall upon due examination by the censors be found to be qualified to practice physic or surgery or both... shall, before they receive the requisite diploma from the President, sign a declaration in the following, viz:
>
> *"I, A. B., do solemnly declare, that I will honestly, virtuously, and chastely, conduct myself in the practice of physic and surgery, with the privilege of exercising which profession I am now to be invested; and that I will, with fidelity and honor, do every thing in my power for the benefit of the sick committed to my charge"* which said declaration so signed by every candidate to practice physic and surgery, shall be filed by the Secretary in the archives of the Society.
>
> And be it further directed, that the President and Secretary is hereby authorized to grant to every such candidate...in the name and under the seal of this said Society, a diploma in the words following, viz:
>
> Omnibus ad quos haec literae pervenerint.... In quorum testimonium hocce diploma, siggillo nostro munitum, donavimus. Datum (*the place, day and year to be inserted*).[31]

Immediately following this section are the bylaws stating conditions under which a *comita minora* may be formed to investigate the credentials of applicants for medical licenses or to investigate accusations of "serious offence[s] against the laws of this State or of the United States or... gross immorality,... improper pretensions to any specific or nostrum, or... improper conduct in the duties of his profession."[32]

"History," as novelist Kurt Vonnegut (1922–2007) had one of his characters remark, "is merely a list of surprises."[33] It is surprising that Manhattanites should turn to Romayne to preside over their medical society after his arrest and exile. Yet it is not surprising that Romayne should be hypersensitive to the intrusive nature of government: his minority Dutch heritage, his trial over violating a loyalty oath, his recent past history as a semi-fugitive, his Edinburgh education, his familiarity with the Edinburgh oath, and his fluency in Latin taken together make it is easy to understand why, under Romayne's leadership, both the MSCNY and the MSSNY mandated swearing a version of the Edinburgh oath—a statement that the physician's primary duty is to the patient, not to the state. New York medical societies had accepted the government's grant of licensing power, but they conjoined it with an official oath justifying members' autonomy in the name of a commitment to "do every thing in their power for the benefit of the sick committed to [their] charge." This odd concatenation—assertions of autonomy in the name of their patients even as they enjoyed governmental licensing authority—would later characterize the American medical profession's generally ambivalent attitude toward governmental authority and regulation.

CODES OF MEDICAL POLICE

The *Boston Medical Police*, 1808–1885

Even as Romayne and his fellow New Yorker's were turning to the Edinburgh oath in reaction to a governmental grant of licensing authority, the Association of Boston Physicians, the Boston branch of the Massachusetts Medical Society (founded in either 1781[34] or 1806[35]), was exploring a different form of self-governance—a medical police—in reaction to the new licensing power accorded them by the Commonwealth of Massachusetts in 1806. Archival sources are mute on why Boston physicians thought that a grant of licensing authority carried with it the obligation to set forth a self-regulatory code of conduct. What is clear is that in 1806 the association's governing or "standing" committee appointed a subcommittee of three members—John Warren, along with Lemuel Hayward (1749–1821) and John Fleet (1766–1815), also associated with Harvard—to draft a code called a "Medical Police." The society approved the code in 1808.

The expression "medical police" has changed its meaning over the course of time. Today, the expression might refer to "a Board of health... brought into action when cholera [or some other epidemic disease] rages,"[36] or it might conjure up images of eugenics courts policing the cribs of newborns to eliminate the genetically unfit; however, in 1808—some two decades before the founding of the Boston police department in 1829[37]—the expression "medical police" meant something quite different. An 1818 American edition of Samuel Johnson's *Dictionary* defines "police" as a noun from the French characterizing "the regulations or government of a city or country, as far as regards the inhabitants."[38] Webster's 1823 dictionary of American usage offers a similar definition, noting that the term derives from the Greek word "*polis*," which means "city":

> POLICE, n. [L. politia; Gr. city.] The government of a city or town; the administration of the laws and regulations of a city or incorporated town or borough; as the police of... Boston. The word is applied also to the government of all towns in New England, which are made corporations by a general statute.[39]

As these dictionaries attest, in Boston in 1808, the expression "medical police" simply described regulations for the self-governance of "medical practitioners."[40]

Fleet, Hayward, and Warren report that in drafting this medical police they drew on the works of "Gregory, Rush and Percival," [41] "select[ing] from them such articles as seemed most applicable to the circumstances of the profession in this place...to form a short system of *policy*, containing general principles... [but] making such alterations...as they thought necessary for rendering them practicable and useful; [and]...adapted to the particular situation of medical practice in America."[42] Five hundred copies of the *Boston Medical Police* were printed: three for each member, with the extra two copies to be distributed to "such other Physicians of the State as [members] may think proper."[43] This code served the association through the 1880s.[44] Its text is available in Appendix I.

Percival's *Medical Ethics* as Ur-Text for the *Boston Medical Police*

The primary source, or ur-text, for the *Boston Medical Police*[45] was a newly published book *Medical Ethics; or, A Code of Institutes and Precepts, Adapted to the Professional Conduct of Physicians and Surgeons* (1803)[46] written by Samuel Bard's classmate at the Edinburgh medical school, Thomas Percival of Manchester, England. Percival's code originated in 1792 as a set of bylaws designed to minimize the likelihood of discord, flytes, and pamphlet wars between practitioners at the Manchester Infirmary (founded in 1752, now the Manchester Royal Infirmary and part of the Central Manchester University System). Over the course of a dozen years, Percival revised these infirmary rules, eventually publishing them as a code for, as he put it in his title, "the professional conduct of physicians and surgeons."[48] The code thus evolved from a parochial discourse of bylaws for a single Manchester hospital into a set of universal rules applicable to anyone playing the professional role of physician or surgeon.

As the quotations opening this chapter make evident, by replicating Percival's language, the authors of the *Boston Medical Police* created a code for anyone acting in the role of physician or surgeon in Boston, not merely for members of their association. This might have been an accident, a product of happenstance that resulted from copying so much of Percival's text verbatim. Yet practical purposes were well served by this shift from parochial bylaws to universal rules. As the case of the wrongdoing Dr. W. illustrates, and as Percival no doubt discovered in his crafting of rules for intrapractitioner conduct, disputes often arise between practitioners affiliated with an institution and those who are not. Consequently, dispute prevention and resolution procedures are most effective if they apply to *all* physicians, irrespective of their affiliation with any particular organization. Peace is most easily achieved if everyone plays by the same set of rules.

Yet asserting authority over nonaffiliates is challenging because it is not clear why an institution like the Manchester Infirmary or the Boston Medical Society may assert authority over nonaffiliated practitioners. Percival addressed this challenge by arguing that since the conduct of anyone acting in the role of physician or surgeon may affect the honor and reputation of everyone acting in these roles, anyone acting in these roles ought to abide by rules insofar as they promote the honor and interests of all practitioners.[47] He also argues that since everyone claiming the title of "physician" or "surgeon" enjoys the benefits of a well-established "brand," so to speak, to maintain and merit these benefits, they ought to abide by rules that support the integrity of the brand. More specifically, Percival offered the following argument, which, although abstruse, was reproduced verbatim in virtually every code of medical police or medical ethics issued by a nineteenth-century American medical society.

> The *esprit du corps* is a principle of action, founded in human nature, and when duly regulated, is both rational and laudable. Every man who enters into a fraternity engages, by a tacit compact, not only to submit to the laws, but to promote the honour and interest of the association, so far as they are consistent with morality, and the general good of mankind.[49]

For Percival, professional ethics emerges at the intersection of occupational solidarity and self-interest on the one hand, and general morality and the public good on the other. Reflecting eighteenth- and nineteenth-century Anglo-American culture, Percival's justification of medical society codes invokes both rationality and sentiments (feelings, emotions), anchoring his intellectual argument for a tacit social compact in natural human feelings of fraternal bonding and social solidarity. Nonetheless, rationality constrains these feelings because professional rules must be "duly regulated" by reason, consistent with morality, and serve "the general good of mankind." Thus, however advantageous or emotively compelling one might find a social contract based on occupational solidarity, such a contract is only binding, Percival contended, if it does not require immoral actions (as a thieves' compact would) and if it promotes some social good (like public health). For Percival, occupational ethics must be grounded in natural human feelings of occupational solidarity *and must also* promote a public good without violating general constraints of morality.

American medical societies also believed that they could justifiably censure any physician or surgeon who breached their codes, not only members of their particular society. Members were clearly accountable because they had signed a pledge accepting the society's authority to arbitrate disputes and to censure, expel, or ostracize them should they be found guilty of violating the society's bylaws or its code of police/ethics. Nonmembers were also censurable insofar as their actions harmed the honor or reputation of fellow practitioners. Thus, in the quotation opening this chapter, the New York *System of Medical Ethics* claims a right to "punish"[50] nonmembers for behavior "which degrades the medical character," stipulating that "medical institutions should always repress and punish by the rejection... those who commit [disreputable acts]."[51] They thus claim a moral right to ostracize miscreant nonmembers who dishonor the profession.[52] As another code put it, "consultations should, under no pretext, be held with... such members of the profession as have, by improper conduct, outraged its dignity and respect."[53]

The *Connecticut Medical Police*, 1817

In 1817, the Connecticut Medical Society[54] published a concise version of the *Boston Medical Police*[55] that was adopted by innumerable municipal, county, and state medical societies from Augusta, Georgia (1822) to Cincinnati, Ohio (1821) to Dover, New Hampshire (1849), and so on down the alphabet. Until 1823, the only codes issued by American medical societies were Boston-style or, more commonly, Connecticut-style codes of medical police.[56] Thus, whereas the New York version of the Edinburgh oath had little impact on American medical morality and was soon relegated to the status of a ceremonial ritual, the Connecticut version of the *Boston Medical Police* became a template for instruments of medical society self-governance in early nineteenth-century America. These Connecticut-style codes of medical police typically consisted of fifteen paragraphs of text, drawn almost verbatim from Percival's *Medical Ethics*, arrayed under seven section headings: Consultations (five paragraphs), Interferences (three paragraphs), Fees (three paragraphs), Differences of Physicians (one paragraph), Discouragement of Quackery (one paragraph), Conduct for the Support of the Medical Character (one paragraph), and Seniority (one paragraph).[57]

The paragraphs on fees were an important aspect of these codes of medical police, taking up six of the nineteen paragraphs in original the *Boston Medical Police* and three of the fifteen paragraphs in the more concise *Connecticut Medical Police*.[58] Although the details vary, they typically offer fee scales indicating a price range for services (e.g., $1–3 for a house call). The amount charged would depend on such things as distance, weather, and the wealth and status of the family: higher fees were charged to wealthier patients, whereas minimal fees, payment in kind, or gratuitous service were for the poor (such as the blind woman whose case will be discussed in the next section). All codes of medical police have some stipulation to the effect that "the characteristic beneficence of the profession is inconsistent with... avaricious rapacity. The poor of every description should be object of our peculiar care."[59]

Only one subject commanded more space in codes of medical police than discussions of cross-subsidizing fee scales: dispute prevention and mediation. Fifteen of the nineteen paragraphs in the *Boston Medical Police* and twelve of the fifteen paragraphs in the stripped-down *Connecticut Medical Police* deal with preventing, assuaging, or resolving disputes between physicians, especially in the context of consults. Consults were considered important "in difficult and protracted cases, as they give rise to confidence, energy, and more enlarged views in practice."[60] Consults are commonplace in "difficult and protracted cases" even today, and they may still become contentious as expertise and egos clash in context of patient care. Yet consults today are typically between physicians with different areas of expertise. An intensivist might consult with an otolaryngologist, an oncologist, or a pediatrician, all specialists, respectively, in a type of medicine (critical care), in diseases of particular parts of the body (ear, nose, and throat), in a specific disease (cancer), or in a life-stage (childhood). What made early nineteenth-century consults particularly combustible was the absence of any comparable level specialization.[61] The consults discussed in codes of medical police and ethics were typically between practitioners claiming the same expertise in competition with each other for the same patients—and even for the business of the specific patient about whom they were consulting. Exacerbating these conflicting economic interests was a nineteenth-century conception of gentlemanly honor that facilitated an easy transition from differences over medical practice to flytes about the honorable character of medical practitioners.

Despite these challenges, colonial and postcolonial American medical practitioners and their patients believed consultation necessary to ensure that no potentially effective treatment had been overlooked. Practitioners also favored consultation because it shielded them against allegations of incompetence or negligence and because they were a source of secondary income. The Boston and Connecticut codes of medical police and their innumerable imitators were drafted in the belief that the procedures that Percival had originally designed to facilitate consultation and prevent flytes at a hospital in his native Manchester were an anodyne and a corrective to the problem of combustible consultations. This was considered important because, as the various codes remark, "the differences of Physicians, when they end in appeals to the publick, generally hurt the contending parties; but, what is of more consequence, they discredit the profession and expose the faculty itself to contempt and ridicule."[62]

As the following passage indicates, consultation rules were also designed to minimize consultants' opportunities to "steal" a patient from the original attending physician:

> The consulting physician is never to visit without the [original] attending [physician], unless by the desire of the latter, or when, as in sudden emergency, he is not to be found. No discussion of the case [between attending and consultant physicians] should take place before the patient and his friends; and no prognostications should be delivered, which were not the result of previous deliberations and concurrence.[63]

These and similar rules encourage the practice of consultation by protecting the original attending physician's relationship with the patient and minimizing the threat that the consulting physician might "steal" the original attending physician's patient.[64]

A RESTORATIVE JUSTICE SYSTEM FOR ADJUDICATING DISPUTES AND ENFORCING ETHICS

During the nineteenth century, American medical societies appropriated aspects of the status-shame morality of gentlemanly honor to enforce their oaths and codes, modifying this morality to create a system of restorative justice (i.e., a system focusing on restoring relationships between practitioners by correcting misunderstandings and righting wrongs). Public apologies, written or oral—supplemented, on occasion, by public humiliations—served to rectify offenses, restore peace between practitioners, and protect the honor and reputation of the medical profession. At issue in these restorative justice proceedings, to quote Alexander Hamilton, were "all the considerations which constitute what men of the world denominate honor."[65] Flyting, duels, and the other conventions of gentlemanly honor center on one's worthiness to be respected and esteemed by one's peers and by one's self. As the philosopher Kwame Anthony Appiah puts this point,

> [H]onor is an entitlement to respect—and shame comes when you lose that title—a person of honor cares first of all not about being respected but about being *worthy* of respect.... For the honorable person, honor itself is the thing that matters, not honor's rewards [i.e., status]. You feel shame when you have not met the standards of the honor code... whether or not anyone else knows you have failed.[66]

To be deemed unworthy of the status of gentleman was so deeply stigmatizing, so profoundly undermining of one's own sense of self-worth that a gentleman would rather face death in a duel, as Hamilton had or accept private or even public humiliation (e.g., by being forced to apologize publicly as the price for readmission to the society of gentlemen) than face the prospect of having one's underlying character condemned or denounced as unworthy of the esteem and respect of one's peers.

The content of these medical apologies was standardized: the offender confessed and explained a transgression, apologized, expressed contrition, was humbled, and then indicated a resolve not to transgress in the future. As one expert observes, "the apology process can be divided into four parts: 1) the acknowledgement of the offense; 2) the explanation; 3) various attitudes and behaviors including remorse, shame, humility, and sincerity; and 4) reparations."[67] In the case of the wrongdoing Dr. W., he (1) "acknowledged to the *Comita* that he has acted indiscreetly and improperly" and (2) explained "that he did not believe at the time... that Dr. M. was a member of this Society."[68] After (3) expressing remorse, he wrote the performative words "I apologize"[69] to Dr. M. and, (4) having made reparations through a humiliating public apology, had his status as a member of the society restored.

Although American medical societies favored restorative justice, they could also mete out punitive justice by expelling members, excluding them from consultation, and generally ostracizing them.[70] Restorative justice was reserved for "gentlemen" involved in breaches of "honor"—terms sprinkled throughout nineteenth-century oaths and codes of medical police and ethics.[71] Insofar as contentions over honor were private matters between two or more gentleman, following a British tradition mentioned in Percival's *Medical Ethics* (chapter II, article XXIV), a *court medical* could be convened to arbitrate the matter. These *courts medical* offer, in the language of one medical society, "formal private arbitration... called in personal misunderstandings not necessarily involving offenses against profession or code."[72] In complex cases, *courts medical* could initiate an inquiry to assess the facts, rectify misinformation, and propose ways of resolving the conflict. As private affairs, however, the proceedings and resolutions of a *court medical* were confidential, but they usually culminated in letters of apology or an oral apology from one or both parties.

When a physician was accused of violating the honor of the profession or of violating a medical society's oath, its formal code of medical ethics, or medical police—as in the case of the wrongdoing Dr. W., who was accused of interfering with another practitioner's practice—the medical society's *comita minora* became involved. The *comita*'s findings and recommendations would be publicly presented to the medical society. As in the case of Dr. W., a standard remedy was to restore the honor of an aggrieved physician or surgeon by publicly notifying the miscreant that he had to apologize to the offended party. If the violation was particularly egregious, this apology had to be read before the medical society or made orally, in person, at a meeting of the medical society. In the most egregious cases, a public apology might be accompanied by public humiliation by the society president or the *comita* chair.

In one case, a famous surgeon actually fled the country rather than make such an apology and face public humiliation at the hands of the president of a medical society. On November 11, 1869, Thomas C. Finnell (1826–1890), head of the Committee on Ethics of the New York Academy of Medicine (NYAM, founded in 1847 and still functioning), charged a famous surgeon, J. Marion Sims, with violating confidentiality at the expense of a celebrity patient, the actress Charlotte Cushman (1816–1876), who was famous for her performances of Shakespeare and notorious for her open lesbianism. The charge read:

> An eminent woman [Charlotte Cushman] applied to Sims for professional advice, the disease is mentioned [in a letter Sims wrote to the New York Times] and the Advice given is fully set forth. It is further stated that the patient "unfortunately followed other Advice"—An unjust and injurious reflection upon the professional advisors under whose care she saw fit to place herself for an operation concerning which there is great latitude of Opinion amongst Surgeons.
>
> A portion of Paragraph 2, Article 1, "On the Duties of Physicians to their Patient," is as follows: "Secrecy and delicacy, when required by peculiar circumstances, should be strictly observed.... The obligation of secrecy extends beyond the period of professional services—none of the privacies of personal and domestic life, no infirmity of disposition or flaw of character observed during professional attendance, should ever be divulged by him except when he is imperatively required to do so."
>
> The undersigned claims that the Code does not allow a physician to announce to the public, the disease of a patient, and that the communications of Dr. J. M. Sims is a violation of these paragraphs from which these quotations were made.
>
> A portion of [Chapter] 3 "Of the duties of physicians to each other and to the profession at large" is as follows: "It is derogatory to the dignity of the profession, to resort to public advertisements."...

> The undersigned claims that it is in violation of this paragraph for a physician to announce publicly that he is the professional Advisor of anyone, and a greater breach is committed, when, as in the present instance, the patient is a distinguished person. It is not improper to state that a leading daily paper in this city [The New York Times] upon the communications that its author made a statement in regard to the lady, entirely uncalled for, and thereby advertised himself as her physician.
>
> The undersigned makes these charges from no malice; it is to him as to many others, a source of deep regret that one whose name is so honorably linked to the fame of our profession [i.e., James Marion Sims], should be placed in such a discreditable position but loyalty to our Code demands that all should be called to account whenever they appear guilty of violating any of its Articles.[73]

After a review of the letter published in the *New York Times* and reflection on the explanation offered by Sims in his defense,[74] the committee "declared that the charges against Dr. J. Marion Sims are fully sustained and [that he be publicly] reprimanded by the President of the Academy."[75] Rather than face such a public humiliation, with its requisite demand for a public apology, Sims took a steamer to London.[76] Sims's expulsion from the NYAM is the earliest known instance in which a physician was censured and ultimately expelled from a medical society for violating patient confidentiality.

Publicly flaunting any medical society's code of ethics usually led to charges and sometimes to expulsion. Another NYAM case is illustrative: the following advertisement about a disease now known as gastroesophageal reflux disease (GERD) but then called "dyspepsia" appeared in New York City newspapers in 1874:

> DYSPEPSIA in its relation to the Liver and Digestive Organs. J. J. Spreng M. D. Member of the New York Academy of Medicine, devotes his special attention to Liver and Stomach diseases. Pamphlet mailed for 10 cents. Address the author, 201 West Twenty-second-st. Consultation 10 to 2, and 6 to 7.[77]

A twenty-four-page pamphlet, *A Synopsis of the Most Important Disease of the Life, their Causes, Symptoms, and Treatments* by Dr. Spreng, which extolled the "superiority and correctness of [Justin J. Spreng's] system . . . proved by its remarkable success" was adduced as evidence. Independently of each other, four fellows of the NYAM filed charges, including Francie D. White, who charged Dr. Spreng:

> Art. 1st "Of the duties of physicians to each other and to the profession at large" is as follows: "It is derogatory to the dignity of the profession, to resort to public advertisements." Sec. 3rd. "It is derogatory to the dignity of the profession, to resort to public advertisements or private cards or handbills, inviting the attention of individuals affected with particular diseases, etc." 1st

> Advertising in the New York Herald...the New York Times...publishing a handbill and a pamphlet.[78]

The president of the Academy informed Dr. Spreng of these charges and summoned him before the Committee on Ethics. In response, Dr. Spreng sent the following note:

> The undersigned respectfully resigns this membership in the N.Y. Academy of Medicine. Said resignation to take effect [immediately].
> Yours Very Respectfully
> Justin J. Spreng. M.D.
> Late member of the N.Y. Academy of Medicine.[79]

Comita could also exonerate the accused. In an 1867 case, the NYAM Committee on Ethics examined charges against one of its members who was accused of "one or more consultations with [a person] well known as a homeopathist, and as an associate of those, 'whose practice is based on an Exclusive dogma' implied in the word 'Homeopathy.'"[80] When the physician explained that the regularly educated former homeopath merely required assistance in a delivery requiring use of an obstetric forceps, he was found not to be in violation. In another case, this time from Massachusetts, a Dr. Robinson was accused of "conduct unbecoming and unworthy of an honorable physician and member of the Massachusetts Medical Society" for "slanderously and maliciously caus[ing] to be published" a report that a Dr. Martin had performed "a surgical operation...improperly and ignorantly."[81] Dr. Robinson's prompt apology earned him a reprieve. As the "trial court" observed in passing judgment, given "his earnest attempts at reconciliation...his free confession of...impropriety, and the full proof produced of his honorable standing and ability as a surgeon...we forbear expulsion, & award on his conduct in those publications the severest censure of this Board, & we confidently hope that his youth and ability will enable him hereafter to maintain an honourable standing in his profession."[82] Like the wrongdoing Dr. .W, the repentant Dr. Robinson underwent the same four-stage apology to earn the censors "forbear[ance] of expulsion." He (1) acknowledged the offense, (2) explained it in terms of his youth and inexperience, (3) exhibited remorse and a desire for reconciliation, and (4) had reparation made by being publicly censured by the society.

As noted earlier, this system of restorative justice was an adaption of the restorative justice conventions of gentlemanly honor. It is also strikingly similar to the forgive-and-remember system of accountability in clinical morality described in the nineteenth century by Percival and in the twentieth century by ethnographer Charles Bosk (see discussion in Chapter 1). Bosk explains differences in the treatment of miscreants in terms of the types of error committed, but if forgive-and-remember accountability is viewed as an outgrowth of the ethics of gentlemanly honor, the real issue is less the type of error than the nature of the miscreant's character. A nineteenth-, twentieth-, or twenty-first-century physician or surgeon who forthrightly admits to an error, who is genuinely contrite and apologetic, and who resolves not to repeat the error in the future displays the character of a true gentleman—or of the gentleman's twentieth-century descendant, the professional. Such a miscreant may be forgiven and readmitted to the company of his or her peers—as were the wrongdoing Dr. W. and the repentant Dr. Robinson. If, however, the miscreant refuses to admit an error or tries to hide it, and/or if the miscreant fails to be contrite or apologetic, he or she is revealed as ungentlemanly or unprofessional in their very character and so cannot be accepted as a peer. Punishment by expulsion or ostracism is thus the only possible resolution, as exemplified in the case of errant intern N from Chapter 1—or the case of another miscreant, one Dr. Bartlett.

For medical societies, expulsion and ostracism are mechanisms of a nonrestorative punishment meted out to those who are demonstrably ungentlemanly (or unprofessional). These mechanisms are exemplified in a well-publicized 1839 case in which the Massachusetts Medical Society expelled and ostracized a physician, Dr. John Stephen Bartlett (1812–1840), for assisting an itinerant quack, known as Dr. Williams, in bilking a blind woman out of her savings. The woman, Abigail Plumer, reported that she went to Boston to seek the care of a specialist. She was a medical indigent, one of "the sick poor" who, as required by the medical morality of the period and by all codes of medical police, was receiving treatment gratis from various medical society members, including a Dr. Abel Peirson (1794–1853). Abigail no doubt expected a similar courtesy when she consulted a visiting eye specialist, Dr. Williams. Williams, however, was not a member of a society and treated her quite differently:

> When I first went to see Dr. Williams he inquired how much money I had, and whether the people I lived with were rich or poor.... He said...that the medicine he gave me would restore my sight. I asked his charge. He said I must pay $50 down, and $50 when cured. He said he could cure me.... He replied [if] I set more by money than my sight he would have nothing to do with me. I told him that I had but $43; that I had a child to support, and could lay by but little. He said he would not take less than $50. [Abigail paid Williams her life savings after being assured of a cure by Dr. Bartlett]. After Dr. Williams' medicines failed to restore her sight, she turned to] Dr. Peirson [who] aided me in getting me into an asylum. Benevolent friends in Salem procured me a loom—I learnt to weave mats and can now earn something for my support.[83]

Dr. Peirson brought the case to the censors of the Massachusetts Medical Society. After a hearing, the censors indicted Dr. Bartlett for consorting with a quack who dispensed secret nostrums. Bartlett was unrepentant. As he later testified before the state legislature: "I admit that the [medical] society acted in good faith in expelling me, under the by-laws. I told the society, I should persevere in violating the by-laws whenever I thought the good of mankind required."[84] The indictment was placed before the membership who voted to expel and to ostracize the unrepentant Dr. Bartlett.

The subsequent ostracism had a dire impact on Dr. Bartlett. In an appeal to the state legislature, Dr. Bartlett was still unrepentant and unapologetic about his conduct. Believing that his Harvard degree gave him a right to practice, Bartlett protested that, "[t]he effects and influence of my expulsion have been highly injurious to my character and prospects.... The influence of the Medical Society is to crush a man down and render him worse than dead... I have had to struggle to sustain myself.... I rely on my professional services for support. I find it necessary to follow other pursuits for a livelihood."[85]

THE MEDICAL SOCIETY OF THE STATE OF NEW YORK'S *SYSTEM OF MEDICAL ETHICS*, 1823–1847

In 1823, the MSSNY became the first American medical society to issue a code bearing the title "medical ethics." This code, like others with the word "ethics" in their title, differs from codes entitled "medical police" because codes of police only address physicians' fees and their conduct toward each other, whereas codes of medical ethics formalize the moral basis of the physician–patient relationship. Codes of medical police pay virtually no attention to patients, except as objects to be fought over or to be charged fees; in contrast, codes of medical ethics place the moral duty of ministering to the sick front-and-center. The MSSNY's *System of Medical Ethics*, for example, expressly states the physician's duty to obey immediately an urgent call for help from the sick.[86] Not one single code among the dozens of codes of "medical police" states any such duty. In another *System of Ethics*, physicians are said to have this duty to obey the calls of the sick because they occupy a role in which they are "intrusted [with] the lives, the honor, and reputation of their *patients*... [who] are... dependent on them for the exercise of their skill and benevolence."[87]

To appreciate the difference between the codes titled "medical ethics" and those titled "medical police," it is helpful to consider the definition of medical ethics that Percival offered in his eponymous ur-text, *Medical Ethics*. Percival characterizes medical ethics as a form of "professional ethics," which states a physician's moral duties toward three other parties: (1) his patients, (2) his brethren, and (3) the public.[88] Codes of medical police address only item (2), a practitioner's duties to fellow practitioners; they do not address items 1 and 3, a physician's duties to the sick or to society. Moreover, unlike codes of medical ethics, codes of medical police never claim that the duties they proclaim are grounded in morality.

From its founding in 1808 through 1822, the MSSNY had been governed solely by its bylaws and its oath (analyzed in Chapter 3). The transition to a code of medical ethics began at its 1821 anniversary meeting (i.e., a general meeting held on the anniversary of a society's founding at which elections were held and that all members were expected to attend). The MSSNY commissioned two members, James Manley (1782–1851) of New York City and John H. Steele (1780–1838), an upstate physician from Saratoga, "to collect and form a system of Medical Ethicks, to govern the profession in their intercourse with each other, and particularly in cases of consultation."[89] Manley and Steele balked at the commission, believing it improper to call such a code an "Ethicks" since it would deal solely with intrapractitioner relations. To resolve the issue, another New York City physician, Felix Pascalis (1762–1833), was added to the committee. This enlarged committee also refused to draft a traditional code of medical police using the title "medical ethics," claiming that such a code would be inadequate because it

> would affect but a small part of the moral duties of physicians and surgeons; and your committee have inferred it to be their duty to embrace all the maxims and precepts of Medical Ethics and Police . . . in relation to the personal character of the profession; to their practical acts; and especially to the information frequently required of them by magistrates and courts of justice.[90]

The authors of the first American code to be denominated "medical ethics" were thus aware of the difference between codes of medical police and a codes of medical ethics, and they declined to draft a code of medical police under the title "medical ethics."[91] (See full text of the New York *System of Ethics* in Appendix II.)

Manley, Pascalis, and Steele appear to have formed a conception of medical ethics from their work as editors of America's first medical journal, the *Medical Repository* (1797–1824).[92] A case in point is an 1820 letter by the editors of the *Medical Repository* that cites Percival's *Medical Ethics* to censure a quintet of physicians.[93] The physicians were condemned for irresponsible conduct of research because they had published a "cure" for a disease in the popular press without first submitting their findings to a professional forum (such as the *Medical Repository*).

> Gentlemen
>
> The following precept is stated by Dr. Percival in the first chapter of his *Medical Ethics*, in relation to the professional conduct of Physicians and

Surgeons, paragraph xii. "Should a case occur in which, ordinary modes of practice having been attempted without success, it would be advantageous to try new remedies, the accomplishment of this salutary purpose requires that we be governed by sound reason, just analogies, and authentic facts, and by a previous consultation of physicians and surgeons," &c.[94]

It appears that you have observed this wise rule in the management of the case of Mary Tice of Milton (related in the *Evening Post* of New York, August 26, 1820), supposed in your certificate to have been hydrophobia in consequence of the bite of a mad dog....

The wound of Mary Tice spontaneously suppurated [discharged pus], and continued to discharge, as late as a month after you commenced her treatment; and by your remedies, of which there was a great variety, her cure was happily effected. So far, gentlemen, you have done well for the safety of the patient...but, furthermore if you wished to benefit the public by the publication of your observations of this case, it would have been highly meritorious,—provided you had forborne your decided opinion of its nature, and of the value of one of the remedies, which, having been used with many others, rendered it difficult to say which was the most efficient. The smallest possible chance of error in your judgment, made it necessary that it should have been previously revised by some regular medical tribunal; for if one or two of you had for the safety of *one* patient to be aided by the consultation of physicians and surgeons, you will readily admit that by giving your opinion to the public on practical points and inferences of such momentous importance, a probable error of danger or misconception, deserved at least to be equipoised by as admissible and weighty authority, as that which you thought proper to exercise. Such a mode of proceeding is clearly marked out by the above rule, which has become fundamental in the code for the regulation of our professional conduct....

We may add another aggravating circumstance, although it was no doubt incautiously overlooked by you, which is, that by a *tacit compact*, you, as members of a fraternity engaged to promote the honour of the association by all those means which are consistent with morality and the general good of mankind.[95] [It is then argued that the Tice case was misdiagnosed, i.e., she did not have rabies.]

Yours respectfully,

THE EDITORS, New York, October 20, 1820[96]

As this letter to a quintet of physicians attests, the editors of the *Medical Repository* were taking responsibility for enforcing the obligations that medical professionals incur by virtue of a tacit compact whose terms Percival had articulated in *Medical Ethics*—and they were doing so, as the date of this letter indicates, well before some of them were charged by the MSSNY with writing a code of medical ethics. The charges against the quintet of physicians should sound familiar: they are similar to those that the College of Physicians of Philadelphia leveled against Benjamin Rush when he hastily published his radical bleed-and-purge cure for yellow fever. Unlike the College of Physicians, however, the editors of the *Medical Repository* could condemn the quintet of physicians by appealing to the authority of a published "precept... stated by Dr. Percival in the first chapter of his *Medical Ethics*, in relation to the professional conduct of Physicians and Surgeons.... Should a case occur in which, ordinary modes of practice having been attempted without success, it would be advantageous to try new remedies... governed by (i) sound reason, just analogies, and (ii) authentic facts, and (iii) by a previous consultation of physicians and surgeons.'"[97]

The physicians were charged with violating all of these precepts: (1) their reasoning was unsound because they used multiple treatments and so there was no way of telling which treatment was responsible for the cure, (2) they did not get their facts straight because they were not actually treating rabies, and (3) they did not consult their fellow physicians before publicly pronouncing a cure. By contrast, when the College of Physicians censured Rush for a similar transgression in 1794—about a decade before the publication of Percival's *Medical Ethics*—they had no such resource. Consequently, because Rush had violated none of the bylaws stated in the College's constitution of 1787,[98] he could reasonably protest to his students and to the world that his expulsion was groundless—a flyte motivated by overly conservative colleagues envious of his success. These physicians, however, were confronted not only with the opinions of the editors, but with the authority of a "precept... stated by Dr. Percival... [in] his Medical Ethics," and so they could not dismiss this accusation as groundless flyte: the grounds had been stated in advance in Percival's code of medical ethics. By appealing to a code, the editors redirected the focus of the censure from personalities to facts: the issue was not a flyte between persons protecting their honor but was based instead on whether, *in fact*, the accused violated a precept stated in an authoritative code drafted independently of particular persons or incidents.

As editors of the *Medical Repository*, Manley, Pascalis, and Steele were well aware that codes of medical police did not address the range of moral issues affecting medical practice in New York. Hence their reiterated insistence that the MSSNY's system of ethics broaden its scope beyond the purview of subjects dealt with in traditional codes of medical police—consultations, interferences, fees, and quackery—by adding three new sections notably absent from medical police: a section on the personal character of physicians, a section on the specifications of medical police/ethics in practice, and a section on forensic medical police dealing with the role of physicians in the courts. (The full text that the MSSNY adopted as its *System of Medical Ethics* is reproduced as Appendix II.)

The Content of the First American System of Medical Ethics

The opening section of the MSSNY's code of medical ethics addresses the character of a physician in a manner that links the new system of medical ethics to the older ethics of the oath. The MSSNY oath committed members to "honestly, virtuously, and chastely, conduct [themselves] in the practice of physic and surgery... [acting] with fidelity and honour, [to] do every thing in [their] power for the benefit of the sick committed to [their] charge."[99] Echoing these ideals, the MSSNY's system of ethics stipulates that physicians must strive for the virtues of "purity, and perfection of personal character" while complying with their "obligations of conscience, honor, and humanity" and maintaining a "personal character... of a perfect gentleman."[100]

Like the MSSNY's oath, the *System of Ethics* addresses the virtue of "honesty" in communicating with patients—a virtue that, like many others involved in patient care, is not mentioned in codes of medical police. Veracity in end-of-life care, however, seems to be as negotiable in the nineteenth century as it proved to be in the twentieth and twenty-first centuries. Then, as now, frank discussions of terminal prognoses are often softened by the liberal dispensation of hope in the form of an experimental drug or a new treatment regimen. The MSSNY's *System of Ethics* portrays end-of-life discussions as a conflict between two duties: the duty of honestly communicating a terminal prognosis and "the duty of administering hope and comfort, without the influence of which, many doubtful cases of disease might at once become positively fatal."[101] The *System* offers the following guidance:

> 1st. Give timely and explicit information of the dangerous situation of the patient to those who have the best right to advise him of his religious and temporal concerns.
>
> 2nd... inform them of a possibility of a change in the prognostic, in order to prevent any relaxation of care on the part of nurses and others....
>
> 3rd... continue... personal attendance... should the physician be dismissed from pecuniary [i.e., financial] motives, his responsibility requires a friendly or gratuitous attention.[102]

It is thus the family or religious advisors who are to be informed of a patient's terminal prognosis, and it is they who bear the responsibility of informing the patient. The patient is not be informed directly. Precedents for this advice are found in both Gregory's *Lectures*[103] and Percival's *Medical Ethics*.[104] Both of these texts assert that physicians have a duty of nonabandonment that obligates them to provide care for terminal patients, irrespective of financial remuneration. End-of-life care involves physiological support in the form of laudanum—a potent analgesic mix of alcohol, herbs, and opium effective in dulling pain—and psychological support in the form of hope.[105] Appropriate parties, such as a "Christian minister," *but not the patient her- or himself*, were to be informed of a patient's terminal prognosis. This party, in turn, had the task of informing the patient of the prognosis at an appropriate moment, so that she or he could put her or his religious or secular affairs in order.

A variant of this division of informational labor is not uncommon in large medical centers even today: physicians who have given patients or families an overdose of hope often outsource the task of conveying a terminal prognosis to an intensivist or to a palliative care service—these parties are tasked with informing patients or their families of the terminal prognosis. Turning back to the nineteenth century, historians are divided over whether, having been informed of a patient's terminal prognosis, clergymen or family members actually informed the patients themselves. Historian Roy Porter (1946–2002) contends that "people were no longer allowed their own deaths; for in the name of sympathy and avoiding distress, their families and doctors were allowing them to slip away oblivious to their fate."[106] Another historian, Pat Jalland, came to the opposite conclusion: that heads of the family and clergymen normally informed patients that their illness was likely to be terminal.[107] Given Americans' Calvinist-Puritan-Presbyterian traditions of facing death, Jalland's account seems more convincing: nineteenth-century Christian ministers and family heads would typically inform patients of their terminal prognoses. Only in the twentieth century, as death rates declined, as the causes of death shifted from infectious illnesses to chronic diseases, and as dying moved from homes to hospitals, did death become so alienated from everyday experience that physicians felt the need to disguise its imminence from the dying patient, forever offering hope in the form of medical miracles.

Another virtue pledged in the MSSNY oath that found its way into its codes was the chaste or pure practice of medicine. The importance of this subject is underlined in the MSSNY's *Medical Ethics* by the remark that although "it is not intended in this system of medical ethics to instruct physicians and surgeons upon every felonious act of infanticide, murder, &c for which the Penal Statutes of this country have made sufficient provision," nonetheless, an exception is warranted with respect to one issue that deserves the attention of "medical authorities," who should "consider, condemn and punish as *criminal*, such acts of medical practitioners as offend the respective obligations of married persons, or the chastity and modesty of the youth of both sexes" by seduction or otherwise "interfer[ing] with marital rights or the observance of a chaste and moral life."[108]

The MSSNY's *System of Medical Ethics* touches on another issue treated in medical oaths but which, like discussions of chastity, was notably absent from systems of medical police—confidentiality or secrecy with respect to information concerning patients. Except for a comment by Benjamin Rush,[109] until the MSSNY's endorsement of the duty of confidentiality, the American medical literature was silent about a physicians' duty to keep patients' medical information secret. This first official statement of a physician's duty of confidentiality in the American medical ethics literature arises in the context of court cases:

> It is a matter of justice, necessity and propriety that the business of a physician and surgeon should be always considered of a confidential nature... *secrecy* in certain circumstances... is the privilege of the faculty, and inviolable even in a court of justice.... XVII. The exposure of the nature of a complaint which a physician is called upon to judge or cure, subjecting the patient to public shame or impeaching his moral character, is an unpardonable breach of medical ethics.[110]

This theme is reiterated emphatically in the section on "Forensic Medical Police," in which the physician's role as an expert witness in courts of law is addressed by "two rules... [first: be] well-informed of all the facts alleged in evidence... [and] decide by known medical principle."[111] The "second rule"

> is that of secrecy upon the facts with which physicians become professionally acquainted... such as whether an apparent pregnancy be real; the gestation and birth of a child; its parentage, colour and age; the judgment and treatment of syphilitic and gonorrheal diseases; the able or disabled state of a person, in limb or constitution; the fallacy [falsification] of virginity and other circumstances, to the confession of which, a degree of shame, and the idea of exposure is attached, and which are never mentioned but with an engagement to secrecy.
>
> This duty has been defined by comparing it to that of the Catholic Confessional, which admits of no disclosures except in cases of treason or murder.[112]

Thus, the MSSNY *System of Ethics* reasserts physicians' oath-sworn duty to prioritize the welfare of the patient by obligating physicians to an absolute duty of confidentiality. Courts may probe for the physician's opinion about infanticide, bastardy, paternity, virginity, sexually transmitted diseases, or malingering, but the physician's duty to his patients, like a priest's duty to protect the secrets of the confessional, overrides his obligation to testify on these issues before a court of law.

The New York *System of Ethics* also addresses fees, but it does not include a fee scale because Article XX of its bylaws prohibits the society, or any affiliated society, from setting a standard fee scale. Elite New York City physicians, led by Nicholas Romayne, three-time President of the MSSNY, had lobbied against a fee scale, noting that physicians with prestigious appointments and honorable reputations justly commanded higher fees from more affluent patrons than did less qualified practitioners. The Third Division of the *System of Ethics* addresses issues of consultation, a traditional focus of codes of medical police. This section asserts a claim, validated by a quotation from Gregory, that distinction between physicians and surgeons "had no foundation"[113]; that is, physicians and surgeons are both equally "doctors" and should not be regarded as practicing different specialties. This point made, the text paraphrases those passages from Percival's *Medical Ethics* that deal with consults: interferences,[114] flyting,[115] pamphlet wars, and quarreling in public newspapers.[116]

On all of these issues, the MSSNY *System of Ethics* initiates discussions that would become the focus of later codes of medical ethics. In one respect, however, the MSSNY code failed to inspire future codes: it abandons the justifying concepts of *esprit du corps* and a tacit social compact that earlier codes of medical police had quoted verbatim from article XXIII, chapter II of Percival's *Medical Ethics*. It invokes instead a more ancient authority, that of Hippocrates and his oath and thus, by implication, its descendant, the Edinburgh-style oath that New York physicians were required to swear.

> XXI. It is enjoined in the sacred obligation which Hippocrates imposed upon the pupils of the noble science of medicine and surgery, which is also the model of the like encouragement... in this and other countries [i.e., in the MSSNY and Edinburgh oaths]; that they shall respect and assist their preceptors and masters... and shall contribute as far as in their power, to the honor, improvement, and utility of their professions. According to this precept physicians and surgeons have something more to do, than to procure their livelihood. As they are indebted to the labors, talents and experience of their predecessors in the healing art for all that constitutes its admirable body of doctrine; so present and future generations look to them for some additional improvement.... [Moreover] this obligation is unbecomingly violated by many physicians who pretend to eminence [but] estrange themselves from medical associations... screen themselves from scientific labors [and] never contribute by any effort... to the advancement of the medical character.[117]

Since other medical societies never required their members to swear a Hippocratic-style oath, this passage was meaningless for them. They therefore continued to look to Percival's concept of a tacit compact as their foundational justification. So, unlike the Boston and Connecticut systems of medical police, this section of the New York *System of Medical Ethics* was not widely imitated except by a transition code drafted by the Baltimore Medico-Chirurgical Society (1832–1848[118]) in its founding year, 1832.

Enforcing Standards: Secret Nostrums, Secret Societies, and Diploma Mills

Setting standards is one thing, enforcing them quite another. Both joint MSCNY-MSSNY standard-setting ventures of the 1820s—the national pharmacopoeia (1818–1821) and the *System of Ethics* (1821–1823)—proved challenging. Emboldened by the new national pharmacopoeia (discussed in the next chapter), on August 9, 1824, the MSCNY voted to confront the issue of adulterated medicines and secret nostrums by commissioning Felix Pascalis (who had also served on the committee drafting the New York *System of Ethics*) to chair a committee "On the Subject of Quack Medicines." In the same period, the *comita minora* of the MSCNY began to enforce the MSSNY's *System of Ethics*. To their dismay, Pascalis and Manley (president of the MSSNY and former chair of the committee drafting the *System of Ethics*) discovered that, in practice, their colleagues were less enthusiastic about enforcing uniform standards than they were in paying lip service to them in principle.

In 1825, a Dr. Cockcroft challenged the MSCNY *comita*'s authority to enforce the MSSNY's *System of Medical Ethics*. Cockcroft had refused to comply with a judgment by the *comita* that he, Cockcroft, had violated the MSSNY's *System of Medical Ethics* and so owed a written apology to a Dr. John Cheesman. Despite the intriguing names of the physicians involved, the particulars of this case are less interesting than the hotly debated jurisdictional issue of whether the *comita* of a county medical society could enforce a system of ethics promulgated by a state medical society. The debate that followed ran the course of several meetings. In the end, Manley and Pascalis convinced the members of the MSCNY to uphold the authority of its *comita* to enforce the MSSNY's *System of Medical Ethics*. Dr. Cockcraft, however, still refused to send the requisite apology to Dr. Cheesman; so the MSCNY voted to expel Cockcroft, who then belatedly apologized in writing to Dr. Cheesman and retained his membership. The upshot of this debate was that the MSSNY's *System of Medical Ethics* could be enforced by the MSCNY's *comita minora*—thus, the state society's system of medical ethics was enforceable at the local level and had real teeth.[119]

Dissident physicians also challenged the reformers with a resolution ordering the dissolution of the Committee on Quack Medicines before it could issue its reports.[120] Reformers beat back the challenge. On August 20, 1827, Manley delivered the report of the Committee on Quack medicine on three secret nostrums: Chamber's Remedy, Le Roy's Medical Curative, and Swaim's Panecea.[121] The reformist *New-York Medical and Physical Journal* lauded the report in an anonymous review (probably written by its editors, John Brodhead Beck [1794–1852] and Daniel Levy Maduro Peixotto [1800–1843]). Their praise was constrained, however, by the committee's finding that so-called quack nostrums offered the same cures as those offered by regulars, except in better tasting formulations and niftier bottles. More embarrassingly still, the committee found that regular practitioners were providing certificates attesting to the efficacy of these secret nostrums.[122]

To deal with the awkward finding that secret nostrums were merely versions of standard prescribed medications, the committee argued that, "any medicine which is beneficially operated, when properly exhibited, must be in the same ratio, injurious if improperly used.... [Moreover] it is necessary to settle the character of that disease."[123] In short, self-diagnosis is problematic, and beneficial medicines may become dangerous precisely because the ingredients are "secret" in these nostrums and thus undisclosed, making it virtually impossible to prevent harmful interactions with other drugs or overdosing. Swaim's panacea for syphilis, for example, was a mixture of sarsaparilla syrup and corrosive sublimate—a medicinal form of mercury chloride—with a tasty topping of oil of wintergreen. Except for the tasty topping, regular practitioners also treated syphilis with mixtures of sarsaparilla syrup and corrosive sublimate. Until the discovery of Salvarsan in 1903, mercury compounds offered the best available treatments for syphilis; however, they had to be prescribed with a watchful eye to prevent overdoses and dangerous side effects.[124] Dispensed as a "secret nostrum," drug interactions and overdosing were unavoidable. (Today, mercury chloride is classified as a poison and used as a pesticide or a wood preservative. As late as 1899, however, *Merck's Manual of the Materia Medica* recommended it for treating syphilitic chancres, the sores that appear on sexual organs during the first stage of syphilis.[125])

Looking on the face of quackery close up, the committee had discovered that "he is us."[126] Despite mouthing agreement with critiques of secret nostrums, the respectable profession was implicated in their legitimization and sale. The committee tried to stop these practices by recommending that

> the Medical Society... forbid Regular physicians to countenance [secret nostrums] by their approbation of certificates—and therefore [we] propose that [1] a copy of the System of Medical Ethics be furnished to every member of the Society, and that [2] a special committee be directed to report what are the nature and effects of certain panaceas now most in "repute"; and that said report be presented at a defined period of time for the Consideration of the Society.[127]

More specifically, the committee had found that members of the MSCNY furnished "certificates" to the purveyors of secret nostrums, such as William Swaim (1781–1846), a bookbinder and manufacturer of Swaim's Panacea.[128] Swain published their testimonials in the public media of the period—magazines, newspapers, and most important, pamphlets—thereby publicizing the names and expertise of the testimonializing physicians.[129] Some physicians received direct financial compensation for their testimonials or for dispensing a panacea at a hospital (a fact that would then appear in print, thereby legitimizing the panacea).

To address these problems, the MSCNY adopted the dual strategy of sending members copies of the *System of Medical Ethics*, which prohibits "producing certificates and signatures . . . in support of the advertiser's skill and success" and calling miscreant members before the *comita*. Although a public apology would usual suffice for first offenses, this transgression was in principle "punish[able] by . . . expulsion."[130] MSCNY also published a series (as it turned out) of reports on the actual contents of these "secret" nostrums.

In 1831, the MSCNY became preoccupied with another issue of secrecy: some members belonged to a "secret medical society," Kappa Lambda. At their December 12, 1831 meeting, the following motion was approved:

> *Whereas* it appears from authentic documents that [twenty-eight members of the MSCNY] are members of a society called *Kappa Lambda*, which imposes on its members obligations of secrecy, and requires members to assist each other in their professional practice and to defend and sustain their respective characters, although it may be prejudicial to the character of other individuals and in direct opposition to the honour and interest of the Profession and *Whereas*, this professional conduct has for some years been highly dishonorable in its character, derogatory to the Profession, in direct violation of our excellent code of Ethics, and in many instances oppressive and injurious to the community; . . . Therefore *Resolved*, that the above named Physicians and all those who are members of the said Kappa Lambda Society shall be considered as excluded from the protection of the code of Ethics of this Society, and from consultation with its members.
>
> *Resolved*, that if they do not on or before the second Monday of January next, 1832, publish a dissolution of the Kappa Lambda Society, and give to the Medical Society a satisfactory pledge, that they will no longer continue to associate under a sanction so dishonorable to the Profession, that a legal prosecution will be instituted. . . . *Resolved* that a copy of these Resolutions be sent by the Secretary to the *Kappa Lambda* Society.[131]

As a consequence of this resolution, all twenty-eight members of the New York section of Kappa Lambda signed these pledges, and the society officially dissolved itself. The event even warranted a poetic epitaph: "Here lies the Kappa Lambda wight! Begot by Selfishness and Night. It was a thing of craft and guile, Which bowed and smiled, and wronged the while. Through dark and sinuous paths, by stealth. It crawled to office, [&] gathered wealth. . . . Exposed at length, to truth's pure ray, It raved, writhed, withered, [&] passed away."[132] Apologies in hand, former members of Kappa Lambda were readmitted to the MSCNY, as they should have been according to its system of restorative justice. Unfortunately, justice did not completely triumph: the New York Kappa Lambda society continued on through the 1860s. (More discussion of Kappa Lambda in the next chapter.)

THE BALTIMORE *SYSTEM OF MEDICAL ETHICS*, 1832

The Medico-Chirurgical Society of Baltimore society was formed to combat a major cholera outbreak in the summer of 1832. Baltimore's physicians and surgeons sought to coordinate their response and to ensure that "information is reciprocally imparted... to the common interest."[133] At its founding meeting, the society charged a committee with drafting a code of ethics.[134] Chairing the committee was Eli Geddings (1799–1838), professor and chair of anatomy and physiology at the University of Maryland. Like the authors of the New York system of ethics, Geddings edited a medical journal, the *Baltimore Medical and Surgical Journal and Review* (1831–1834[135]). In drafting a code for the new society, his committee drew from the writings of Percival, Gregory, Rush, and, adding a new name to the pantheon of valorized physicians, Michael Ryan. The Americanized edition of Percival's *Medical Ethics*, published by the Kappa Lambda Society of Hippocrates of Philadelphia (1823–1835), also served as a source of its text.[136] (The Baltimore *System of Ethics* is reprinted in Appendix III.)

Influenced by southern literary culture and preoccupied with the cholera epidemic that prompted the society's formation, the preface to the Baltimore *System of Ethics* is written in a floridly morose language inspired by the King James Bible and a season of cholera.

> In the hour too, "when pestilence walketh in darkness,"[137] [physicians and surgeons] are seen mingling familiarly in scenes of death and despair, and like ministers of good, dealing out the balm of health and consolation to the sorrowing and the afflicted. The couch of splendor and the squalid cot are alternatively the scenes of their benevolent actions; and calls of distress, from whatever quarter they emanate, are obeyed with alacrity, regardless of all personal considerations of comfort, fortune, health, or even life.[138]

By contrast, the same precept is parsed more matter of factly in the MSSNY codes as follows:

> [Division IV] Art. XIX. In urgent cases of sickness or of injuries occasioned by accidents, a call for medical or surgical help should be obeyed immediately, unless such compliance be to the detriment of some other sufferer.[139]

The Baltimore prose may be melodramatic, but the point is clear: during epidemics, physicians are obligated to attend to those stricken, even if doing so disturbs their comfort and jeopardizes their finances, their health, and their very lives. This same point is reinforced elsewhere in the Baltimore code in more matter-of-fact language:

> Sec. I, Art. VIII. It should be remembered, that the office of a physician is not exclusively one of emolument [i.e., motivated by money, prestige, and privilege], but also of benevolence and humanity. As, therefore, he may be often summoned, in haste, to offer assistance in urgent cases of sickness, or of recent accidents and injuries, it always behooves him to obey such calls with promptitude.[140]

The background context of the cholera epidemic not only explains the repeated emphasis on the duty to respond to the calls of the sick as integral to "the office of a physician," it also frames the code's characterization of another professional duty: attending to public health by giving "salutary instructions, by the adoption of which mankind may be secured against the incursions of disease and death, and by which health . . . may be preserved. [And] warn[ing] us of the dangers which surround us, and devis[ing] means for their avoidance."[141]

Drawing on language from the Kappa Lambda edition of Percival's *Medical Ethics,* the *Baltimore System of Medical Ethics* parses the prohibition against associating with quacks in a precedent-setting way. Percival had expressly recommended that regularly educated practitioners, or "regulars," *should* willingly consult with irregularly educated practitioners, known as "irregulars," because a regular medical education is "not indispensably necessary to the attainment of knowledge, skill and experience." Consequently, practitioners "who have acquired, in a competent measure, such qualifications without [the] advantages [of a regular education] *should not be excluded from fellowship [or] consultations*, especially as the good of the patient is the sole object in view."[142] The Baltimore code inverts Percival's meaning prohibiting consultations with irregulars:

> X. As a regular medical education furnishes the only presumptive evidence of professional abilities and acquirements, and [ought to be] the only acknowledged right of an individual to the exercise and honors of the profession, no consultation should be held with any individual who has not complied with the laws enacted for the proper regulation of medicine in the State in which he resides, or who is not in possession of a diploma from some medical college or university of known and acknowledged respectability. Consultations

should, under no pretext, be held with unqualified persons, or quacks, or with such members of the profession as have, by improper conduct, outraged its dignity or respect.[143]

This radical departure from Percival's ur-text threatens regular practitioners who consult with irregulars with the same punishment that Dr. Bartlett suffered for consorting with the quack who bilked a blind woman out of her life savings—expulsion and ostracism. Such an adamant rejection of any form of consultation with irregulars may have made sense during a season of cholera—when desperate patients were buying useless remedies from unscrupulous scam artists—but insofar as it was extended to normal periods, it excluded any form of cooperation between regular and irregular practitioners. A decade and a half later, when the newly formed AMA appropriated this radically exclusionist passage for its code of ethics, a rigid line would be drawn between regular practitioners and all others, thus providing a framework for politicizing licensure, internal inquisitions, and campaigns to delegitimize alternative schools of medicine.[144]

The Baltimore code also introduced a new twist on Percival's tacit social compact by asserting that a community has obligations to the medical profession and by further adding Rush's view that patients have obligation to their (demigod-like) physicians. These added sections reflect notions of reciprocity. Thus, in reciprocity for a physician's obligation to answer the calls of the sick "when the pestilence walketh in the darkness,"[145] even at jeopardy of their lives, "how great are the obligations of the community to the profession, and how well earned the high and unlimited respect and confidence which it has at all times secured whenever its duties have been exercised with honor, integrity, and humanity."[146] Communities should thus reciprocate for physicians' sacrifices by bestowing respect and confidence on their physicians.

Following the same logic of reciprocal obligation, the code argues in a section aptly titled *Duties of Patients toward their Physician* that patients have obligations to their doctors:

> The members of the medical profession, upon whom are enjoined so many important and arduous duties towards the community, and who are required to make so many sacrifices of comfort, ease and health, for the welfare of those who employ them, certainly have a right to require and expect, that their patients should entertain a due sense of the reciprocal duties which they owe to their medical attendants. These have been very clearly detailed by the celebrated Rush, than whose authority none could be of greater weight on such a subject, and more entitled to confidence.[147]

Rush's list of patients' duties toward their physicians follows, commencing with the first commandment, the rule of medical monotheism, "to select no person as [your] medical advisor, who has not received a regular professional education."[148] The fifth and ninth commandments follow in due course: prompt and implicit "obedience . . . to the prescriptions of [your] physician;"[149] and, since this emanates from Rush's businesslike pen, the commandment to "remunerate [your] physician properly."[150] These statements of the reciprocal obligations of physicians and the community to each other and of physician and patient to each other are effectively a tacit contract—a notion that the AMA would refine and develop when it integrated this language of reciprocal duties of patients, community, and physicians into the code of ethics that it adopted a decade and a half later.[151]

THE CODIFICATION AND PROFESSIONALIZATION OF AMERICAN MEDICAL MORALITY

Codes of medical ethics and other aspects of the professionalization of American medicine are commonly presented as a response to regular medical societies' loss of licensing authority in the 1830s and 1840s,[152] when Thomsonians—herbal healers who followed the teaching of a self-taught New Hampshire healer, Samuel Thomson—launched campaigns that effectively stripped regulars of licensing authority in states like Connecticut and New York.[153] As one historian observed, "[b]etween 1833 and 1844, nearly every state repealed or reduced the penalties for unlicensed practitioners. . . . Only New Jersey refused to repeal its medical act."[154] The chronology of code development outlined in this chapter suggests that a different account of the professionalization process is needed, since the major period for developing medical society oaths or codes of medical ethics or police was from 1806 to 1832—a period when regular medical societies still enjoyed undisputed licensing authority. In the case of the Boston and New York medical societies, it was not the loss of licensing authority but the opposite—conferral of licensing authority—which led these medical societies to develop a medical police or an ethics oath.

New York City practitioners, moreover, never sought licensing authority. The history of licensure in the state and its capital city indicates that, as often as not, medical practitioners and their societies opposed governmental licensing as an intrusion on their autonomy. Under British colonial authority, in 1665, the Duke of York's laws came into force empowering professional self-regulation because would-be practitioners had to obtain the "consent of such as are skillful in the same art (if such may be had)" before commencing their practice.[155] Governmental authority over licensing was first asserted in a 1760 New York City licensing law (discussed in Chapter 2) that required anyone seeking to practice midwifery, physic, or surgery to present evidence of their training to a judge or governor.[156] A trio of lawyers had lobbied for governmental regulation of the medical professions, stating their case in a 1753 issue of a New York City reformist journal of opinion, *The Independent Reflector* (1752–1754).[157] Their call for regulation opens with a portrayal of what it would be like to be cared for by a " good physician" who would act as a

> Friend [or] Father... [who the sick person] could scarce refrain from adoring... as a Deity.... 'Tis his Office to relieve the Sick, assuage our Pain, and distribute Health, Felicity, and Joy: He even combats for us the greatest of all Evils, and, for a While, retards the mortal Attacks of the *King of Terrors*. This is his proper Duty; but he may at the same Time... support our Patience, banish our Fears, or improve them to our best Interests, by raising our Hop es... and... if... Death must come, he can soften us into a Compliance with, and Resignation to, the Will of our Common Creator.[158]

Having deified the good physician as friend, father, and virtual demigod, the lawyers warn that in the absence of proper governmental regulation such physicians were rare in eighteenth-century New York City. Instead,

> the greatest Part [of New York practitioners] are meer [sic] Pretenders to a Profession, of which they are entirely ignorant.... How many Lives of the good People of this city, must annually fall a Sacrifice to those Pests of Society, those merciless Butchers of Human Kind.... By the Law of the Land, a Person is guilty of Murder, for killing a Man, by throwing a Stone from a House into the street.... And shall an illiterate Mountebank, who deals about the Instruments of Destruction, escape with Impunity, when 'tis demonstrable, that he has often deprived his Patients of Life, as if he had stabb'd them to the Heart?...
>
> In most of the well-regulated Cities in *Europe* the Practitioners of Physic are under the Regulation of the Law: that Profession, above all others, ought to be under its Direction, as it is more dangerous to Mankind than any [other]. Thousands may be poison'd, and the Doctor pass unpunished.[159]

Persuaded by these lawyers—not by medical practitioners—New York City authorities passed the 1760 licensing law. A 1797 New York State law, formulated in similar terms, extended these regulations to the entire state,[160] thus establishing a pattern in which government officials, untrained in medicine, oversaw the licensing of physicians, surgeons, and midwives.[161] Moreover, in 1797, over the objections of the MSCNY—albeit at the request of upstate medical societies—state legislators gave medical societies the power to license medical practitioners and required all proper practitioners to become members of a county medical society. This requirement brought an unsought intrusion of outsiders into the convivial group of gentlemanly practitioners of the MSCNY and was a likely the precipitating factor in prompting the society's leader, Nicholas Romayne, to require a standard oath of all members, in which they asserted the autonomy of medicine in the name of duties to their patients. Thus, insofar as standardizing ethical conduct by means of an oath can be considered a step toward professionalization, this step was prompted in reaction against an unwanted imposition of licensure. Professionalization arose as an alternative to governmental authority, not as an attempt to appropriate this authority. A similar story can be told with respect to the *Boston Medical Police*, which was prompted not by loss of licensing authority, but in response to a grant of licensing authority that prompted the medical society to adopt a medical police—a set of dispute mitigation rules—to put their own house in order lest the government impose regulations on physicians as a condition of licensure.

Perhaps the theoretical model most helpful in understanding why medical societies should perceive grants of licensing authority as threats is offered by sociologist Andrew Abbott's analysis of the system of professions.[162] Abbot's richly complex analysis of professions portrays them as occupations that seek to control their abstract knowledge base, skill set, and practices. To oversimplify one aspect of Abbot's analysis: professions evolve as practitioners attempt to assert control over their knowledge base and its practical application. Thus, they develop educational standards to control practitioners' knowledge base, and they implement oaths, codes, and "standards of care" to control professional modes of practice. A profession's control over its forms of knowledge or modes of practice can be threatened by consumers' economic power, by competitive systems of practice—or by governmental regulations. Consequently, as Romayne clearly appreciated, grants of licensure carry with them the implicit threat that outside bureaucrats will take control of a profession. In reaction to this perceived threat, a society may try to prevent such a takeover by putting its own house in order by writing an oath or a code to prevent uncontrolled flytes and pamphlet wars that might invite governmental intervention. Similarly, courtroom intrusion into the core of the physician–patient relationship can also threaten a profession's control over that relationship, prompting professional self-regulation through a system of ethics that asserts an absolute duty of confidentiality to protect the patient.

Extending Abbott's analysis in directions not explored in his writings, it should be clear that, insofar as ideals of gentlemanly honor provided the core of the concept of professionalism, any self-regulatory apparatus created by professions would prohibit threats to the gentlemanly status of professionals. The apparatus—the oath or code—would naturally be deployed to thwart commercialization of the practice by such "vulgar" activities as advertising or self-promotional letters in newspapers, and it would exclude the uncouth and ungentlemanly—foreigners, former slaves, women—from joining the gentleman's club known as a professional society.

Abbot's analysis can also offer insight into the correlation between epidemics and professionalization. The deadly outbreaks of yellow fever (New York, 1795) and cholera (Baltimore, 1832) demonstrated the fecklessness of physicians' claims to knowledge. Frustrated, seeking to bring a measure of order out of chaos and to assert some measure of control, practitioners became better organized in order to lobby the government to control miasmatic conditions associated with epidemics, and they began to take actions—expelling Benjamin Rush, for example—to prevent practitioners from profiting by selling or endorsing ineffective nostrums. They also tried to tighten control over practitioners' conduct, emphasizing their duty to provide the epidemic-stricken with care, even if they could not cure them "when pestilence walketh in darkness" and to do so "regardless of all personal considerations of comfort, fortune, health, or even life."[163]

Abbot's fundamental insight is that, insofar as professions are occupations that seek control over their knowledge base and skill set, they will resist other occupations offering to apply a different knowledge base and skill set in the same domain. This explains why practitioners developed educational and practice standards, oaths and codes, and other hallmarks of professionalism—and why they would reject "irregulars," "homeopaths," and other modes of alternative practice. What I am suggesting here is that this same quest for control illuminates a link between failure to control disease and professionalization. In the eighteenth and nineteenth centuries, American medical practitioners were frustrated by their patent failure to treat, cure, or prevent epidemic diseases. Unable to control the diseases themselves, they asserted control where they could: over members' conduct, their education, and their modes of practice—and over sanitary conditions.

The pull of professionalization, that is, the movement toward standardizing abstract knowledge and ethical and technical practices, was neither uniquely American nor was it confined to regular practitioners. In America, eclectics, homeopaths, osteopaths, and other irregular practitioners also formed municipal, county, state, and, eventually, national medical societies, setting standards of practice and conduct for their practitioners. Leading the way were the Thomsonians, who formed a national society, the Friendly Thomsonian Botanic Society, in 1832. About a decade later, in 1843–1844, homeopaths formed the American Institute of Homeopathy (AIH), thus setting a precedent that the regulars would follow by founding the AMA in 1846–1847. As historians have noted, the AIH was founded for much the same reasons as the AMA, "[r]eformation and augmentation of the Material Medical," and the "restraining of Physicians from pretending to practice Homeopathy who have not studied it in a skillful manner."[164] To reiterate, the professional organizations of alternative practitioners set standards of practice and conduct for their members—and excluded those who practiced or conducted themselves differently. The Thomsonian Test Resolution of 1837, for example, stipulates, "we will not use, or admit into this Institution, anyone who uses, or intends to be used as medicine, any mineral or vegetable poisons; or practices contrary to the system of practice as laid down by Dr. Samuel Thomson."[165]

The phenomenon of professionalization was not restricted to American practitioners. Through the nineteenth century, irregular and regular practitioners throughout Europe—including Britain,[166] France,[167] and Germany[168]—formed medical societies that defined educational and technical standards, as well as standards of conduct, for their members.[169] Any analysis of professionalization or of oaths and codes of medical ethics and medical police that focuses exclusively on regular practitioners or that ignores the international sweep of the phenomenon of professionalization—any account that, for example, focuses primarily on such parochial events as American regulars' loss of licensing authority in the 1830s—is bound to misrepresent the phenomenon. The forces impelling professionalization were not constrained by forms of medical practice or by national boundaries. The professionalization of the healthcare occupations is best understood as a quest for control over abstract knowledge, practical skills, and forms of conduct that is designed to achieve the goals shared by all forms of medical practice: comfort or cure for the sick, disease prevention, and health promotion—as well as financial security and public respect for practitioners.

6

A NATIONAL CODE OF MEDICAL ETHICS

CHAPTER I. Of the duties of physicians to their patients, and of the obligations of patients to their physicians. . . .

CHAPTER II. Of the duties of physicians to each other, and to the profession at large. . . .

CHAPTER III. Of the duties of the profession to the public, and of the obligations of the public to the profession. . . .

Code of Medical Ethics, American Medical Association, 1847

PRECONVENTIONS AND PRECURSORS

A Reiterated Proposal: Albany 1844

It was an inauspicious start. Something so small it might have been nothing at all. Two physicians from backwater counties, Broome and Cayuga, were complaining about the inadequacies of medical education. Having been rebuffed in their efforts to hold a national conference on the subject just four years earlier, the delegates to the 1844 meeting of the Medical Society of the State of New York (MSSNY) were uninterested in new ventures in that direction. So they sent the complainants off to form a committee and assumed that would be the end of the matter. It might well have ended there had not one of the delegates, the young physician from Broome county, Nathan Smith Davis caught the attention of the society's leading upstate voice, Alden March (1795–1869), founder and chair of surgery at Albany Medical College (founded in 1839). With March's support, Davis cajoled delegates to the MSSNY's next anniversary meeting into approving a resolution inviting a "National Convention of Delegates from Medical Societies and Colleges in the whole Union"[1] to New York City on May 5, 1846, to address the subject of medical education. When that day dawned, 122 delegates gathered in New York City—and out of their failure to reach agreement, the American Medical Association (AMA) was conceived and born.

Precursor National Conventions: Forming a National Pharmacopoeia,1806–1820

New Yorkers had experience in organizing national conventions. In 1817, physicians in the Medical Society of the County of New York (MSCNY) noticed that some vaccines were failing to immunize New Yorkers against smallpox. An investigative committee found that, because of the variety of pharmacopoeias used in New York City, vaccines and other medicines were not being prepared in a uniform fashion.[2] Having identified the cause of the problem, the committee collaborated with the state society to hold a conference on creating a uniform pharmacopeia,[3] that is, a standard formulary for the preparation of medicines and vaccines.[4] Lyman Spalding (1755–1821) a sixty-two-year-old Harvard graduate with a thirst for fame, had an ingenious plan for developing a national consensus statement on pharmaceuticals.[5] In the 1820s, when travel was a matter of foot, horse, or steamboat and communication was based on letters carried by horse, communication across the nation was a daunting challenge. Spalding met that challenge by designing a plan by which local societies would convene regional meetings to determine the most common formulations used in regional pharmacopoeia. Representatives from these meetings would then convene in a national meeting—the first national meeting of American medical societies—to compare and reconcile differences in formulations. His plan worked. On December 15, 1820, Spalding held in his hands a copy of the dual-column Latin-English *Pharmacopoeia of the United States of America* "published by the authority of the Medical Society and Colleges." (Its descendant, *The United States Pharmacopoeia,* is still used today.[6]) Ambition fulfilled, Spalding died the next year, but the tradition of decennial national conventions to revise the pharmacopeia survived him, and a precedent for national medical conventions was established.

The Education Convention: New York 1846

New Yorkers would next convene a national conference in the 1840s. In 1834, the New York state legislature, responding to effective lobbying by Thomsonians—reportedly half the counties in New York state submitted petitions supporting Thomsonians' demands—rescinded most of the laws criminalizing the unlicensed practice of medicine. Consequently, a medical degree became the only discernible difference between a regular practitioner and a quack. Yet, because there were no accreditation standards for a medical degree, diploma mills and fly-by-night medical schools proliferated, rapidly depreciating the value of an M.D. Facing a similar challenge, in 1835 the Medical College of Georgia sent a note to the MSSNY and other medical societies inviting them to a national meeting on standards for medical education.[7] No society accepted. In 1839, Dr. John McCall of Utica (1787–1867) revived this proposal.[8] Again, no medical society accepted. In 1845, with the backing of Alden March, the young Nathan Smith Davis again proposed a national meeting on education. This time, 122 delegates responded, convening on May 5, 1846, at the medical school of the University of the City of New York (now New York University, NYU).

The New York convention opened unpromisingly. Davis's enthusiastic invitation had been addressed to "Medical Societies and Colleges in the whole Union." Having second thoughts, however, the MSSNY narrowed its invitation to exclude delegates from "mere local" county or municipal societies, except in states that lacked a state society.[9] In an era in which letters traveled at a leisurely pace,[10] delegates from local societies, having never learned that they were disinvited, innocently presented their credentials—diploma-like signed documents bearing seals that functioned as "ID cards" for the nineteenth century—to the credentials committee. Pragmatism prevailed, and they were accepted, thereby quite inadvertently setting a precedent that would be followed by AMA conventions for the next quarter century. This odd combination of accident and precedent meant that the AMA was founded as a broadly democratic organization, accepting representation from all regular medical societies, dispensaries, hospitals, and mental institutions in the United States and its territories.

No rest for reformers! Even as the credentialing crisis was being resolved, the anatomist-duelist Granville Pattison and a colleague, both professors at NYU, the conference's host institution, proposed its dissolution on grounds that it had "failed in a representation from one half the United States—and from a majority of the Medical Colleges."[11] Their motion was defeated 74 to 2. After some discussion about moving the conference away from its reluctant hosts, the delegates got down to business: setting standards for American medical education.

Reflecting on the conference about a half-century later, Nathan Smith Davis described the challenge confronting the conferees:

> The college degree of M. D., being almost everywhere accepted as authority to practice without other examinations, the college that offered to confer [an M.D. degree] after attendance on the shortest annual courses of instruction and the lowest college fees could generally draw the largest class. Under these conditions…the [tuition-funded] annual courses of medical college instruction were progressively shortened from six months…to sixteen weeks or less; all semblance of a requirement of suitable preliminary education was omitted; and before the middle of the century had been reached the number of medical colleges had increased from four to forty, and the annual aggregate number of medical graduates from fifteen to more than one thousand.… [Moreover, if any state acted alone to increase] the requirements of a fair standard of education or a longer annual college term with proper grading of the curriculum, and independent examinations for license to practice…student[s would] abandon her colleges for those of [other] states.[12]

To sum up, in the absence of national standards, regular medical schools were forced to compete on the price of tuition alone. In their efforts to lower the cost of education, colleges shortened their courses by eliminating such ancillary activities as clinical rounds, dissections, and laboratory work, and/or by admitting larger classes with less qualified students. The result was a viciously downward spiral, eroding educational content as more and more students paid less and less for an ever-skimpier education. Inevitably, the quality of graduates' knowledge declined. Yet, no matter how minimal an education it represented, the Medical Doctorate, M.D., or Medical Bachelors, M.B. degree gave every graduate the same right to practice as the few students who had undergone a full Edinburgh-style education. Regular medicine, as the conferees to the 1846 New York convention understood all too well, was on the brink of self-deprofessionalization.

The conferees appreciated the evident and imperative need to reprofessionalize medical education by developing uniform and rigorous standards for medical and premedical education, but they failed to agree on any specific proposal for reform.[13] In desperation, Davis turned the conference over to Dr. Isaac Hays of Philadelphia, who, as the saying goes, snatched victory from the jaws of defeat by proposing "to institute a *National Medical Association*…[to develop] a uniform and elevated standard of requirements for the degree of M. D., [that] should be adopted by all the Medical Schools…and [also standards for] a suitable preliminary Education and [a national] code of Medical Ethics."[14]

Davis's agenda had not included establishing a national medical society or a national code of medical ethics, but these were long-time ideals of Isaac Hays and his fellow Philadelphian, John Bell. Seizing the opportunity, Hays folded their plan for a national code of medical ethics into Davis's education initiative and, with this dual agenda, an organization conceived at the 1846 New York conference was born in Philadelphia, in May 1847, where it was named the "American Medical Association."

John Bell and Isaac Hays

Bell and Hays were the odd couple of Philadelphia medicine. Born around the same time (1796), they met as the sole students in a private course on the theory and practice of medicine taught in 1820 by an Edinburgh-educated William Hunter student, Nathanial Chapman, professor of medicine at the University of Pennsylvania and, at the time, Philadelphia's leading physician. Bell was an Irishman forced to flee his native land because of English repression in the wake of the Irish rebellions of 1798–1810. The City of Brotherly Love did not welcome such immigrants. Rapid industrialization and immigrant waves from the 1820s through the 1840s had unsettled the city's inhabitants who often reacted viscerally to the intrusion of alien cultural and religious traditions. Nativist, specifically anti-Irish riots—some culminating in the burning of Catholic Churches—periodically rocked the city.[15] Having already studied at the University of Pennsylvania and in Paris and other European centers, Bell likely viewed a stint with the eminent Professor Chapman as an avenue of entrée, assisting him to surmount anti-Irish chauvinism.[16]

Hays, too, confronted prejudice and probably enrolled in the course for similar reasons. He was a Sephardic Jew from a well-known merchant family whose members were treated as model minorities by their Christian friends. Yet their acceptance was always provisional, set against a background of ethnic stereotypes and bias.[17] A letter between two self-described liberal Christians discussing Hays's aunt captures the environment in which Bell and Hays functioned. Hays's aunt, the wealthy and beautiful Rebecca Graz (1781–1869), was the best-known Jewish-American woman of her era. In this letter, she was described as a "sensible and amiable woman" who, "like the few righteous persons [that] saved the city of Nineveh from destruction[18] ... save[s] her family from that scorn and contempt which we *liberal* Christians generally attach to Jews."[19]

Even though self-described "liberal" Christians of enlightened Philadelphia regarded Jewish Americans—and, one might add Irish Americans and African Americans—with "scorn and contempt," they exempted "sensible and amiable" model minority members and their families. As these model minority members appreciated all too well, however, should they cease to be "sensible and amiable," should their conduct be considered "uppity," they could lose their exempt status.[20]

So, in writing critical letters to the press, Rebecca Graz was careful to use her initial, "R," as a signature.[21] Hays, who knew his aunt well and who provided medical services for some of her charities,[22] followed this precedent. When he edited *The American Journal of the Medical Science* (1827 and still publishing),[23] Hays kept his name off the journal's masthead. Yet the journal was deemed "by far the best periodical (before us),"[24] according to the *Lancet*, and "the most important journal" of its age, according to John Shaw Billings (1838–1913), founder of the National Library of Medicine and the New York Public library system.[25] Billings chided Hays to abandon anonymity, observing that, "Dr. Isaac Hays...took charge of the Journal and gave it its present name [*The American Journal of the Medical Sciences.* It] contains many original papers of the highest value; nearly all the real criticisms and reviews which we possess.... It is evident that its editor has exercised a careful supervision over every part but his personality is nowhere apparent, there being no editorial articles, and very few papers appearing over his signature."[26] In 1841 Hays finally claimed editorship of the journal, which had gone unannounced for fourteen years. Memorial notes on Hays speak openly of his life-long struggle against anti-Semitism. "By birth a Hebrew...[Hays] through long life adhered to the ancient faith...often quoting [Alexander] Pope's lines: 'For modes of faith let graceless zealots fight: His can't be wrong whose life is in the right.'"[27]

Hays penchant for avoiding the limelight and for preferring that public attention fall on others made him an ideal companion for the loquacious Irishman, John Bell. After meeting in Chapman's course, Bell, who was broadminded for the period (entering into an interfaith marriage with Jewish-American Phoebe Israel, in 1841) found common bond with Hays. The grandiloquent Irishman and the diffident Jew became life-long friends and allies. So, in 1822, after Bell had become an initiate of the elite Kappa Lambda Society of Philadelphia, he proposed Hays for membership. Hays became a member of the Society in January 1823.[28]

The Kappa Lambda Society of Hippocrates: The AMA's Fraternity Precursor

The AMA is such an august and respectable presence on the American institutional landscape that its origins as a medical fraternity, the Kappa Lambda Society of Hippocrates, are seldom recounted—even though these origins have been well documented in the scholarly literature.[29] Kappa Lambda was a medical fraternity founded in 1819 by Dr. Samuel Brown (1769–1830), a professor at the Transylvanian University medical school in Lexington, Kentucky (1799–1857, America's fifth Edinburgh-style medical school). A fad for founding fraternities gripped American higher education around this time. The Greek letter fraternities Kappa Alpha, Sigma Phi, and Delta Phi were founded at Union College (Schenectady, New York, founded in 1795) between 1825 and 1827; the Skull and

Bones society was founded at Yale in 1832.[30] Like other fraternities of the period, the Kappa Lambda Society of Hippocrates was a secret society with secret symbols and a secret handshake. It appears to have been founded in response to drunken revels, flytes, fights, and duels among the medical students at the college, and to impart an idealistic conception of medicine. Pledges to the fraternity were inducted with a form of Hippocratic oath and swore to abide by the rules of conduct in Percival's *Medical Ethics*. Imitating the organizational pattern of medical societies, Kappa Lambda had censors, called "guardians," who were responsible for bringing students accused of violating the conduct code to trial, where they faced penalties of censure or expulsion.

In founding Kappa Lambda at his medical school, Samuel Brown had, in effect, replicated a traditional medical society in a fraternity format. Another Samuel—Samuel Jackson (1787–1872), professor of *materia medica* at the Philadelphia College of Pharmacy—was to reverse this transformation by bringing Kappa Lambda to Philadelphia as a medical society. Since that city was already well populated with medical societies, Jackson decided to recruit the founding members of the Philadelphia branch of Kappa Lambda from the practicing professionals of the American Philosophical Society. So, where Samuel Brown's version of Kappa Lambda had transformed a medical society into a student fraternity, Samuel Jackson's version of Kappa Lambda inverted this process, transubstantiating a fraternity into a medical society. Jackson thereby created a curious hybrid: a secret fraternity-like medical society, not for students, but for practicing physicians, pharmacists, and medical scientists.[31]

As in any fraternity, members of the Philadelphia branch of Kappa Lambda were required to swear an oath "to keep the secrets, guard the reputations and advance the interest of this Society" and to advance the interest of "each of its members" as fraternal brothers. This oath also committed members to such high-minded ideals as "exalt[ing] the character of the Medical Profession by a life of virtue and honour" and "never encourag[ing] any one to devote himself to the Study of Medicine whose learning, talents, and honourable qualities are not such as to render him respectable in his Profession."[32] The society's constitution required members to "support the dignity, and extension of the usefulness of the medical profession, [by] the encouragement of virtue and science.... To this end [members should] engraft medical ethics on moral precept."[33]

The Kappa Lambda Editions of Percival's *Medical Ethics*

In pursuit of this last goal, "engrafting medical ethics on moral precept," in 1821, the parent Kappa Lambda society in Lexington published a fifteen-page pamphlet, *Extracts from the Medical Ethics... by Thomas Percival, MD*,[34] distributing packets of twenty copies to the Philadelphia society and to the Kappa Lambda branches that had sprouted in Baltimore, the District of Columbia, and New York City. In 1822, a committee of Philadelphians consisting of Bell, who was then the treasurer, and the chemist-pharmacist Franklin Bache (1792–1864), was charged with reprinting 500 copies of the *Extracts from Percival's Medical Ethics*. Finding "several inaccuracies existed which it was desirable to correct [they] were... authorized to make... emendations."[35] Once begun, this "emendation" process would initiate a decade-long project of revising Percival's *Medical Ethics*—a code originally intended for British practitioners—into a code suitable for American physicians. All references to "hospital patients," for example, were changed to "patients" since American physicians attended patients in their homes, not in hospitals.

In 1823, a revised Philadelphia Kappa Lambda edition of 500 copies of the *Extracts* was published, and each Kappa Lambda member received three copies: two to be distributed to nonmembers and one for their own personal perusal.[36] A committee of three, chaired by Bell with Hays acting as secretary, was then commissioned to prepare another edition for publication in the *National Gazette and Literary Register* (a Philadelphia newspaper publishing from 1820 to 1841).[37] This committee, which met from 1823 though 1826, continued the project of Americanizing the *Extracts*. Each proposed revision was submitted to the Kappa Lambda membership for approval. On January 8, 1823, for example, the Bell-Hays committee revised the section dealing with fees. Article 18 of earlier Kappa Lambda editions of the *Extracts* had replicated a passage from Percival's *Medical Ethics* stating that clergy should be treated without charge, except for those who can "make a reasonable remuneration."[38] The committee held that the wording was the wrong way around, "clergy should be placed upon the same footing as any other class of people; that is, when able to pay the charges for medical attendance, they should be presented with their respective bills for payment, but if poor, to be treated as any others who may be poor [i.e., at no charge]." The revisions were approved.[39, 40]

On September 13, 1826, "Percival's Medical Ethics... as amended [was] adopted and considered as part of the Ethical Code of the [Philadelphia Kappa Lambda] Society."[41] As it turned out, the emended version of the *Extracts* would guide the conduct of an even larger society than the Kappa Lambda Society of Philadelphia. Over half of the text of the Code of Ethics that the AMA would adopt two decades later would be drawn, verbatim, from the 1826 version of the *Extracts*. This replication is perhaps not surprising since Bell and Hays played the same roles on the committee drafting the AMA code of ethics that they had played on the Kappa Lambda committee: Bell serving as chairperson, Hays as secretary.

Another member of the Philadelphia chapter of Kappa Lambda, Gouverneur Emerson,[42] would also serve on the AMA code-drafting committee. Emerson, a public health reformer and pioneer public health statistician, served on the

Philadelphia Board of Health during the 1820s. He also assisted Hays in providing medical care at Rebecca Graz's charities, and the two became close friends. During the Philadelphia cholera epidemic of 1832, they worked as a team to provide healthcare to the epidemic-stricken. After Emerson's death, "a note written by him on the cover of a copy of" the AMA code of ethics was discovered in which Emerson "claims that the *Code of Medical Ethics* was compiled exclusively by Dr. Isaac Hays and himself."[43] Evidence supporting Emerson's claim is offered by the order of signatures on the code-drafting committee's report: they appear in nonalphabetical order, with Emerson's following immediately after the signatures of Bell and Hays.[44] This suggests that the three people most responsible for the text of the AMA code were Bell, Hays, and Emerson.

By 1830, the Kappa Lambda society of Philadelphia had more than ninety dues-paying members. Nonetheless, Kappa Lambda's dual functions as secret fraternity and reformist medical society would soon be undone by flytes, pamphlet wars, and lawsuits between members and former members[45]; by their own reformist zeal to expel misbehaving members[46]; by the anti-Masonic fervor sweeping America; and—the *coup de grâce*—by the MSCNY's 1830–1831 public campaign against the New York branch of Kappa Lambda, in which Kappa Lambda was branded a self-serving Masonic-style secret society (see Chapter 5). The Philadelphians had a propensity for issuing publications, which is a rather public undertaking for a society that was supposedly secret. After publishing 500 copies of the *Extracts*, the Philadelphians founded a medical journal, *The North American Medical and Surgical Journal* (1826–1831). Finally, in 1826, the Philadelphia branch of Kappa Lambda petitioned the parent chapter in Lexington about "whether secrecy was still enjoined upon the members."[47]

In 1827, Philadelphia Kappa Lambda finally revoked the secrecy provision, but it was too late.[48] A tell-all book, *Illustrations of Masonry by One of the Fraternity*, by William Morgan (1774–1826?), became a bestseller on rumors of Morgan's alleged kidnapping and murder by Masons.[49] Consequently, in the 1830s, when the MSCNY publicly classified Kappa Lambda as a Masonic-style secret society, the now public Philadelphia branch of Kappa Lambda lost its cachet and its members abandoned it.[50] John Bell was among the ten remaining members of the Philadelphia Kappa Lambda who met on February 5, 1835 to dissolve the society.[51]

Although it disappeared in a cloud of opprobrium, Kappa Lambda was America's first national medical society. Even after its official demise, Kappa Lambda left behind the ideal of "unit[ing physicians] ... to be governed by ... [a common national] constitution ... directed to the support of the dignity, and extension of the usefulness of the medical profession."[52] Hays would reiterate this proposition almost a quarter of a century later, when he recommended to the failed New York convention of 1846 the formation of a national society "for the protection of [physicians'] interests, for the maintenance of their honour and respectability, for the advancement of their knowledge, and the extension of their usefulness."[53]

In proposing a common code of medical ethics for this new national medical society, Hays echoed another Kappa Lambda ideal, that "the Medical Profession in the United States should be governed by the same code of Medical Ethics."[54] Moreover, by placing Bell, other former Kappa Lambda members, and himself on the code-drafting committee, Hays ensured that the code that emerged would be based on those extracts from Percival that Bell and he had revised for the Kappa Lambda society of Philadelphia. In a sense, the successful conference that founded the AMA in May 1847 merged the failing dreams of two different sets of visionaries—Davis and March, who sought a uniform standard of medical and premedical education, and Bell, Emerson, and Hays, who envisioned a national medical society unified and regulated by a common Percivalean code of ethics.

THE AMERICAN MEDICAL ASSOCIATION'S 1847 CODE OF MEDICAL ETHICS

Crafting a Code of Medical Ethics for the AMA

Committees get little respect in the American pantheon. Ours is a culture with a penchant for individuals—for founding fathers, however mythic. So, in a mythic tale told by the AMA, Nathan Smith Davis is its founding father,[55] but, in reality, a series of committees fleshed out Hays's proposal—note, *not* Davis's proposal—to form a national medical society.[56] From May 1846 to May 1847, committees met across the country to draft a plan for the new organization and to propose national standards: standards for medical and premedical education, standards for official registers of birth and deaths, a standard "nomenclature of diseases . . . [for a] general registration of deaths," and a standard code of medical ethics for all regular medical societies.

The seven-member committee drafting the code of medical ethics was chaired by Bell. Hays served as secretary. All members save one, Vermont-born New Yorker Alonzo Clark (1807–87), were alumni of the University of Pennsylvania.[57] Three former Kappa Lambda members—Bell, Emerson, and Hays—created the code by supplementing a Kappa Lambda edition of Percival's *Medical Ethics* with material from various other codes. Bell presented the result to the AMA's 1847 founding convention, delivering an introductory speech and reading a short note from Hays. In that note, Hays indicated that the proposed code is "based on [that by] Dr. Percival," whose "phrases . . . were preserved, to a considerable extent, in all" medical society codes. So, "having no ambition for the honours of authorship, the Committee which prepared this code have followed a similar course, and have carefully preserved the words of Percival wherever they convey the precepts it is wished to inculcate."[58]

The committee thus seems to abdicate all claims of authorship, having merely followed tradition by parroting Percival's words and borrowing a few lines from Rush and some other notables. On careful reading, however, Hays's note indicates that the committee made emendations: "in all cases, wherever it was thought that the language could be made more explicit by changing a word, or even a part of a sentence, this has been unhesitatingly done; and thus there are but few sections which have not undergone some modification; while, for the language of many, and for the arrangement of the whole, the Committee must be held exclusively responsible."[59] Hays thus diplomatically represents the Americanization and updating of Percival's text as, "making" Percival's thought "more explicit," thereby disguising innovation as editing. (The text of Hays's note, Bell's Introduction, and the 1847 Code of Ethics are in Appendices IV, V, and VI.)

The 1847 AMA Code of Ethics as a Social Contract

Hays credits the code-drafting committee with "the arrangement of the whole." This overly modest characterization disguises a fundamental transformation: the reformulation of Percival's code of ethics as a formal social contract. This structure is laid bare in the code's table of contents, viz.:

CODE OF MEDICAL ETHICS

CHAPTER III. Of the duties of the profession to the public, and of the obligations of the public to the profession.
article I. Of the duties of the profession to the public.
article II. Of the obligations of the public to the physicians.

Res ipsa loquitur—the table of contents outlines a tripartite social contract: each chapter a different set of reciprocal duties and obligations: chapter I states the duties and obligations of physicians and patients to each other; chapter II states the duties of physicians and the profession at large to each other, and chapter III the duties and obligations of the profession and the public to each other. A close reading of the language of the code and its table of contents reveals that, whereas patients are said to have "obligations," physicians are characterized as having "duties." To appreciate the "obligation/duty" distinction it is helpful to turn to the Webster dictionaries.[60] A legacy of Noah Webster's (1758–1843) postcolonial nationalist pride, these dictionaries record *American*, in contrast to British, usage and spelling.[61] According to the 1828 edition of Webster's dictionary, the term "obligation" can refer to the "binding force of civility, kindness or gratitude, when the performance of a duty cannot be enforced by law. Favors conferred impose on men an obligation to make suitable returns." A *duty*, in contrast, is "[t]hat which a person owes to another; that which a person is bound, by any natural, moral or legal obligation, to pay, do or perform." Understood in the latter sense, the code of ethics stipulates duties that physicians were bound to perform by virtue of their role and the obligations that patients and society incur by virtue of "the binding force of civility... or gratitude," which require them "to make suitable returns," to physicians individually and collectively.

Lest these linguistic nuances seem overly subtle, Bell spelled them out in his speech introducing the code of ethics to the 1847 convention. After first characterizing "[m]edical ethics, as a branch of general ethics... rest[ing] on the basis of religion and morality," Bell observed that medical ethics "comprise[s] not only the duties, but, also, the rights of a physician."[62] Bell then observes that

> Every duty or obligation implies, both in equity and for its successful discharge, a corresponding right. As it is the duty of a physician to advise, so has he a right to be attentively and respectfully listened to. Being required to expose his health and life for the benefit of the community, he has a just claim, in return, on all its members, collectively and individually, for aid to carry out his measures.[63]

The AMA's *Code of Medical Ethics* is thus a statement of physicians' duties *and* of the reciprocal obligations that the community, "collectively and individually," owes to its physicians. Bell stipulates further that "Medical ethics cannot be so divided as that one part shall obtain the full and proper force of moral obligations on physicians universally, and, at the same time, the other be construed in such a way as to free society from all restrictions in its conduct to them."[64] Patients and the public were thus under an obligation to their physicians and to the profession at large.

Because patients might be surprised to learn that in visiting a physician they are obligated to do more than pay for services rendered, Bell explains by drawing on the distinction made in nineteenth-century discourse between a *duty* and an *obligation*:

> In thus deducing the rights of a physician from his duties, it is not meant to insist on such a correlative obligation, that the withholding of the right exonerates from the discharge of the duty... [N]o medical man can withhold his services from the requisition either of an individual or of the community.... In the discharge of their duties to Society, physicians must be ever ready and prompt to administer professional aid to all applicants, without prior stipulation of personal advantages to themselves.[65]

Physicians, therefore, are duty-bound to serve the community and individual patients and, in doing so, they thereby obligate individual patients and society collectively to reciprocate with respect and support. However, just as physicians are duty bound to provide urgent care even to ungrateful patients, so too they are duty bound to serve even unappreciative communities that renege on their obligations to the profession.

The Physician–Patient Contract

The first line of article I of this physician–profession–patient–public contract guarantees that physicians will be "ever ready" to "obey the calls of the sick." This unequivocal statement of the physician's duty to *obey* the calls of the sick is characteristically American. No such duty is mentioned in Percival's writings. One might speculate that the duty to obey the patient's call traces to America's origins as a frontier society with a Calvinist heritage. In fact, the earliest known American formulation of a duty to obey the calls of the sick are found in colonial -era documents, the New York Midwives' Oath of 1716[66] and the *Instruments of Association* of the New Jersey Medical Society of 1766.[67] A more general statement of obligation to obey the calls of the sick was issued in the postcolonial era by the MSSNY in its *System of Ethics* of 1823.[68] These themes are reiterated in the Baltimore *System of Ethics* of 1832,[69] and, to reiterate, the duty to obey the calls of the sick is the first physicians' duty stated in the 1847 AMA code of ethics.

The doctor's duty to obey the calls of the sick was deleted from the AMA code in the twentieth century, and American medical practitioners today no longer consider themselves duty bound to answer urgent or emergency calls by visiting the sick in their homes or by rushing to the scene of an accident. To fully appreciate the value of the right accorded to patients by the 1847 AMA *Code of Medical Ethics* (and, prior to that, by the codes of the Baltimore, New Jersey, and New York medical societies and by midwives' oaths), one has to envision a medical era without ambulances or emergency departments,[70] in which no person of means would use a hospital, since, to quote Thomas Jefferson (1743–1826), "it is poverty alone which peoples hospitals."[71] In this era, urgent and emergency medical care were provided by midwives and physicians responding to "calls" to attend to people in their homes or at the scene of an accident. The oaths and codes of that era guaranteed that *anyone* issuing such a call, irrespective of socioeconomic status, would be attended to "with promptitude."[72]

As in earlier statements of traditional American medical ethics, the AMA *Code of Medical Ethics* reaffirms the physician's duty of providing medical care to poor and rich alike, and it stipulates that this duty remains in force even "when pestilence walketh in darkness." Thus, article I, chapter III of the 1847 AMA code restates the physician's "duty to face the danger" during times of pestilence "and to continue their labors for the alleviation of the suffering, even at the jeopardy of their own lives." As to "poverty," the code stipulates that it "should always be recognized as presenting valid claims for gratuitous services." Moreover, echoing the language of the 1766 New Jersey *Instruments*, it states that professional services to "individuals in indigent circumstances... should always be cheerfully and freely accorded."[73]

Validating and reinforcing the imperative nature of these duties are appeals to ideals of character. Appropriating a line from John Gregory (referenced in the New York *System of Ethics*),[74] the AMA *Code of Medical Ethics* emphasizes that obedience to the calls of the sick is a matter of moral character because "no other tribunal" sits in judgment of the physician's performance in discharging this duty, viz.: "A physician should not only be ever ready to obey the calls of the sick, but his mind ought also to be imbued with the greatness of his mission, and of the responsibility he habitually incurs in its discharge. Those obligations are the more deep and enduring, because there is no tribunal other than his own conscience, to adjudge penalties for carelessness or neglect." Today, of course, the claim that "there is no other tribunal but [the physician's] own conscience to adjudge penalties for carelessness or neglect" no longer rings true. American physicians are held accountable in a variety of ways, ranging from quality assurance mechanisms to malpractice suits; however, neither quality assurance[75] nor malpractice suits were issues in the medical world of the 1840. As one historian observed, "malpractice suits were virtually nonexistent... between 1790 and 1840. [Although] the United

States population grew 334 percent, from 3,929,214 to 17,069,453, during this period, the number of appellate malpractice decisions remained almost constant: 7 decisions were scattered over fifty years."[76] When the AMA *Code of Medical Ethics* was written, there actually was "no tribunal other than [the physician's] own conscience, to adjudge penalties for carelessness or neglect" in responding to the urgent and emergency calls for medical care.

Hays and his colleagues were responding within the context of American medicine during the 1840s. With characteristic diffidence, however, Hays's note to the convention understates the committee's role in shaping the *Code of Medical Ethics*, seemingly attributing primary authorship to Percival. Yet the committee did not simply parrot Percival, as Hays's note seems to imply. From the very first passage in the code (chapter I, article I, section 1), Percival's words had been edited and Americanized. The following extract shows this first section of the code with the text from Percival's *Medical Ethics* in plain script, deletions represented by crossed out words and additions italicized.

> ~~A Hospital~~ [P]hysician~~s and surgeons~~ should *not only be ever ready to obey the calls of the sick, but his mind ought also to be imbued with the greatness of his mission, and of the responsibility he habitually incurs in its discharge. Those obligations are the more deep and enduring, because there is no tribunal other than his own conscience, to adjudge penalties for carelessness or neglect.* Physicians should, *therefore*, minister to the sick with due impressions of the importance of their office; reflecting that the ease, the health, and the lives of those committed to their charge, depend on their skill, attention and fidelity. They should study, also, in their deportment, so to unite tenderness with firmness, and condescension with authority, as to inspire the minds of their patients with gratitude, respect and confidence.[77]

As the italicized words indicate, the editors added substantially to the text. Of the 131 words in this paragraph, about half, sixty-nine, are drawn from Percival, and even these had been Americanized. Thus, the word "hospital" was deleted because American physicians usually treated the sick in their homes. "Surgeon" was deleted as redundant in American usage[78] because, in contrast to nineteenth-century British usage, in nineteenth-century American usage the term "physician" was used broadly to encompass surgeons.[79]

The retention of some of Percival's original wording has led to a common misreading of this text by later commentators. In discussing physicians' "deportment" toward patients, article I requires physicians to "unite tenderness with firmness" and to combine "condescension with authority." This advice is easily misread today because, as current editions of Webster's dictionaries indicate, today the term "condescension" means "patronizing"—and in egalitarian America, no one believes that physicians should patronize their patients. In the status-oriented world of the nineteenth century, as the 1828 edition of Webster's explains, "condescension" is the opposite of patronizing.

> CONDESCENSION, n. Voluntary descent from rank, dignity or just claims; relinquishment of strict right; submission to inferiors in granting requests or performing acts which strict justice does not require. Hence, courtesy. It forbids pride and commands humility, modesty and [requires] behavior, as are suitable to a superior.

Thus, in nineteenth-century American usage, to condescend to one's patients was not to look down on them but just the opposite: to relinquish prerogatives of status, to refuse to patronize, and to treat one's patients as courteously as one would treat one's superiors.

The AMA code accorded patients the right not to be patronized and as article I, section 1 continues, in "every case" to be treated "with attention, steadiness and humanity." The code also recognizes patients' rights to confidentiality (section 2) and not to be overcharged for unnecessary visits (section 3). Physicians, moreover, were forbidden to magnify the importance of their services by making "gloomy prognostications" and then taking credit for the patient's recovery (section 4). Breaking with Bard and Rush's emphasis on directly communicating a terminal prognosis to patients themselves (discussed in Chapter 4), section 4 reiterates Gregory and Percival's position that patients must be buffered against the emotional impact of a terminal prognosis. This prognosis "is so peculiarly alarming when executed by [a physician], that it ought to be declined whenever it can be assigned to any other person of sufficient judgment and delicacy." So, physicians are to play the role of "minister[s] of hope and comfort to the sick [bringing] cordials to the drooping spirit... smooth[ing] the bed of death... and counteract[ing] the depressing influence of those maladies which often disturb the tranquility of the most resigned, in their last moment." The next section prohibits physicians from abandoning their patients (section 5) and requires them to seek consultation in difficult cases (section 6). The final section (section 7) is frankly paternalistic, obligating physicians to offer moral counseling to their patients, motivated by a love of virtue and a "sincere interest in the [sick person's] welfare."

In return for these commitments, article II stipulates patients' reciprocal obligations toward their physicians: "The members of the medical profession, upon whom are enjoined the performance of so many important and arduous duties... certainly have a right to expect and require, that their patients should entertain a just sense of the duties which they owe to their medical attendants."[80] What follows in the rest of article II is an edited version of the section of the Baltimore *System of Ethics* on the patient's duties toward physicians. The Baltimore

System had simply replicated, verbatim, parts of Rush's 1808 lecture, "On the Duties of Patients to Their Physician."[81] Bell, Hays, and Emerson pruned the text substantially, as this sample from section 2 indicates (plain text is replicated verbatim from the Baltimore *System*; italics indicates additions; struck-through text indicates deletions):

> The first duty of a patient is, to select ~~no person~~ as his medical adviser *one* who has ~~not~~ received a regular professional education. In no trade or occupation do mankind rely on the skill of a*n* ~~self~~ untaught artist; ~~while~~ *and* in medicine, confessedly the most difficult and intricate of the sciences, *the world* ~~appears to think~~ *ought not to suppose* that knowledge ~~may be~~ *is* intuitive. ~~That astonishing cures have been performed by quacks, is readily admitted, but these have always been accidental, and the disastrous consequences of their blind ignorance and rash presumption, although carefully concealed from the public eye, far outnumber the records of their success~~.

Turning from text to context, it is important to note that, as in Rush's text, patients' obligations to their physicians often reciprocate physicians' duties toward patients. Thus, patients are obliged to "faithfully and unreservedly communicate to their physician the supposed cause of their disease . . . [because—note the reciprocity] a medical man is under the strongest obligations of secrecy" (section 4).[82] Moreover, just as a physician is duty bound to "obey" a patient's calls promptly, so too, "[t]he obedience of a patient to the prescriptions of his physician should [also] be prompt and implicit."[83] The tenth and final obligation is also reciprocal: just as a physician is bound to serve the patient irrespective of financial rewards or—to use an expression preferred by Percival and echoed in the AMA code, irrespective of "pecuniary acknowledgements"[84]—so, too, the patient should "entertain a just and enduring sense of the value of the services rendered him by his physician; for these are of such a character, that no mere Pecuniary acknowledgement can repay or cancel them."[85]

The Intraprofessional Contract

Intraprofessional conflict and its resolution is a primary focus of all nineteenth-century Anglo-American codes of medical police and medical ethics. The AMA *Code of Medical Ethics* is unexceptional in this regard. At 2,854 words, chapter two "The Duties of Physicians to Each Other and to the Profession at Large," constitutes over half the words in the AMA code, dwarfing all other chapters. It opens with a justification of physicians' duties "to each other" and to "the profession at large." The distinction between duties "to each other" and to "the profession at large" is important. The AMA code distinguishes between physicians as a collection of individuals owing duties "to each other" and physicians as corporate body, "the profession at large," empowered by this group of individuals to enact "laws for the government of its members." Individual physicians may have duties to this corporate body, "the profession at large," in the same way that they have duties to their patients. The concept of a profession thus becomes transformed, reified, to refer to a corporate entity. This transformation, and the notion that members have obligations to the profession at large, is justified in article I, "Duties for the support of professional character."

> article I. *Duties for the support of professional character* 1. Every individual, on entering the profession, as he becomes thereby entitled to all its privileges and immunities, incurs an obligation... he should therefore observe strictly, such laws as are instituted for, the government of its members.

By virtue of this claim, because individual physicians inherit a set of "privileges and immunities" by entering a profession, they incur five reciprocal obligations: to maintain the profession's dignity, to uphold its honor, to exalt its standing, to extend its usefulness, and to hold themselves to a higher standard of "moral excellence" than is required of ordinary people. Article II states that physicians are duty bound to respect senior physicians (section 1), to practice soberly (section 2), to eschew advertising (section 3), to abstain from holding patents, and to refuse to prescribe secret nostrums or provide certificates of their efficacy (section 4).

After a discussion of physicians' obligations to each other (article II), which, it should be reemphasized, is here distinguished from a physicians' duties to the corporate body known as the profession at large, the code moves to physicians' duties in substituting for each other (article III). It then turns to one of the central issues preoccupying all nineteenth-century codes of medical ethics and medical police: Consults and Interferences. In conjunction with article VI, "On difference between Physicians," these twenty-one sections distill a half-century of American medical society experience in dealing with intrapractitioner disputes. Consults are to be exclusively held with regular physicians (article IV, section 1), they are to be attended punctually (section 5) and conducted in confidence (section 7) with "candor, probity and due respect" between physicians (section 2)—especially with respect to the attending physician (sections 3, 4, and 10).

Article V, "Interference," deals with tricky situations like that of the wrongdoing Dr. W. (discussed in Chapter 5), in which a physician provides care for a patient who another physician considers "his." After reminding physicians (section 1) that theirs is a "liberal profession" based on "qualifications, not on intrigue or artifice" and warning them not to "meddle" with other practitioners' patients (sections 2, 3), the code states forthrightly that, "[a] physician ought not to take charge of or prescribe for a patient who has recently been under the care of another member of the faculty in the same illness, except in cases of sudden emergency, or in consultation with the physician previously in attendance, or when the latter has relinquished the case or been regularly notified that his services are no longer desired" (sections 4 and 5). Special cases are then discussed: for example, how to behave when "a number of physicians are simultaneously sent for" (section 6). Finally, article VI stipulates that when physicians' differences seem irreconcilable they "should be referred to the arbitration of…a *court-medical,*" that is, a private version of the *comita minora*. The findings of such a court-medical should be considered confidential; that is, "the adjudication of the arbitrators should [not] be made public" since "publicity in a case of this nature may be personally injurious to the individuals concerned, and can hardly fail to bring discredit on the faculty."

The Professional–Public Contract

In the final provisions of the AMA's 1847 *Code of Ethics*, chapter III, the section specifying the reciprocal "Duties of the Profession to the Public, and…the Obligations of the Public to the Profession" are some of the most demanding and wistful sections of the social contract. Originating from the minds and pens of Bell, Emerson, and Hays, this section stipulates the duties of the corporate body designated as "The Profession" and the reciprocal obligations of the corporate body designated as "The Public." Article I states that "as good citizens," physicians have a "duty to be ever vigilant for the welfare of the community and to bear their part in sustaining its institutions and burdens." In addition, in parallel with their duty to be ready to serve the individual patient, physicians have a role-specific professional duty of "be[ing] ever ready to give counsel to the public in relation to matters especially appertaining to their profession, as on subjects of medical police, public hygiene, and legal medicine." Physicians also have a duty to offer advice "in regard to measures for the prevention of epidemic and contagious diseases" and in epidemics like cholera and yellow fever (with which Emerson had extensive experience as a member of the Philadelphia Board of Health and as a pioneering public health statistician and reformer). Moreover, "when pestilence prevails [they must] face the danger, and…continue their labors for the alleviation of the suffering, even at the jeopardy of their own lives"—as Emerson and Hays had done during the cholera epidemics of the 1830s. [86]

Article I, section 3 turns to "eleemosynary" (i.e., charitable) services.[87] Here, another line is drawn since "justice requires that some limits should be placed to the performance of such good offices"; more specifically, although physicians have a professional duty to provide eleemosynary services "to *individuals* in indigent circumstances,"[88] to whom, the section reiterates, "professional services should always be cheerfully and freely accorded," they have no such duty to provide unpaid services to institutions or organizations, such as hospitals and insurance companies. The profession, however, is duty bound to protect the public against "the injury to health and even destruction of life caused by the use of quack medicines" by enlightening it as to the perfidious nature of quack remedies and lobbying against their manufacture and sale.

The "Obligations of the Public to Physicians" are stipulated in article II, which opens with a reminder that "[t]he benefits accruing to the public . . . from the active and unwearied beneficence of the profession, are numerous and important." Therefore, since individual patients should "entertain a just and enduring sense of the value of the services rendered," the public, too, owes physicians "the utmost consideration and respect" and (1) "ought . . . to entertain a just appreciation of medical qualifications" (by restoring the profession's control over licensure); (2) ought to "support . . . medical education" by legalizing the dissection of cadavers, which "the statute books [prohibit], under liability to heavy penalties"; and (3) make "a proper discrimination between true science and the assumption of ignorance and empiricism" (i.e., by distinguishing between science-based medicine practiced by regular physicians and the unscientific medicine of homeopaths, Thomsonians, and the like).

Legalizing Dissection

The meaning of chapter III, article II, section 1 is a cipher; a cryptic message dancing around a subject that can only be referenced obliquely. Here is the text:

> The benefits accruing to the public . . . from the active and unwearied beneficence of the profession, are so . . . important, that physicians are justly entitled to . . . every . . . facility for the acquisition of medical education—and [the public should] no longer allow the statute books to exhibit the anomaly of exacting knowledge from physicians, under liability to heavy penalties, and of making them obnoxious to punishment for resorting to the only means of obtaining it.

Some of the wording of the text is drawn from a famous editorial by Thomas Wakely (1795–1862), founding editor of *The Lancet* (founded in 1823 and still publishing) in which he states bluntly, "If dead bodies can not be procured, it will be impossible for the pupils to learn anatomy, and without anatomy neither surgeons nor physicians can practice with the least prospect of benefitting their patients."[89]

Wakely's editorial in the *Lancet* of January 1824 continues:

> If a surgeon commits an error in the practice of his profession from a deficient knowledge of anatomy . . . it is perfectly right to visit such gross ignorance with punishment; but . . . [it is a] ridiculous *anomaly of first making*

> *laws to punish medical practitioners if they do not possess a knowledge of their profession, and subsequently passing other laws which deprive them of the only source from whence it is possible that knowledge can be obtained.*[90]

Bell, Emerson, and Hays echoed the italicized section of the text when they wrote "the anomaly of exacting knowledge from physicians, under liability to heavy penalties, and of making them obnoxious to punishment for resorting to the only means of obtaining it."

Wakely states the case plainly enough, so why couldn't Bell, Emerson, and Hays be as blunt? The answer is that they are alluding to something extremely controversial. As the English physician Thomas Southwood Smith (1788–1861), a Unitarian minister and a friend and disciple of the utilitarian philosopher Jeremy Bentham (1748–1832) argued, "the basis of all medical and surgical knowledge is anatomy," but "obstacles... at present oppose the acquisition of [anatomical] knowledge."[91] Since "anatomy ought to form an essential part of medical education, [and since] anatomy cannot be studied without the practice of dissection; [and since] dissection cannot be practiced without a supply of subjects, [and since] the manner in which that supply is obtained in England is detestable" (i.e., grave robbing and body snatching—see Chapter 3), it "ought immediately [to] be changed." [92]

Smith proposed an anatomy act that addressed what he took to be the morally disruptive element in the use of human anatomical dissection for purposes of medical education—"exhumation," or, to a use the less euphemistic common name for this morally disruptive element "grave robbing."[93] As Smith put the point:

> Much of the opposition on the part of people, arises from the present mode of procuring subjects [i.e., body snatching before burial, grave robbing after burial]. Fortunately, there is... no custom, no superstition, no law, and we may add, no prejudice against anatomy itself... [although] there may be a feeling that it is a repulsive employment, but it is commonly acknowledged that it must not be neglected. The opposition which is made, is made not against anatomy, but against the practice of exhumation: and this is a practice which ought to be opposed. It is in the highest degree revolting; it would be disgraceful to a horde of savages; every feeling of the human heart rises up against it; [however] so long as no other means of procuring bodies for dissection are provided, it must be tolerated; but, in itself, it is alike odious to the ignorant and the enlightened, to the uncultivated and the most refined.[94]

Having identified the morally disruptive element, Smith urged reform. Bringing his argument home to American readers, Smith cites cases from Connecticut and New York State, which, like most American jurisdictions, had laws making it a felony to dig up or remove a dead human body with the intent to dissect it. In New York, a medical student found guilty of grave robbing was sentenced to six months imprisonment. At his sentencing, the court warned "the young gentlemen attending the medical school of this city [to] take warning from this man's fate . . . that justice will be executed on any man, whatever may be his condition in life, who is found violating the law and the decency of Christian burial."[95] In the Connecticut case, two ladies taking a walk found that the body of a young woman had been hauled out of her grave by a rope around her neck. Smith notes, "The circumstances produced a great excitement in the public mind [and] *the citizens turned out in a body . . . and interred the corpse again.*"[96]

Smith joined with the judge and the citizens in condemning these incidents as disgraceful. He did not "blame the Americans for abolishing the practice of exhumation; but [he] blame[s] them for stopping there." Employing language similar to Wakely's and that of the authors of the AMA code, Smith maintained "that it is absurd and criminal, to make this practice [a] felony without providing . . . some other method for the cultivation of anatomy."[97] Worse yet,

> unless some other means for affording a supply [of cadavers for dissection] be adopted; whatever the law or the popular feeling [nothing] can or will put a stop to the practice [of grave robbing]. . . . What is the consequence? So long as the practice of exhumation continues, a race of men must be trained up to violate the law. These men go out in company for the purpose of nightly plunder, and plunder of the most odious kind, tending in a peculiar and most alarming measure to brutify the mind and to eradicate every feeling and sentiment worthy of a man. . . . It is an odious thing that the teachers of anatomy should be brought in contact with such men: that they should be obliged to employ them.[98]

To remedy the situation, Smith proposed legalizing medical schools' right to procure, for purpose of dissection, "the bodies of all persons dying . . . *unclaimable by their immediate relatives, or whose relatives decline to pay the expenses of interment* [to be used for medical education and after dissection to be] placed in a coffin . . . and decently buried."[99] Thus, bodies that might otherwise be abandoned or dumped in a potter's field would be given a decent burial, no family that claimed a body for burial would be deprived of their right to the body, and, since a legitimate supply of cadavers would be available for medical education, the market for illegally obtained cadavers would vanish, as would financial incentives for grave robbing—so graveyards would be undisturbed.[100]

A philosophically sophisticated minister and physician, Smith combines, in one person, the elements that would later constitute bioethics: expertise in medicine, moral philosophy, and religious ethics. His diagnosis of moral disruption was astute. After the enactment of Smith-style anatomy acts in Massachusetts in 1831 and Britain in 1832,[101] the morally disruptive act of grave robbing ceased to be a major social problem in those jurisdictions—as it did in all jurisdictions that enacted Smith-style anatomy acts.[102] Yet, in 1846–1847, when the AMA *Code of Medical Ethics* was being drafted, Massachusetts was the only state in the union to have enacted a Smith-style anatomy act. Attempts to pass such acts in Maine, New York, Ohio, Pennsylvania, and Vermont had repeatedly met with failure. Connecticut and New Hampshire had enacted such acts, but their anatomy acts had been repealed by 1847.[103] In 1847, no legal supply of cadavers was available in any state other than Massachusetts, and so the cadavers dissected in every anatomy course taught in every state in the United States, save Massachusetts, were supplied illegally, by grave robbers or bodysnatchers. Thus, in the cryptic lines in the code that they drafted for the AMA, Bell, Emerson, and Hays were claiming that the public in every state in the union owed the medical profession the enactment of a Massachusetts-Smith-style anatomy act.

DISTINGUISHING TRUE SCIENCE FROM EMPIRICISM: THE CONSULTATION CLAUSE

Article IV, section I of chapter II, which came to be known as the "consultation clause," restricts consultation and membership in the AMA to regular practitioners, stipulating that "[n]o one can be considered as a regular practitioner...whose practice is based on an exclusive dogma, to the rejection of the accumulated experience of the profession, and of the aids actually furnished by anatomy, physiology, pathology, and organic chemistry." Such clauses were a standard feature of American codes of medical police and systems of medical ethics, oaths, and bylaws—including those of homeopathic and Thomsonian societies. The AMA version differs from its precursors in specifically mentioning the basic medical sciences and invoking the notion of an "exclusive dogma." By contrast, the comparable section of the 1832 Baltimore *System of Medical Ethics* reads, "no consultation should be held with any individual...who is not in possession of a diploma from some medical college or university.... Consultations should, under no pretext, be held with unqualified persons."[104] By the mid-1830s, however, the Baltimore wording had been obsolesced by the willingness of state legislatures to recognize the legitimacy of alternative medical colleges. Pennsylvania had incorporated a homeopathic college in 1836, and Ohio had chartered a botanical college in 1839. Moreover, a national homeopathic organization, the American Institute of Homeopathy, was founded at national homeopathic conventions in New York City in 1843 and 1844. Since irregulars could now earn medical diplomas—and since some degree-holding regulars were now prescribing homeopathic treatments—new criteria were needed to exclude botanicals (i.e., Thomsonians and eclectics) and homeopaths from the AMA.

In 1842, the Philadelphia County Medical Society, to which Hays belonged, simply prohibited its members from "practicing or sanctioning any system of quackery or imposture, including what is known as homeopathia."[105] Significantly, the authors of the AMA did not adopt a similar clause (i.e., one that excluded eclectics, homeopaths, or Thomsonians by directly branding them "quacks" and "imposters"). Instead, they crafted a complex exclusionary clause in which irregulars were characterized as practitioners who subscribe to an "exclusive dogma" that "reject[s]...the accumulated experience of the profession, and...the aids actually furnished by anatomy, physiology, pathology, and organic chemistry." By the 1870s, this clause—and this word choice—would become a focal point of discontent within the AMA that would culminate in a secession crisis. Not surprisingly, the consultation clause is the subject of extensive commentary, and no review of the 1847 AMA code would be complete without an analysis of it.

Some commentators view the consultation clause as a mechanism for monopolizing the medical marketplace.[106] This reading is plausible if one thinks of the AMA as the behemoth it became in the twentieth century. By the 1840s, however, Thomsonian antimonopoly campaigns had deprived regular medical societies of the licensing authority they once enjoyed, and legislatures were increasingly willing to charter botanical, eclectic, and homeopathic colleges. Moreover, had regulars sought to monopolize the medical marketplace, their best strategy would have been to follow the model set by John D. Rockefeller's Standard Oil (formed in 1870; it was split into thirty-one companies by the Sherman Antitrust act in 1911) and other nineteenth-century monopolies: amalgamate, co-opt, and absorb the competition. Yet the consultation clause was designed to do just the opposite, to prevent the incorporation of alternative practitioners into the AMA; it could be characterized as an antimonopolization measure. As a leading scholar observed, "the consultation clause was not expected to seal the lid on the coffin of homeopathy. Rather, it was to prevent the orthodox profession from giving 'support' to the homeopathic 'quacks.'"[107] It was a purity clause.

Commentators exploring the interplay between heterodoxy and orthodoxy offer more plausible analyses of the consultation clause as an avowal of faith in science that evolved into a test of orthodoxy. The clause would serve as a loyalty oath enabling regular practitioners to close ranks in the face of competition from popular but heterodox forms of medicine. Such avowals of faith in science, sociologist Paul Wolpe observes, have "been traditionally used by the American medical profession as a wedge (and sometimes a club) to denigrate, exclude, or deny the efficacy of alternative models of healing."[108] The threat of homeopathy, comments historian John Harley Warner, "transform[ed] regulars' confidence in their heritage into a dogmatic ideology of orthodoxy, and this strengthening impulse to orthodoxy [led] regular physicians...to set themselves apart from heterodox healers and to purify their own ranks."[109]

The Warner-Wolpe stigma-purity analysis of the consultation clause is insightful for the period 1870–1910, when homeopaths were treated as if they were irredeemable sinners rather than subscribers to an alternative but erroneous medical theory. By this time, English-language translations of the homeopathic literature had become widely available to non–German-speaking regulars who could and would defect to homeopathy in significant numbers. By 1900, the U.S. population had grown to 76 million people served by 123,553 physicians, of which 9,664 physicians admitted to practicing homeopathy—approximately one in every thirteen practitioners (8 percent).[110] Homeopathy had become a temptation and a threat by the 1870s, and the AMA reacted by rejecting anyone who succumbed to its wiles or who contaminated himself by association with it.

In 1846–1847 when the text of the AMA code of ethics was being drafted, however, homeopathy was a faltering movement. The homeopathic literature and language of instruction was still primarily in German, the first homeopathic college in America had closed its doors in 1842,[111] and the American Institute of Homeopathy (AIH) represented only a handful of American physicians, mostly of German background. According to the 1850 census, only about 600 of the 40,000 physicians serving an American population of 23.5 million practiced homeopathy—fewer than 1.5 percent of physicians. When the code was drafted, homeopathy was neither a temptation nor a threat to the AMA, so the motive for the exclusionary consultation clause is neither stigma nor purity; it is more plausibly a rejection of a pseudoscience.

The Scientific Status of Homeopathy in 1846–1847

As Warner suggests, "the debate over the [consultation clause in the] Code of Ethics cannot be fully comprehended without recognizing it as part of a large debate over newly emerging ideals of science and the place that science should occupy in a rapidly changing medical world."[112] Wolpe agrees but contends that:

> [H]omeopaths [were] no less scientific than regulars by the standards of the nineteenth century... [with] their own scientific methodology, a system they called "proving," whereby they took scrupulous notes of all symptoms and remedies... [which] were used as empirical justifications of homeopathic validity.... Homeopathy was not a pseudoscience of the nineteenth century; it was a science of the nineteenth century.[113]

Wolpe here voices an important assumption underlying both the monopolization and purity interpretations of the consultation clause: that in 1847 the authors of the AMA code should have regarded homeopathy as legitimately "a science of the nineteenth century" and that in writing homeopathy off as a pseudoscience the authors of the clause were acting for some ulterior motive, such as monopolization or purification. To assess this assumption, it is helpful review the character of medical science and the dominant philosophy of science in the 1840s and to reappraise the reasons offered in the medical literature of that period for treating homeopathy as pseudoscientific or "popular delusion," rather than accepting it as a legitimate science of the nineteenth century.

The leading philosophy of science text in the English-speaking world in the 1840s was written by Cambridge don William Whewell (1794–1866),[114] who actively collaborated with working scientists like Michal Faraday (1791–1867), the discoverer of electro-magnetic induction, for whom Whewell invented such terms as "anode," "cathode," and "ion." Whewell also coined the very words "physicist" and "scientist" that we still use today, believing that the older expression, "natural philosopher," misrepresented the experimental nature of the sciences. Most importantly for our purposes, Whewell based his analysis of scientific methodology on a careful study of the practices of successful scientists in his own era and in the past.

Recognizing that science, much like philosophy, begins with conjecture and imagination,[115] Whewell differentiates between these fields by observing that, unlike philosophers, successful scientists turn their conjectures into hypotheses whose truths can be assessed through experimentation:

> The framing of hypotheses is, for the enquirer after truth, not the end, but the beginning of his work. Each of his systems is invented, not that he may admire it and follow it into all its consistent consequences, but that he may make it the occasion of a course of active experiment and observation. And if the results of this process contradict his fundamental assumptions, however ingenious, however symmetrical, however elegant his system may be, he rejects it without hesitation.[116]

Mere empirical data and simple experience, moreover, is *not* a suitable basis for true science. "In order that the facts obtained by observation and experiment may be capable of being used in furtherance of our exact and solid knowledge, they must," Whewell contended, "be apprehended . . . according to some Conceptions which . . . give distinct and definite results, such as can be steadily taken hold of and reasoned from."[117] Thus, for empirical data to confirm or disconfirm a hypothesis it must yield results that are "distinct," "definite," and "steady" (i.e., replicable). Whewell also found that hypotheses are most likely to be accepted as valid science if they predict phenomena *beyond* those they were invented to explain. As he put it, valid hypotheses "ought to explain phenomena which we have observed. But they ought to [also] . . . foretell phenomena which have not yet been observed."[118]

Finally, Whewell found that "the best established theor[ies] that the history of science contains" predict or explain "classes of facts altogether different" from those that "the hypothesis was originally intended to explain." He called this sort of interlocking confirmation of causal explanation "consilience."[119] Whewell's claims about the nature of valid scientific practice were recognized by leading Anglo-American scientists of the day, including his student and mentee, Charles Darwin, who prefaced *Origin of Species* with a quotation from Whewell.[120]

In the mid-nineteenth century, France, and especially Paris, was the center of medical science. John Bell had studied there; so, too, had the authors of the two major English-language critiques of homeopathy published prior to 1847, John Forbes (1787–1861) and Oliver Wendell Holmes Sr. (1809–1894). Forbes and Holmes built their careers around the dissemination of French medical science into English-speaking medicine. Like Bell, Forbes was editor of a journal dedicated to bringing the latest in European medicine into the English-speaking cultural sphere, the *British and Foreign Medical Review* (1836–1847). Forbes's 1821 translation into English of Parisian physician, René Théophile Hyacinthe Laënnec's (1781–1826) classical 1819 work, *A Treatise on the Diseases of the Chest and on Mediate Auscultation*[121]—the book that introduced the stethoscope to medicine—was the turning point of Forbes's career. An Edinburgh medical college alumnus, Forbes would eventually rise to the top of his profession, becoming physician to Queen Victoria and Prince Albert of Britain.

Coincidently, Holmes also wrote about the stethoscope in an essay that won him Harvard Medical School's coveted Boylston Prize in 1837. From 1833 to 1835, Holmes studied in Paris with Pierre Charles Alexandre Louis (1787–1872). He was in Paris during the period when Louis was developing "the numerical method" for evaluating alternative therapies. Here is Louis's description:

> [I]n any particular epidemic, let us suppose five hundred of the sick, taken indiscriminately, are subjected to one kind of treatment, and five hundred others, taken in the same manner, are treated in a different mode; if the mortality is greater among the first than among the second, must we not conclude that the treatment was less appropriate, or less efficacious in the first class than in the second? It is unavoidable; for among so large a collection, similarities of conditions will necessarily be met with, and all things being equal, the conclusion will be rigorous.[122]

In the 1830s, Louis applied this method to assess the efficacy of a common treatment for pneumonia—bloodletting. Retrospectively reviewing the records of seventy-seven previously healthy patients admitted with pneumonia, Louis found that whereas 44 percent (18/41) of patients bled within the first four days died, only 25 percent (9/36) of those bled at a later date died. These data indicate that bloodletting impeded rather than facilitated recovery from pneumonia; that is, that the form of treatment preferred by regular physicians in the treatment of pneumonia was ineffective or deleterious.[123]

Applying this evidence-based numerical method to homeopathic therapeutics, in 1834, Paris Professor Gabriel Andral (1797–1876) conducted a prospective study of homeopathic remedies on patients at the *Hôpital de la Pitié*; the next year, homeopathic physicians were invited to a repeat experiment at *Hôtel Dieu*, another Parisian hospital. Both sets of experiments involved administering homeopathic remedies to large numbers of patients; neither experiment found that homeopathic medicines had any visible effect on the progress of disease symptoms.[124] Thus, a large-scale, replicated, prospective clinical trial had demonstrated the ineffectiveness of homeopathic remedies. Holmes was present to observe the inefficacy of homeopathic remedies during the *Hôtel Dieu* experiments.[125]

In 1843, Holmes adapted Louis's techniques to perform what would today be considered a meta-analysis of the literature on puerperal fever (childbirth fever). The analysis commenced with a description of a 1795 study by Scottish physician Alexander Gordon (1752–1799). Gordon had discovered that puerperal fever was contagious and that physicians, midwives, and nurses were transmitting the disease to pregnant women. Conducting a prospective study, Gordon "arrived with certainty in the matter [i.e., that puerperal fever was contagious since he] could venture to foretell what women would be affected with the disease, upon hearing by what midwife they were to be delivered... and in almost every instance [his] prediction was verified."[126] After citing Gordon's study, Holmes found multiple accounts in the published literature confirming it. He concluded that a physician who practiced "midwifery should never take any active role in the post-mortem examination of cases of puerperal fever" and should abstain from midwifery for "some weeks" if any of his patients contracted puerperal fever because other patients are "in danger of being infected by him, and it is his duty to take every precaution to diminish [patients'] risk of disease and death."[127]

It was against this background, as part of their ongoing efforts to bring the latest in Parisian medical science—the stethoscope, the numerical method, Louis's critique of bloodletting—into the English-language medical sphere that these reformers, Forbes and Holmes, wrote about homeopathy. Holmes published, "Homeopathy and Its Kindred Delusions" in 1842[128]; Forbes published "Homeopathy, Allopathy, and Young Physic" in his journal in 1846. When they published their critiques, Hahnemann was still a respected world-renowned physician who, in 1832, had been awarded an honorary membership in the MSSNY.[129]

Forbes and Holmes were not particularly interested in homeopathy; their interests lay in establishing the need for an evidence-based review of medical practices using the numerical method and other scientific techniques developed in Paris. Implicit in their writings on homeopathy was the reformist contention that practices found wanting by scientific standards ought to be abandoned. Forbes says precisely this:

> In finishing our examination of the writings of the Homeopathists... we do not shrink from adopting inferences—however unfavorable to Allopathy [i.e., regular medicine][130]...
>
> 1. That in a large portion of the cases treated by allopathic physicians, the disease is cured by nature, and not by them.
> 2. That in a lesser, but still not a small proportion, the disease is cured by nature in spite of them....
> 3. That, consequently, in a considerable portion of diseases, it would fare as well, or better, with patients, in the actual condition of the medical art, as more generally practiced, if all remedies, at least all active remedies, especially drugs, were abandoned.[131]

As Holmes memorably put a similar point, "if the whole *materia medica*, as now used, could be sunk to the bottom of the sea, it would be better for mankind—and all the worse for the fishes."[132] Forbes and Holmes critiqued homeopathy not only to demonstrate its unscientific nature and to argue for the inadvisability of incorporating homeopathy into regular medicine, but primarily because they were trying to alert regulars about the unproven nature of their own practices: bloodletting[133] and the prescribing of purgatives like calomel. The regulars clearly understood this and retaliated by flyting with Holmes[134] and shutting down Forbes's journal.[135]

By the 1840s, "true" medical science, as practiced by Louis and the Paris school, required the confirmation of homeopathic hypotheses by experiments that yielded, to use Whewell's turn of phrase, "distinct and definite results, such as can be steadily taken hold of and reasoned from."[136] The large-scale Paris experiments repeatedly found that homeopathic results could not be "steadily taken hold of" because they were not in evidence. As Holmes remarks in his essay, when Professor Andral "experimented on the effects of cinchona[136]... and other highly extolled [homeopathic] remedies [in Paris he found that] they never produced the slightest appearance of the symptoms attributed to them."[137]

Moreover, the interrelated homeopathic hypothesis about the effectiveness of *simillimum* (minute doses of a substance causing similar symptoms) did not cohere with the laws of chemistry, physics, or even common sense; it lacked "consilience."[138]

> So extraordinary would be the fact, that a single atom of substances which a child might swallow without harm by the teaspoon could, by an easy

> mechanical process, be made to develop such inconceivable powers, that nothing but the strictest agreement of the most cautious experimenters, secured by every guaranty... appealing to repeated experiments in public, with every precaution to guard against error, and with the most plain and peremptory results, should lead us to lend any credence to such pretensions.[139]

Holmes and Forbes recognized that failure to cohere with everyday experience or with other scientific theories does not disprove a hypothesis, but they argued that it does require a higher level of experimental confirmation to be accepted as "true" (or well-confirmed) science. Yet, Holmes emphasizes, "repeated experiments in public" did not confirm the homeopathic hypotheses. Clinging to conjectures despite failing to produce the predicted results in "repeated experiments in public, with every precaution to guard against error," reduced homeopathy to, as Holmes put it, a "medical delusion."[140]

Because homeopathy was a medical delusion, Forbes argued, regulars could not introduce homeopathy into their practice or accept homeopaths into their organizations without endangering their claims to practicing scientific medicine:

> The guiding principles of homeopathy appear to us to be of that character which must render its exercise very injurious to medicine as a branch of science... we cannot but regard it as calculated to destroy all scientific progress in medicine and to degrade the minds of those who practice it. Its direct tendency seems to be that of severing medicine from the sciences.[141]

Forbes and Holmes would willingly jettison the entire *materia medica*, "all active remedies, especially drugs," on the basis of Louis's experiments and comparable empirical data. Yet the homeopaths seemed unwilling to change any aspect of their theory on the basis of empirical data. So, Forbes argued that, "until the proof is obtained, it behooves all who regard the prosperity and dignity of the true art, to resist [homeopathy's] progress."[142] Homeopathy could not be accepted as scientific medicine because, to quote the wording of the *Code of Medical Ethics*, homeopaths "reject the accumulated experience of the profession, and... the aids actually furnished by anatomy, physiology, pathology, and organic chemistry."

Hays had followed the debate over Forbes's essay, reprinting one of the *Lancet* critiques almost immediately after the essay's publication in 1846.[143] Bell, Emerson, and Hays would also have been aware of Holmes's work because of a very public flyte-like dispute that their Kappa Lambda brothers, Hugh H. Hodge (1796–1873) and Meigs were having with Holmes over the contagious nature of puerperal fever. In fact, the year after Holmes's essay on homeopathy was published, in 1843, Hays created a new journal, *The Medical News and Library*, as a supplement to the *American Journal of the Medical Sciences*. This new journal would challenge the "medical delusions of the day... [which] will receive due attention and be fully exposed... [in an] effort... to arrest it, and [so that] medical men are furnished with the means of refuting the numerous falsehoods and absurdities daily propagated" (note Holmes's terminology "medical delusions").[144]

The first issue of *The Medical News*, published in January 1843, contained an ironic (but characteristically unsigned) article by Hays, lampooning homeopaths' use of testimonials rather than empirical data as evidence for scientific theories:

> *Homeopathic Fictions*. The very *weighty* reasons adduced by the advocates of this humbug in support of their doctrines are sufficiently amusing.... Thus as incontestable proofs of the soundness of their theory, statements are constantly put forth that some privy counselor, or grand chamberlain, or duke's valet, of grand duchess's maid, or some equally elevated character and competent judge has become a convert; or that a chair of homeopathy has been created in some German principality, or the practice legalized by some formal audience.[145]

Similar articles appeared in virtually every issue of *The Medical News*, including those published between May 1846 and May 1847, the period during which the AMA *Code of Medical Ethics* was being written.

Bell's journal was less aggressive in its treatment of homeopathy but, as he argued in his introduction to the 1847 AMA code, the unscientific nature of such "delusions" made it imperative to refuse to extend to its practitioners the "slightest countenance."

> Adverse alike to ethical propriety and to medical logic, are the various popular delusions.... Although it is not in the power of physicians to prevent, or always to arrest, these delusions in their progress, yet it is incumbent on them, from their superior knowledge and better opportunities, as well as from their elevated vocation, steadily to refuse to extend them the slightest countenance, still less support.[146]

Later in his introduction to the code, Bell characterizes physicians as:

> trustees of science and almoners of benevolence and charity [who] should use unceasing vigilance to prevent the introduction into their body of those who have not been prepared by a suitably preparatory moral and intellectual training.... Human life and human happiness must not to be endangered by the incompetency of presumptuous pretenders. The greater the inherent difficulty of medicine, as a science... the more necessary is it... to unravel its mysteries and to deduce scientific order from apparently empirical confusion.[147]

Writing in the context of the Forbes-Holmes critique, Bell and Hays rejected homeopathy as unscientific. In this they had a cause that paralleled the Davis-March campaign of reinstituting the medical sciences as the basis of American medical education. Hays expressed this unity of purpose in a ten-column lead article in the May 1847 issue of his journal, *The Medical News*—the same issue parodies the homeopathic doctrine of infinitesimal doses—explicitly championing Davis's educational reforms.[148] Yet, in the code, Bell, Hays, and Emerson did not have ten columns to express their belief in scientific medicine and medical education or their correlative rejection of unscientific medicine. They needed a succinct statement, parsed in regulatory language, which would be acceptable to other members of the drafting committee and would be uncontroversial when perused by delegates to the AMA's founding convention.

As with Hays's note to the convention, every word in the consultation clause appears to have been carefully chosen to offer a sophisticated reading to the cognoscenti and a simpler reading for those less knowledgeable. The exclusion of those "whose practice is based on an exclusive dogma to the rejection of the accumulated experience of the profession" as not a "fit associate" could be read simply as a fraternity blackball. The original Kappa Lambda oath rules permitted the exclusion of anyone whose practices were "not such as to render him respectable in his Profession, [since they were not] worthy to be distinguished as a member of this society";[149] and, similarly, the consultation clause could also be read as excluding anyone who rejected "the accumulated experience of the profession" since those excluded had excluded themselves through a "practice . . . based on an exclusive dogma."

The term "dogma" also sustains multiple readings. In the 1823 edition of Webster's dictionary, "dogma" designates "[a] settled opinion; a principle . . . a doctrinal notion, particularly in matters of faith and philosophy; as the dogmas of the church." The 1913 edition extends this definition: "A doctrinal notion asserted without regard to evidence or truth; an arbitrary dictum. . . . A dogma is that which is laid down with authority as indubitably true." Homeopathic and Thomsonian societies often treated the writings of their founding fathers, Samuel Hahnemann and Samuel Thomson, as dogma in precisely this sense. All Thomsonians and some major homeopathic organizations required members to sign test resolutions, comparable to *sponsio academica*, in which they pledged "[t]hat we consider the Thomsonian System and Practice of Medicine the best in our knowledge for the removal and cure of disease. We know of no other Medicines equal to those recommended by Doctor Samuel Thomson."[150] Some homeopathic societies also required pledges stating that, "[w]e believe the *Organon of the Healing Art* as promulgated by Samuel Hahnemann to be the only reliable guide in therapeutics. . . . That as some self-styled homeopathists have taken the occasion to traduce Hahnemann . . . and his teaching as 'not being the standard of homeopath today,'... we denounce all such as being traitors to our cause and recreant to its interests." [151] Anyone familiar with Thomsonian medicine or with some forms of homeopathy would know that their societies were dogmatic, treating the writings of their founders as "settled opinion; a principle... a doctrinal notion [like] the dogmas of a church."

On another level, those cognizant of the Forbes-Holmes critique of homeopathy could reject homeopathy as dogmatic for different reasons: homeopaths persisted in their beliefs even in the face of the disconfirming Parisian experiments. The difference between a scientific hypothesis and a dogma, to use Whewell's criterion, was that scientific hypotheses generate "active experiment and observation. And if the results of this process contradict [a theory's] fundamental assumptions, however ingenious, however symmetrical, however elegant his system may be, [the scientist] rejects it without hesitation."[152] Homeopaths chose the ingenuity of the theory over the results of the experiment, and thus, as Forbes and Holmes argued at length, they thereby converted their theories into a dogma. To the most knowing eyes, therefore, the words "exclusive dogma" taken in conjunction with the statement "to the rejection... of the aids actually furnished by anatomy, physiology, pathology, and organic chemistry" encapsulated the Forbes-Holmes critique. The clear implication of that critique was that the AMA, as an organization committed to regrounding medicine and medical education in the sciences, had to reject homeopathy and homeopaths because homeopathy was predicated on a pseudoscience, a medical delusion incompatible with the basic medical sciences.

The consultation clause had been carefully crafted to serve, on one level, as a fraternity-style pledge for "fit associates" that rejected the heterodox simply because they were heterodox; on another level, it was a rejection of alternative medicine as simply dogma; and, at the deepest level, as a sophisticated statement of commitment to the AMA's educational and scientific agenda. These multilevel readings of the clause facilitated the unanimous passage of the code at the AMA's founding meeting in 1847. However, as Warner and Wolpe argue persuasively (and as we shall see in Chapter 8), by the 1870s, those who read the clause as a simple test of orthodoxy would turn medical practice from science to faith—converting homeopathy into a form of heresy.

On the Relevance of the 1847 Code of Ethics

Some historians question the relevance of the AMA code of medical ethics. As one historian wrote in a leading journal, "One can write very interesting pieces on the topic [of American medical ethics], with nary a mention of the 1847 AMA code."[153] Yet most of the issues that nineteenth-century American practitioners considered matters of medical ethics—advertising, antivivisectionism, confidentiality, consultations, contract practice, fee splitting, health insurance, patents and patent medicine, prescribing quack remedies and secret nostrums, public health initiatives, pure food and drug legislation, recognizing African-American and female practitioners, research on human subjects, specialization, and so forth—would be discussed within the framework and the language of the AMA's code of ethics or reports of the AMA's committees on ethics. The AMA code was so iconic, in fact, that, in 1884, the AIH adopted a version of this code;[154] so too did the American Osteopathic Association (AOA) in 1904.[155] To be sure, a history of American medical ethics should focus on more than medical society codes, yet any history that neglects these formalized statements of medical morality would be substantively incomplete.

REPUTATIONS OF THE REFORMERS: BELL, EMERSON, AND HAYS

Until the AMA's sesquicentennial celebrations of 1997, the standard scholarly view of the AMA code took Hays's note to the convention literally, and so the code was treated as a reiteration of Percival's *Medical Ethics*, with some minor emendations. Consequently, Bell and Hays were viewed as mere couriers for Percival. Their role in formulating the code and founding the AMA faded quickly in historical and institutional memory even though Hays remained active in AMA affairs until his sixties, serving as treasurer until 1852 and chairing the committee that edited official AMA documents, including its journal, *Transactions*, until 1853. Davis took over the latter role after Hays retired, renaming the AMA's journal the, *Journal of the American Medical Association* in 1883. Moving into other spaces vacated by Hays and his Kappa Lambda brethren, in 1897, on the fiftieth anniversary of the AMA's founding, Davis accepted the title "Father of the AMA," assuming credit as the society's sole founder.

Davis was an ideal hero for a nineteenth-century American foundation narrative: a lone, young (white, eminently Christian) idealist (of Protestant American-born stock) who came out of the backwoods to call forth the better nature of his brethren by founding a national medical society committed to scientific medical education. It remains the AMA's foundation narrative to this day, retold in the organization's literature and on its website.[156] Lest members forget, at the very entrance to the AMA's Chicago headquarters, a tableau is dedicated to celebrating the life and work of its founder, Nathan Smith Davis. Commendably, as their real roles emerged from historical documents examined in preparation for the AMA's 1997 sesquicentennial, the AMA's Institute for Ethics established an Isaac Hays and John Bell award for Leadership in Medical Ethics, commemorating the authorship of the AMA's code in a manner that Bell, Hays (and Emerson) would have welcomed.

Unlike the AMA, other Philadelphia institutions—the Academy of Natural Sciences, the American Philosophical Society, the College of Physicians of Philadelphia, and the Franklin Institute (which regards Hays as a founder)—honored Hays in life, memorialized his death, and preserved his papers and his portrait.[157] As one memorialist notes, Hays died with a medical journal in his hands: a fitting death for "a man so industrious, zealous, steadfast, wise, and pure, whose long life had been devoted to promoting the noblest of sciences and the most beneficent of arts, and cleansing them from the blight of ignorance and the strain of falsehood... its natural and necessary ending... he clung most fondly at last to that work which he had reared as the fittest monument to perpetuate his memory," that is, the journals Hays edited.[158]

Bell garnered fewer memorials and was remembered less fondly than the affable but diffident Hays. The loquacious Irishman disdained anonymity and readily forgot his minority status, getting "uppity" from time to time. Bell protested publicly and in print when the trustees passed him over for two chairs vacated at the University of Pennsylvania by the retirement of his teacher and mentor, Nathanial Chapman. He characterized one appointee as a lecturer so bad that "the soporific influence which he might desire to exert over his patients with ether or chloroform overspreads his class when listening to his sedative discourses."[159] Kappa Lambda founder Professor Samuel Jackson, who had chaired the selection committee, wrote a public rejoinder emphasizing that the committee opted to give the position to an empirical researcher.[160] Jackson also publicly demeaned Bell's achievements as an educator and an author:

> Dr. Bell has been ambitious of the reputation of authorship. He is no more than a book-maker.... But when the principal alteration and addition consists in the erasure of an author's name on the title page, and the substitution of his own, some other appellation might be given to the act. In all the books he has made, not a single thought is his own, not an idea germinated in his mind... giving this merit justly due to Dr. Bell, he remains no more than a maker of books, not a writer.[161]

Publicly humiliated by one of the Philadelphia medical elite, Bell fled to Ohio—only to return sheepishly to Philadelphia a few years later. On his return, he remained active in a few organizations but never regained his former stature. His obituary portrays him as an "old and eminent Philadelphia physician [who] was at one time editor of a Philadelphia journal... for one session Professor of the Theory and Practice of Medicine in the Ohio Medical College, and one of the authors of 'Stokes and Bell's Practice,' a standard work in its day, and winner of a prize essay"[162]—a sad and somewhat pathetic memorial for an author of the AMA's code of ethics.

Emerson fared better than his co-authors. As was customary in the American Philosophical Society, after his death in 1874 another fellow, naval surgeon W. S. W. Ruschenberger (1807–1895), was commissioned to write Emerson's obituary. Finding that "materials for a suitable memoir could not obtained," Ruschenberger never wrote the memorial. About a decade and a half later, however, he was approached by members of the family who "kindly opened sources of information." Consequently, in 1891, Ruschenberger published a twenty-six-page memorial, *A Sketch of the Life of Dr. Gourverneur Emerson*, paying tribute to Emerson's pioneering work in public health and vital statistics. Ruschenberger also reported on "a note written by [Emerson] on the cover of a copy of the [1847 AMA Code] in which he claims that the code... was compiled exclusively by Dr. Isaac Hays and himself."[163]

Ruschenberger further observed that "Dr. Emerson, by invitation, began to live with Mr. Henry Seybert at No. 926 Walnut Street, in May 1856." Reassuring readers that the two bachelors "kept separate apartments," Ruschenberger noted that, rather than engaging a housekeeper "Dr. Emerson was the caterer" (i.e., he cooked for both of them).[164] This relationship puzzled Ruschenberger, who noted that

> Mr. Henry Seybert and Dr. Emerson were warm friends. Their close relationship is notable because their pursuits and aims in life were wide apart. Their mental characteristics were quite different. They were alike in condition. Both were unmarried and both in [financially] easy circumstances. Yet "they lived together in perfect harmony eighteen years, until Dr. Emerson died."[165]

Ruschenberger could not articulate what puzzled him by the enduring "warm friendship" of two affluent bachelors who chose to live together despite their differences in "mental characteristics"—one even playing a feminine role of cooking for the other. In the twenty-first century we could affix a label to an affluent, same-sex couple enjoying a relationship in which one plays a traditionally feminine role.

Schleiner hypothesized that empowered members of disempowered groups created renaissance medical ethics. Perhaps not surprisingly, a similar characterization applies to the Kappa Lambda trio responsible for the AMA's code of ethics: Bell, the exiled Irishman; Hays, the Sephardic Jew (a descendant of Schleiner's Lusitani, in fact); and Emerson, who, in all likelihood, would today characterize himself as "gay." In their lives, they felt the frustrations of disempowerment and, in the words that they added to those previously penned by Percival, they expressed a deep concern for other disempowered groups: for the poor, to whom "professional services should always be cheerfully and freely accorded"; for the epidemic-stricken, who should be cared for "even at the jeopardy of [physicians'] own lives"; and for the ordinary patient whose calls the "physician should . . . be ever ready to obey." The AMA of the nineteenth—and even the mid-twentieth century might reject a foundational narrative that imputes authorship of its code of ethics to such a diverse trio, but it is a fitting narrative for twenty-first-century American medical ethics.

7

PROFESSIONAL MEDICAL ETHICS, 1848–1875: ABORTION, INQUISITION, AND EXCLUSION

What virtuous woman, nay, what woman, with whom, though fallen, there yet linger the instincts of maternity, would be accessory to so foul a deed as the destruction of her offspring?

AMA Presidential Address, Henry Miller, Obstetrician, 1860[1]

If, then, woman is unfitted by nature to become a physician, we should, when we oppose her pretensions, be acquitted of any malicious or unkindly spirit.

AMA Presidential Address, Alfred Stillé, 1871[2]

For the American nation and for its regular medical profession, the second half of the nineteenth century was, to paraphrase Dickens, "the best and the worst of times." Progress was everywhere: a transcontinental railroad connected a nation that could navigate its rivers by steamboat, could write its thoughts on a typewriter, and could communicate them across the continent via telegraph. Whitney's cotton gin made cotton clothing available worldwide, enriching the bank accounts of plantation owners and making slave labor an even more profitable investment in the American South. Edison and Otis illuminated and elevated the world, and Crapper's plumbing changed everyday life by making it practical to bring outhouses indoors—toilet paper was invented by the end of the century.

Progress in medicine was just as dramatic: modern urban sewage systems were installed (first in Boston, then in other urban centers), public works made potable water commonplace, and the pasteurization of milk and other sanitary and public health reforms reduced the frequency of epidemics. After the germ theory of disease was confirmed in the 1870s, vaccines were developed for five major diseases: bubonic plague, cholera, rabies, tetanus, and typhoid. The application of germ theory to the operating theater led to aseptic surgery which, when coupled with anesthesia (a neologism invented by Oliver Wendell Holmes Sr.), transformed the nature, efficacy, and locus of surgery—moving it from the patient's kitchen or dining room table to the hospital operating theater and thereby giving affluent patients a reason to be treated in hospitals. The clinical thermometer, the sphygmomanometer (for measuring blood pressure), the hypodermic syringe, the stethoscope, and other instruments were finding their way into the doctor's medical bag, and, at the end of the century, a new wonder drug for controlling fever was introduced—the aspirin tablet.

Mid-century was also a time of despair, dissension, and conflict as secession from the national political union, driven by the South's "peculiar institution,"[3] slavery, led to civil war. An estimated 600,000–700,000 combatants died in the conflict, more than in all of America's other wars from the revolution of 1776, through to the First and Second World Wars, and on to the Asian and Middle Eastern wars of the twentieth century. It was against this backdrop of carnage, this wartime legacy of death and dying, that the American Medical Association (AMA) would undertake to criminalize prequickening abortion.

THE AMERICAN MEDICAL ASSOCIATION'S CAMPAIGN TO CRIMINALIZE PREQUICKENING ABORTION

In antebellum nineteenth-century America, menstrual extraction—a procedure that would today be known as a first-trimester abortion—was socially, religiously, legally, and medically accepted, widely practiced, and profitable for a wide range of practitioners. Home medical manuals offered recipes for using herbals such as black hellebore and savin (made from the common juniper bush) to make teas and powders, known as "emenagogues" to induce menstruation flow—that is, to self-administer a first-trimester abortion. "Remedies" to induce menses were also advertised in newspapers and readily available.[4] Midwives, herbalists, and every form of medical practitioner—from irregulars to respectable regulars—performed prequickening abortions.

Then, as now, Anglo-American law and morality considered the Sixth Commandment—which Samuel Bard rendered as "Thou shalt do no murder"[5]—just as applicable to midwives, physicians, and surgeons as it was to butchers, bakers, and candlestick makers. Webster's 1823 dictionary defines "murder" as "[t]he act of unlawfully killing a human being with premeditated malice, by a person of sound mind." The verb "kill" is defined as "to deprive of life, animal or vegetable, in any manner or by any means." Killing an infant, infanticide, was then, as it is now, a paradigm case of an immoral and an illegal act. Neither mothers, nor midwives, nor physicians had a moral or legal right to kill an infant *ex utero*. Killing a fetus *in utero* was a more complex matter—and remains so today. Nineteenth-century American law and medical morality held that it was permissible and lawful to kill a fetus for only one reason: to save the life of its mother. However, since one can only deprive of life something that is alive, and since, (as discussed in Chapter 2) the moral, legal, religious, and medical consensus in antebellum America was that a fetus was *not* alive prior to quickening, the destruction of a prequickened embryo was not considered an act of killing, and thus was not considered murder or any other form of homicide.[6] From the 1840s onward, however, some regular physicians had argued against the practice of killing the prequickened fetus and, in the aftermath of the Civil War, they were able to persuade the AMA to lend its imprimatur to a campaign against prequickening abortion, eventually persuading every state in the union to criminalize abortion at any stage of fetal development.

The movement to criminalize prequickening abortion was not uniquely American. It swept across the Western world during the nineteenth century as a consequence of the morally disruptive effects of the developing technologies of the microscope, the stethoscope, and the emerging science of embryology.[7] This broad history, however, is beyond the scope of this book. In America, the ethical saga attaching to prequickening abortion originates, as so much in American medical ethics does, with Percival's *Medical Ethics*. Percival offered a "life stage" argument to show that inducing a miscarriage of a prequickened fetus was manslaughter. "To extinguish the first spark of life is a crime of the same nature, both against our Maker and society," Percival contended, "as to destroy an infant, a child, or a man; these regular and successive stages of existence being the ordinances of God, subject alone to His divine will."[8] Percival followed this invocation of divinity by citing Hippocrates, "the father of physic,... [who] enjoined on his pupils, an oath which...obliged them solemnly to abjure the practice of administering the *pessary*... to procure an abortion."[9]

Percival's observations on prequickening abortion had little impact in either Britain or America—except among the Kappa Lambda brotherhood. One of the Kappa Lambda brethren, Hugh L. Hodge, a professor at the University of Pennsylvania and a founding member of the Kappa Lambda fraternity and of its descendent, the AMA, cited Percival's arguments at length in the lectures on obstetrics that he offered from 1839 onward. Hodge supplemented Percival's arguments with the observation that "[t]he practitioner of Obstetrics has his duties and responsibilities necessarily enlarged. He must regard the infant, as well as the mother, from the period of conception to delivery; and is generally called upon to be its medical attendant during the first few weeks or months of its independent existence."[10] However, when an obstetrician finds himself conflicted between his duties to mother and infant, Hodge taught his students that "the absolute necessity of the science and practice of obstetrics [is] to detect...dangers, and to protect and to preserve a being so wonderfully constructed, so beautiful, so interesting, so moral, so intellectual, and so influential for the good over the bests interests of man, and over the destinies of nations, as woman, 'the last, best gift of Heaven to man.'"[11] Consequently, obstetricians are obligated to perform embryotomies; that is, to destroy the fetus *in utero* to preserve "the mother; her life is to be secured, if possible, even by the sacrifice of her infant."[12]

Hugh Hodge's Lectures: The Refutation of Quickening as a Criterion for Life

Hodge goes to great lengths to demonstrate the inadequacy of quickening as a criterion for the commencement of embryonic life.

> The usual impression, and one which is probably still maintained by the mass of the community, is that the embryo is perfected at the period of quickening.... When the mother first perceives motion, is considered the period when the fetus becomes animated; when it receives its spiritual nature into union with its corporeal. These, and similar suppositions are, as has already been shown, contrary to all fact...and if it were not for the high authorities, medical, legal and theological, in opposition, we might add to common sense.
>
> What, it may be asked, have the sensations of the mother to do with the vitality of the child? Is it not alive because the mother does not feel it?...how can a fetus be termed *inanimate* when it grows is nourished, and manifests all the phenomenon of life? The supposition of inanimate embryos capable of being developed is, at the present day, an absurdity. From the moment of conception it must be alive, for immediately it begins to be developed; it is separated, as you will hereafter learn, from the ovary, where it was generated and travels, some three or four inches, through a narrow tube or canal, to the uterus, as much disconnected from the mother as the chick in ovum is separated from the parent hen. Its subsequent attachment to the mother, by means of the placenta and uterus, are so indirect...that we are justified in

asserting that the mother has little more influence upon the child in utero than the parent bird has upon its offspring in the egg.

If the question, therefore, be returned upon us, when does that mystical union between our corporeal and spiritual nature, between the matter and spirit, body and soul occur? We answer, at the time of *conception*.[13]

After reviewing legal and moral opinions on abortion, Hodge concluded by reminding his medical students of their ethical commitments as obstetricians:

> [M]edical men, must be regarded as the guardians of the rights of infants. They alone can rectify public opinion; they alone can present the subject in such a manner that legislators can exercise their power aright in the preparation of suitable laws; that moralists and theologians can be furnished with facts to enforce the truth on this subject upon the moral sense of the community, so that not only may the crime of infanticide be abolished, but that criminal abortion be properly reprehended, and that women, in every rank and condition of life may be sensible of the value of the embryo and fetus, and of the high responsibility which rests on the parents of every unborn infant.[14]

Hodge's positions on criteria for fetal life were strongly influenced by the development of more powerful microscopes and by the invention of the stethoscope. As two quite different historians, Stanley Reiser and Michel Foucault (1926–1984),[15] separately observed, the stethoscope became the hallmark of a transformation in clinical modes of perception (the medical "gaze") and the patient-physician relationship. As physicians shut their eyes to focus on the information audible through the stethoscope, or turned their head from their patient to read a sphygmomanometer, the patient's narrative was relegated to secondary status, and patient reports became secondary to the signs revealed by instruments. A similar phenomenon was occurring in nineteenth-century obstetrics. Maternal narratives, mothers' perceptions of quickening, were being obsolesced as criteria of life as the stethoscope revealed the presence of a fetal heartbeat well before maternal sensations of "quickening" and as the microscope revealed that the fetus "is separated…from the ovary…and travels…through a narrow tube or canal, to the uterus, as much disconnected from the mother as the chick in ovum is separated from the parent hen." This new perception of the fetus *in utero* as a separate living entity was disruptive to the conventional moral, ethical, and legal view of the prequickened fetus as a nonvital, nonliving entity. New knowledge, Hodge informed his students, created a moral imperative for obstetricians to inform their patients that by undergoing a prequickening abortion they were naïvely killing their children. It also obliged obstetricians to urge changes to moral opinion and obsolete laws that failed to recognize the vital status of the prequickened fetus as revealed by modern embryology. Thus, the conjoined evidence of the stethoscope and microscope were profoundly disruptive to the moral and legal consensus that had legitimated prequickening abortions.

David Storer's 1855 Lecture

Although Hodge gave a version of his 1839 lecture annually, he first allowed it to be published in 1854. He may have gauged medical hostility to his views on prequickening abortion accurately, since, in the next year, 1855, the *Boston Medical and Surgical Journal* (1828–1928, precursor to the *New England Journal of Medicine*) censored a lecture by Harvard obstetrician David Humphries Storer (1804–1891) by expurgating Storer's critique of prequickening abortion on the grounds that it was "injudicious."[16] This act of censorship was imposed over the objections of the journal's editors, at the insistence of the Harvard faculty, led by the eminent surgeon, Henry Jacob Bigelow (1818–1890), son of self-limiting disease theorist, Jacob Bigelow.

David Storer's censored statement on abortion differs from Hodge's in two significant respects. Hodge had held blameless those women who sought abortions, attributing their decisions to a misunderstanding about the status of the prequickened fetus. Consequently Hodge's remedy was to enlighten the profession, society, and women about the findings of modern embryology. Yet, as sociologist Kristin Luker has observed, holding women blameless "meant that American women who practiced abortion…could be defined as *inadvertent* murderesses…thus, a physician could condemn the 'sin' without condemning the 'sinner.'"[17] David Storer, in contrast, uses the rhetoric of moral scorn to condemn women who seek abortions:

> The fashionable young bride, accustomed to adulation, is reluctant to forego at once the excitement of society…wishing still to enjoy the immunities of unmarried life—to be as free, as unshackled as ever—she will not endure the seclusion and deprivations necessarily connected with the pregnant condition, but resorts to means, readily procurable, to destroy the life within her, apparently unconscious that she is not only committing a crime in the sight of the law, but also a sin in the sight of her Maker.
>
> The mother, too…not unfrequently is willing, anxious, to pursue a similar course to produce a similar result. Unfortunate, perhaps pecuniarily unable to have her family provided for in the manner in which they have been accustomed to live, her pride will not allow her to see those already dependent upon her, appearing less "respectable," to use a word thus applied

> in common parlance, as she thinks must be a necessary consequence upon the introduction of every addition to the circle; or learning from others that woman was born for higher and nobler purposes than the propagation of her species, that it is unreasonable that so large a portion of her life should be yielded to its drudgery, or, imagining, from some misinterpreted remark her physician may have carelessly made, that it would really be dangerous for her again to be called upon to give birth to a mature child, and even that it would certainly cause her death, she persuades herself into the belief that it is not morally wrong, that it is really her duty, to destroy her unborn child.[18]

Having so flagrantly moralized, David Storer employs a rhetorician's trick: he denies what he is doing, proclaiming "I do not presume to stand here as a moralist," even as he expresses "*horror*, that a female can so completely unsex herself, that her sensibilities can be so entirely blunted, that any conceivable circumstances can compel her to welcome such degradation!"[19]

David Storer thus informed his students that married women "should forego the excitement of society," that a woman's place is in the home, adoring her husband and bearing his children, even if she is "pecuniarily unable to have her family provided for in the manner in which they have been accustomed to live"; that is, even if she cannot afford to support them. Women, moreover, should ignore their physician's advice that "it would really be dangerous for [them] again to be called upon to give birth to a mature child, and even that it would certainly cause her death." These are not, David Storer informed his medical students, good reasons for a woman "to destroy her unborn child."[20]

It is not clear why Henry Jacob Bigelow considered these passages so "injudicious"[21] that they had to be expurgated.[22] Whatever motivated the censorship, if the intent was to silence Storer Sr., Bigelow succeeded; if the intent was to squelch discussion of prequickening abortion, it failed. After the censorship incident, David Storer's son, obstetrician Horatio Robinson Storer (1830–1922), would publish the deleted section of the lecture in an 1872 issue of the *Journal of the Gynecological Society of Boston*. Storer Jr. also became America's leading campaigner for criminalizing prequickening abortion.

Horatio Storer's Campaign to Criminalize Prequickening Abortion

At the time of the censorship incident, Horatio Storer (hereafter Storer Jr., to distinguish him from his father, David, referred to as Storer Sr.) was a young man in his mid-twenties. He studied with and idolized his teacher, Oliver Wendell Holmes Sr.[23] As Holmes's student, the younger Storer "strongly believed in the high reliability of the fetal heart rate," detected by stethoscope, as a criterion for fetal life, rejecting such criteria as "active movements of a child, unequivocally detected by another."[24] Storer Jr. was reared on the new technology, on the numerical method, and on the data-driven critique of the iatrogenic harms taught by Jacob Bigelow and Holmes. In carrying forward his father's work—in speaking where his father had been silenced—the younger Storer eschewed his father's moralist rhetoric, preferring instead to elaborate on data about declining rates of population increase and the iatrogenic harms inflicted on women by abortionists and abortifacients.[25] Storer Jr., in short, stripped the antiabortion campaign of its misogynist rhetoric and reconfigured his father's views in the language of Harvard Medical School's doctrine of evidence-based scientific medicine.

His campaign against prequickening abortion began in 1857 when, in a possibly planned outburst at a meeting of the Boston-Suffolk Medical Society, instead of delivering the advertised talk on the methods he had used to cauterize a Jewish infant hemorrhaging after a circumcision, Storer Jr., with his father sitting before him in the audience, suggested that "a committee be appointed to consider whether any further legislation is necessary in the Commonwealth [of Massachusetts] on the subject of *criminal abortion*, and to report to the Society such other means as may seem necessary for the suppression of the abominable, unnatural, and yet common crime."[26] The motion was approved and a committee of three, chaired by Storer Jr., was set up to implement it. The meeting then returned to its normal business—Storer's Jr.'s self-disrupted report on treating a hemorrhaging circumcision.

In the spring and summer of 1857, Storer Jr. presented his committee's report at a series of meetings of the Boston Society. The report recommended a radical revision of existing law to make it a felony, punishable by three to ten years imprisonment, to intentionally cause or procure a miscarriage—except if, after consultation, the procedure was deemed necessary to preserve the life of the mother. Penalties were to be doubled if the abortionist was a medical professional. The report also incorporated Storer Sr.'s views on the culpability of mothers, making it a misdemeanor, punishable by fines and/or as much as a year's imprisonment, for a woman to knowingly procure, receive, or submit to an abortifacient or an abortion—except to save her own life. Advertising or selling abortifacients would also be a misdemeanor.[27] These proposals catalyzed a roaring debate and the Boston-Suffolk society refused to endorse them. It did, however, pass a resolution, by a close vote (14 to 13), to bring the report to the Massachusetts Medical Society, where it proved just as controversial.[28]

So it happened that, in 1857, when the young Storer made his entrance into the AMA's Tenth Annual Meeting in Nashville, the brouhaha that his abortion report had stirred up in Massachusetts and the articles on abortion that he was publishing in various medical publications made him something of a celebrity. Such celebrities were often given the opportunity to deliver special reports at national

AMA meetings. Consequently, Storer Jr. was commissioned as a committee of one to report "On Criminal Abortion," with a view toward its suppression at the next AMA meeting.[29] His report, however, was delayed until 1859. In the interim, Storer Jr. recruited a regionally diverse group of seven physicians (from Alabama, the District of Columbia, Missouri, New York, Pennsylvania, South Carolina, and Wisconsin) to co-sign his report on criminalizing abortion. The signatory from Pennsylvania was Hugh Hodge. Other distinguished signatories were Charles A. Pope (1818–1870), president of the AMA 1854–1855; Thomas Blatchford (1794– 1866), past president of the Medical Society of the State of New York (MSSNY) and former vice president of the AMA; another former AMA vice president, the Southern medical educator Edward Hall Barton (1796–1857); and William Henry Brisbane (1806–1878), a physician and former slaveholder turned abolitionist preacher.

Their 1859 special report[30] opened with a statement about the falling rates of population increase and the rising rates of fetal deaths. It attributed both to an iatrogenic cause: the widespread increase in abortions. This increase, in turn, was attributed to three primary causes: "popular ignorance of the true character of the crime," "the fact that the profession themselves are frequently… careless of fetal life" (i.e., to put the same point less diplomatically, the embarrassing fact that regular practitioners provided abortions to their female patients), and "grave defects in our laws."[31] The report proposed "enlighten[ing] this ignorance" by "establish[ing] an obstetrics code [to] prevent such unnecessary and unjustifiable destruction of human life" and reforming the law. Three resolutions were then put before the AMA delegates: (1) that the AMA "enter an earnest and solemn protest against [this] unwarrantable destruction of human life," (2) that it present an agenda for reform to all the state legislatures in the Union, and (3) that it enlist the assistance of state medical societies to do so.[32] The resolutions passed unanimously. There was no debate.[33]

As it happened, the president of the AMA for 1859–1860 was Henry Miller (1800–1874), a former professor of obstetrics at the University of Louisville. Collaborating closely with Storer Jr., he implemented the resolutions, sending letters and supporting documents to state and federal legislators, to President James Buchanan (1791–1868, president 1857–1861), and to the governors of every state and territory in the Union. Since this was the AMA's first national lobbying campaign, as President Miller notes, "a little embarrassment was experienced, arising from the want of information touching these organizations"; that is, the AMA had not yet developed a database of contact information for its lobbying campaign.[34]

The Civil War disrupted normal routines throughout the United States, and the AMA held no national meetings until 1863. It reconvened in Chicago, at the very moment when the Confederate and Union armies under the commands of Robert E. Lee and Ulysses S. Grant were slaughtering each other in Virginia. With this bloodshed as a backdrop, the AMA passed a resolution stating that "[w]hereas, Criminal abortion has become an alarming common evil, we need some means to educate the community as to its criminality and physical evils; therefore... the [AMA]... offers a [prize] for the best short and comprehensive tract calculated for circulation among females... designed to enlighten them upon the criminality and physical evils of forced abortion."[35] Storer Sr. headed the Committee on Prizes, which, as it happened, awarded the gold medal for best essay to none other than Storer Jr. Irrespective of whatever nepotistic connivance occurred between the Storers, the essay merited the medal. Storer Jr. had honed and simplified his arguments. Citing stethoscopic evidence that "sounds [from the fetus] may sometimes be heard several weeks before the usual period of the mother's becoming conscious of the motion of the child, [or] the pulsations of the fetal heart," Storer Jr. argued that this "proved life and independent life... of a child."[36] Then, after wrapping his claims in the mantle of ancient authority provided by the Hippocratic oath[37] and citing Percival in a scholarly footnote, Storer Jr. devotes over ten pages—the paper's longest section—to the "Inherent Dangers of Abortion to a Woman's Health and to Her Life."[38] The persuasiveness of Storer Jr.'s essay lay in its frank description of the impact of abortion on women's health. Then, having dealt at length with abortion as a threat to women's health and fertility, Storer Jr. observes "that abortions are infinitely more frequent among Protestant women than among Catholic; a fact, however, that becomes less unaccountable in view of the known size, comparatively so great, of the families of the latter—in the Irish, for instance."[39] Worse yet, in Storer Jr.'s view, "induced abortion... is proportionately much more common in the married than in the unmarried."[40]

Married women, Storer argued, have a moral obligation to reproduce to repopulate the nation with the right sort of children after the devastation of the Civil War. "All the fruitfulness of the present generation, tasked to its utmost, can hardly fill the gaps in our population that have of late been made by disease and the sword.... Shall they be filled by our own children or by those of aliens? This is a question that our own women must answer; upon their loins depends the future destiny of our nation."[41] These passages reflect a powerful pronatalist desire to repopulate typical of postwar periods. The contrast between "our own children" and "those of aliens" indicates that Storer Jr. shared the anti-immigrant, anti-Catholic, anti-Irish bias commonplace among white Anglo-Saxon Protestant Bostonians during this period—biases reiterated, word-for-word, in Storer Jr.'s bestselling popular version of his essay, published in 1866 as *Why Not? A Book for Every Woman.*[42]

It should be noted that no such comments appear in Storer Jr.'s 1867 book *Is It I? A Book for Every Man,* written after Storer Jr. became an attending surgeon at the Franciscan Hospital for Women, a Catholic medical institution. In that book, Storer Jr. commends the emigration "of the Irish, the English, and the modern

Jews" as an example that other "older nations" should have followed.[43] No anti-Catholic, anti-Irish, or anti-Semitic comments appear in Storer's final book on abortion, a careful policy analysis of criminalizing abortion written with lawyer Franklin Fiske Heard (1825–1889) and published in 1868.[44] In 1872, after the death of his second wife, Storer Jr. married the founder of the Franciscan Hospital, Sister Superior Francis Sophia MacKenzie (?–1910) and converted to Roman Catholicism. Storer's views on religion had evidently changed.

THE CRIMINALIZATION OF ABORTION: THE IMPACT OF MORALLY DISRUPTIVE TECHNOLOGIES

By the end of the nineteenth century, every regular medical society supported prohibitions on prequickening abortions, public opinion stigmatized abortion at any stage as immoral, and every state in the reunited United States had enacted, or would soon enact, a statute criminalizing prequickening abortion. This transformation was not uniquely American. Moral, ethical, and legal views of the prequickened fetus changed throughout the Western world, commencing in Britain in the 1830s and ending with changes at the Vatican in 1869. The phenomenon is particularly striking because the moral, ethical, and legal status of first-trimester abortion would be revised again in the latter half of the twentieth century in most of the Western world—with the sole exception of areas in which the Catholic Church predominates. The Church has never reversed its position on prequickening abortion, and it has sufficient political clout to impose its ethical stance as public policy in many countries. So the abortion issue is a case study in moral and ethical change, which is why one must ask: Why did doctors condemn prequickening abortion in the mid-nineteenth century? Why were their campaigns to criminalize it successful? Why did they change their position in the mid-twentieth century?

In the American context, the short answer to the first question, as is evident in passages cited earlier from Hodge and the Storers, is that a new understanding of embryological development—revealed and confirmed by the microscope and the stethoscope—had the morally disruptive impact of obsolescing quickening as a criterion for fetal life. If cardiopulmonary criteria were used to assess life, then a prequickened fetus *in utero* was as alive as a newborn babe. Medical school professors engaged in applying the new sciences of embryology and physiology to transform traditional midwifery into the specializations of obstetrics and gynecology felt that they could not ignore this scientific evidence. So they undertook the role of public health reformers, educating the public about the status of the prequickened fetus and the deleterious impact of abortifacients and abortions on women's health. Lobbying in the name of the new sciences, they upended customary morality, ethics, and laws condoning the termination of first-trimester pregnancies.

The stethoscope and microscope are thus paradigm cases of morally disruptive technologies that transformed medical morality, medical ethics, and the law. Yet the morally disruptive dimensions of these new technologies in and of themselves may not have sufficed to effect a change in ethics and law. Science is inextricably intertwined with normative issues, and the early rhetoric of the Storers reflected the prejudices of the urban Northeast: a deeply felt need to repopulate a war-ravaged country with properly white Anglo-Saxon Protestant stock. So, medical science and medical ethics, aligned with social need, popular prejudice, and professional pride, supported by a public education campaign and persistent lobbying by local medical societies, changed public policy, criminal law, and popular morality in America. As to the reasons why all of this was reversed in the twentieth century—the answer would appear to involve a similar combination of factors: morally disruptive medical technologies, most notably Bjorn Ibsen's ventilator, which obsolesced cardiopulmonary criteria of life; the transformational impact of a war; the changing role of women in the workplace and at the voting booth; and the sociopolitical impact of feminism. In combination, these forces changed public morality, medical ethics, and, eventually, the law.

THE AMERICAN MEDICAL ASSOCIATION'S EXISTENTIAL DEFINITION OF PROFESSIONALISM

Antiabortion arguments were not the sole Percivalean legacy that the Kappa Lambda brethren transmitted to American medicine: they also imparted a vision of a national code of ethics. By craftiness and stagecraft—by resorting to an old vintner's trick of repackaging new wine in old bottles—Bell and Hays persuaded the AMA to adopt a national code and created a pseudo-consensus around a code whose central concept, the notion of a "profession," was essentially undefined. It was thus an open question how the AMA's new code of *professional* ethics would mesh with traditional concepts of gentlemanly honor. For Percival and for the Kappa Lambda brethren, the term "professional" was a value-laden concept inextricably connected to role-related duties. Ordinary AMA members, however, had no reason to understand the term in any but the standard sense defined by Webster's (1828) as "[t]he business which one professes to understand and to follow for subsistence; calling; vocation; employment; as the learned professions. . . . But the word is not applied to an occupation merely mechanical"; it also means "[t]he collective body of persons engaged in a calling. We speak of practices honorable or disgraceful to a profession."[45] So, to ordinary AMA members, the term "profession" was not value laden; it merely referred to a nonmechanical occupation that one could practice, honorably or disgracefully. As a synonym for "occupation," the term carried no normative weight: consequently, the expression "unprofessional practice," which today would be understood as condemnatory, would have made no more sense in the nineteenth century than the expression "unoccupational occupation." A normative notion of "unprofessional practice" first surfaces in the 1913 edition of the Webster's dictionary, which characterizes "professional conduct" as "conforming to the rules or standards of a profession."[46] Understood in this sense, "unprofessional practices" are those that violate the standards of a profession. In the nineteenth century, however, the notion of a profession, the concept of professionalism and professional conduct, were as yet undefined; they had no normative weight. The AMA would ultimately define these expressions not through an academic exercise, but existentially, through decisions that effectively defined a medical professional as a secular, scientific, ethical gentleman. The first existential defining point was at the AMA's 1855 meeting.

Professional Ethics as Secular Ethics

Some 528 delegates from twenty-six states attended the AMA's eighth annual meeting, convened in Philadelphia in 1855. Charles Pope was president, Nathan Smith Davis was one of his vice presidents, and Isaac Hays played host as chair of the committee on arrangements. Davis complained that partying seemed to preoccupy most delegates, who were more interested in celebrations, balls, and dinners than in scientific presentations. Nonetheless, a trio of issues were debated at that meeting that would inform the interpretation of the code of ethics and the meaning of American "professionalism": religion, patents, and specialization. At the previous meeting, New York physician James L. Phelps, an officer of the American Bible Society (founded in 1816 and still functioning), raised an issue about the relationship between professionalism and religion. In a controversial paper, "Religion, as an Element in Medicine; or the Duties and Obligations of the Profession," Phelps advanced the theory that it was consistent with the AMA's *Code of Medical Ethics* for physicians to view the inculcation of religious beliefs, specifically "the truths of the Gospel," as a professional duty.

As textual support for his interpretation of the code, Phelps cited John Bell's Introduction, which opens with the line that "[m]edical ethics, as a branch of general ethics, must rest on the basis of religion and morality."[47] Further evidence for his view could be found in the section of the code stating physicians' duty to their patients (Rush's patrimony), the paternalist imperative that a physician's "counsels or even remonstrances, [to patients] will . . . not [give] offense, if they be proffered with politeness, and evince a genuine love of virtue, accompanied by a sincere interest in the welfare of the person to whom they are addressed" (chapter I, article I, section 7). In carefully enumerated theses, Phelps argued that medical paternalism should extend beyond care for the body to encompass care for the soul and, thus, the inculcation of the gospel should be integral to the practice of medicine:

> 13. That hence we deduce inferentially, the solemn and responsible professional relation existing between the physician and his patients, and that in consonance both with the requirement or our code of ethics...it is obligatory on the practitioner in grave disease, seasonably to take the initiative demanded...leading to that consolation which religion can afford.
>
> 14. That the prudent and discreet inculcation of the truths of the Gospel and the method of man's redemption by a Mediator...begetting trust, confidence and joy and often ending in fatal cases in a peaceful and triumphant death.
>
> 15. [T]he paramount duty of the profession to their patients not only as regards their body in disease, but also the higher interests of the immortal soul. And hence, also the just claim of religion, the great anesthetics of the immortal mind, to be considered an element of medicine or the healing art.[48]

Since *Transactions* was an official publication of the AMA, the question raised at the 1854 meeting was whether to appear to give official sanction to Phelps's religious interpretation of the AMA code by publishing it in *Transactions*. The issue was placed in the hands of three rising stars, all future presidents of the AMA, John Atlee (1799–1885), Alden March, and Lewis Sayre (1820–1900). This committee determined that

> the principles promulgated by this code have been assumed as a common ground upon which every member of the Association may stand, without reference to distinctive principles or doctrines which distinguish the various religious societies existing among the vastly extended and diversified population of our country.[49]

Consequently, the committee concluded, the AMA is

> bound to regard the religious sentiments of every medical brother, and to withhold their assent from any publication which does not strictly belong to the declared objects of the Association, and which would be in derogation of the rights, or conflict with the sentiments of any...who have united with us.[50]

Respect for religious diversity, assisted no doubt by the gracious hosting of Isaac Hays, an affable Sephardic Jew, as chair of the meeting's Arrangements Committee, thus justified the committee's decision to declare the autonomy of professional medical ethics from religious belief. Autonomy from religion thereafter became a fixed principle of American medical professionalism, and intruding religious beliefs or religious ethics into professional decision making came to be considered "unprofessional." Yet there was nothing predetermined about this separation of religion from profession. A different committee, meeting in a less pluralistic environment than Philadelphia, whose host happened not to be a well-liked and highly respected Sephardic Jew—who also happened to edit the field's leading journal—might well have welcomed discussion of integrating Christian ideals into medical professionalism. Happenstance helped to integrate secularism into the American concept of professionalism.

Patents and Gentlemanly Honor

At the same 1854 AMA convention, delegates from the Ohio medical society, having passed a resolution permitting the patenting of medical instruments in their own code of medical ethics, proposed deleting the words "for any surgical instrument" from chapter II, article I, section 4 of the AMA's Code of Medical ethics. The deletion would alter the language as follows: "Equally derogatory to professional character is it, for a physician to hold a patent ~~[for any surgical instrument]~~, or medicine; or to dispense a secret nostrum." The Ohio proposal raised three questions: first, since the drafters of the AMA code made no provision for its amendment, may the code be amended? Second, what is the AMA code's relationship to state and local society codes? And, more substantively, should the traditional prohibition against secret nostrums be extended to cover patents?

The Massachusetts Medical Society was moving in the same direction as the Ohio society. In 1846–1847, it had ruled that it was permissible for regular physicians to hold a patent on either a medicine or on a surgical device. An editorial in the February 1847 edition of the *Boston Medical and Surgical Journal* reported that the society had stipulated that once a medicine or an instrument is "patented—it is no longer a secret and therefore using it is no longer an offense, "and those who are curious to know what their neighbors are doing in the matter, may ascertain [it] by writing to Washington."[51] The editorial continues,

> no wrong against the Society is done in securing one's self behind the broad parchment of the patent law, [nor any] sin [in] the exclusive enjoyment of any income which those laws grant.... [T]his...law will unquestionably give scope to genius, hitherto constrained from extraordinary manifestations of tact and enable it to keep the medicine-taking multitude of New England well supplied with patented preparations.... [P]eople in this blessed country may do as they like, and who has the right to complain? [52]

The stage was thus set for a confrontation over the process of amending the national code of ethics, its status with respect to state and local codes, and over the propriety of patents. In the end, these questions were answered by passage of a single resolution stating that

> [n]o State or local society...shall hereafter be entitled to representation in this Association, which has not adopted its Code of Ethics. No State or local society which has violated or discarded any article or clause in said Code of Ethics shall any longer be entitled to representation in this body. The Secretary of this Association [is] directed to inform the officers of the State Medical Society of Ohio, that unless [its position on surgical patents] be rescinded, it cannot hereafter be represented in this Association.[53]

As historian Samuel Haber has astutely observed, ideals of gentlemanly honor would be conserved in the American concept of professionalism. Because commercial conduct had always been anathema to the ideals of gentlemanly honor, the AMA's approval of this resolution reasserted it as inimical to the ideals of professional conduct as well.

The vote on the Ohio patent proposal also resolved questions about the relationship between local and national codes of ethics: all state and local societies were hereafter required to adopt the national code as their own. This jurispathic edict inadvertently froze ethical and moral innovation at the state and local level, forcing almost all ethical issues to be debated in terms of the national code of ethics. Yet, even as ethical issues were being uploaded to the national level, there was still an astonishing lacuna in the code itself: its framers had never formulated a process for interpreting, amending, revising, or enforcing it. The AMA thus fell into a pattern of appointing ad hoc committees to investigate and arbitrate ethical controversies—and, since no procedures were in place to guide these committees, ethical issues became matters of medical politics, hostage to such happenstance events as the inclinations of the physicians who served on these committees. By 1858, these ad hoc committees had become so commonplace that they became a standing "Committee on Medical Ethics," whose members were appointed annually.[54]

Specialists, Advertising, and Exclusive Practices

Twenty years after Nathan Smith Davis first enticed his colleagues in the MSSNY to hold a national conference on medical education, he presided as president over the AMA's seventeenth national convention, held in Boston in 1865. For the nation and for the AMA, the mood was a mix of celebration overlaid by grief. "Peace," was upon the land, Davis proclaimed: "Our National Union unbroken," and "[t]he cherished *flag* of our country again waves in triumph over every part of our boundless domain."[55] Yet "a deeper, more enduring sadness," casts a pall, because of "the darkest crime... the deliberate murder of the Chief Magistrate of this great Republic," the assassination of President Abraham Lincoln (1808–1865, president 1861–1865). Davis called on the delegates to reunite and "to make our reunion one of hearts as well as States."[56]

Ironically, the theme of "unity of hearts" became the backdrop for a divisive debate over advertisements indicating physicians' areas of specialization (as, for example, an ophthalmologist). The issue had been raised two years earlier, in 1863, when a specialist's advertisement in the *New York Evening Express* was brought to the attention of the *comita* of the Medical Society of the County of New York (MSCNY). Contrition, apology, in conjunction with a commitment to never repeat the "accident," secured the forgiveness of the miscreant. Nonetheless, since medical ethical policies now had to be determined at the national level, the *comita* asked the MSSNY to raise the issue at the next national meeting of the AMA.[57] The MSSNY offered a resolution at the 1865 national meeting, "[t]hat all reference to special branches of medical practice as extra inducements to patronage should be deemed violations of the code of medical ethics."[58]

The MSCNY's concerns were exacerbated by advertisements in a journal published by a Brooklyn-based immigrant German-Jewish ophthalmologist, Julius Homberger (1838/9–1872). On arriving in New York City in 1861, Homberger founded the *American Journal of Ophthalmology* (1862–1864)—often described as the first American journal of specialty medicine.[59] Following a standard practice of Berlin ophthalmologists, Homberger published this notice in the journal's first issue:

> CLINICAL EYE INFIRMARY
> The undersigned is prepared to receive at his private
> surgical home a limited number of patients requiring
> the performance of operations on the eye.
> J. Homberger M.D. 39 West 23rd Street, N.Y.[60]

The policy proposed by the MSCNY/MSSNY to the AMA would require deletion of the words "eye" from this advertisement, as a reference to a "special branch of medical practice" and an improper "extra inducement to patronage"; that is, as a form of unfair competition. This prohibition would deprive specialists of the right to notify colleagues and the public of their expertise, treating specialized expertise as an "extra inducement to patronage," rather than significant information about a surgeon's expertise and skills.

In 1864, Homberger established the American Ophthalmological Institute and joined the AMA, becoming secretary of its Section on Surgery. In the latter capacity, he was commissioned to chair a committee to report on the relationship of specialty to general practice medicine. He ended up being the sole signatory to the report; the three other members of the committee—Hooker, Storer Jr., and another physician—refused to sign. Both MSCNY/MSSNY's proposed prohibition on specialty advertising and Homberger's report defending it were presented at the AMA's 1865 national meeting.

Homberger's report opens with a gratuitous polemic against the AMA's *Code of Medical Ethics*. "We do not think," Homberger wrote, "that there was a physician, who, being at the same time a gentleman, needed the recommendations in [chapter I of the Code, the physician–patient contract] to be written out for him[61]. . . . Whoever is fit to be a physician must certainly know from intuitive knowledge of propriety which a gentleman possesses, how to behave himself at the bedside; and only gentlemen can be physicians deserving of the name."[62] With sarcastic but scathing logic, Homberger then skewers the "paragraphs on the duties of patients towards their physicians . . . as ludicrous."[63] He then turns to the prohibition against advertising. Invoking the right of a well-educated physician "to reap the fruits of a special study in a special branch"[64] and observing that the economics of specialty practice dictate a need to inform a large patient base through advertising,[65] Homberger asserts the moral basis of specialists' claims, competency: "no physician has a right to attend to any case, unless he is satisfied that he can do it full justice."[66]

> [I]t is an abuse of his confidence and a breach of trust reposed in him, if the physician undertakes the operation if not fully competent for the task. It cannot be denied then that it is the duty of the practitioner to send the patient to a specialist in order to discharge his obligations to his patient.[67]

Specialists, Homberger claims, thus have expertise that enables them to perform specialized procedures, like eye surgery, more competently and safely than general practitioners. Hence, Homberger argued in his report, it is an "abuse of confidence and a breach of trust" for a general practitioner to fail to refer patients to specialists. Such referrals require that general practitioners know specialists' names and locations.

Probing deeper, Homberger asks a fundamental question: Why should medicine be considered different from any other commodity?

> A physician gathers his knowledge of disease as an engineer gathers his knowledge of the laws of mechanics. . . . They sell to their clients, patients . . . those special inferences which their general knowledge enables them to draw. They are paid according to the value of their services. Such transactions the public justly considers commercial. . . .

> There is no reason why the laws of free trade should not be applicable to medical services, as to all others. The plea that the public must, in its ignorance, be protected against quacks and empirics, is no more valid than the laws which in despotic countries protect the people from liberal newspapers and "dangerous" religious dogmas.... There is no valid argument which can be advanced to prohibit the [general] practitioner of medicine, as well as the specialist, from proceeding with a view of securing practice in the same way as dealers in commodities or vendors of other services [i.e., by advertising].[68]

Homberger acknowledges that the initial prohibition against advertising was reasonable because "[t]he Code of Ethics was drawn up at a time when scientific specialization was in its infancy, [when it was] perhaps proper [to look with] disfavor and distrust" on such claims. So, "by means of your code, [you] attempted to combat what you feared would eventually flower into charlatanism. But continuing...prohibitions originally directed against charlatans, against a class of men who you must confess to be scientists...must prove...inoperative and injurious."[69] Homberger then predicts that "within a few more years [specialists] will form a strong minority.... [T]hey may, in the larger cities, at least, form a strong majority." "What," he asks, presciently, "will be the necessary consequence of an increase in their numbers if the profession continue by legislation to interfere with their interests?... [W]e do not make the demand unadvisedly or inconsiderately for the recognition of the right of the specialist to advertise" because specialist advertising is economically essential.[70]

On a motion from Storer Jr., Homberger's report was referred to the Committee on Ethics, chaired by Hooker (who had opposed the report.)[71] The upshot of this diversion was that Hooker's opinion of Homberger's report was debated at the convention—the report itself was neither presented at the convention nor published in *Transactions*.[72] Storer Sr. used his 1865 presidential address to rebut Homberger's report—which, to reiterate, was never made available to the delegates. A master of Orwellian doublespeak, Storer Sr. reframed the debate over whether the AMA should censure or expel specialists who advertise as the question: Shall specialists "voluntarily" "alienate" themselves from the AMA. Advertising was not "gentlemanly and honorable" since to claim special expertise is to "assume an ideal superiority over [one's] brethren and thus...an undeserved reward." The claim that specialists have expert knowledge and superior special skills was thus reconceived as a breach of "professional etiquette."[73]

Defending Homberger in a minority report was Henry Ingersoll Bowditch (1808–1892). Henry Ingersoll, a committed abolitionist who had lobbied successfully to introduce an ambulance service into the Union Army during the Civil War, was a Harvard lecturer, a public health reformer, and a male feminist who served as an attending physician at the first American hospital for women, the New England Hospital for Women (NEHW). He was also a future president of the AMA. Bowditch argued that specialists did not seek "exclusive" privileges; they merely wished to inform fellow practitioners and the public of the nature of their training and practice.

> The specialists never claim anything further than that they...have decided to devote themselves to the study and treatment of diseases of the head, chest, or abdomen, &c.... [N]o association of physicians have any reason for expressing an opinion [on this], unless the advertisement is evidently of the mountebank character—claiming for the advertiser extraordinary powers and facilities, &c, and then an association may discard the quack from its body, or punish him until he repents.[74]

A hubbub arising after delegates learned that Homberger had advertised in local newspapers soon drowned out Henry Ingersoll Bowditch's careful analysis. One Homberger advertisement published in a Philadelphia newspaper read:

> SURGICAL OPERATIONS ON THE EYE.
> DR. JULIUS HOMBERGER, OCULIST, editor of the American Ophthalmic Journal, informs the public that he is prepared to perform all SURGICAL OPERATIONS, necessary to restore SIGHT or correct DEFORMITY. In no case will he make a charge unless perfectly SUCCESSFUL. DR HOMBERGER can be seen at Dr. VON MOSCHZISKER'S office, No. 1031 Walnut Street, Hours from 11. A.M., to 2 P.M."[75]

Outraged, members voted, "without dissent,"[76] to expel the unrepentant,[77] hence ungentlemanly, Homberger from the AMA.

The next year (1868), the Committee on Ethics recommended "rigid observance of the general laws of professional courtesy and etiquette which have hitherto governed us...under the established Code." Specialists, the committee concluded, have an unjustified tendency to "assume to themselves the privilege of advertising...[and] the Committee think that this great evil should be corrected. They cannot see the justice of permitting the specialist to advertise, while withholding the privilege from the general practitioner."[78] Based on this report, the AMA reaffirmed its position "recogniz[ing] specialties as proper and legitimate forms of practice...governed by the same rules of professional etiquette as have been laid down for general practitioners [which means] that it shall not be proper for specialists to advertise themselves as such, or to assume any title not specially granted by a regularly chartered college."[79] Thus "private handbills addressed to members of the medical profession, or cards in medical journals, calling attention to themselves as specialists, [were] declared in violation of the Code of Ethics of the American Medical Association."[80] The next year, after Storer Jr. objected on behalf of the American Gynecological Society, this resolution was rescinded, legalizing specialist advertising in informational ads directed toward other physicians.[81]

So it came to pass, through happenstance, xenophobia, and habits of conservatism, that another feature of gentlemanly honor was incorporated into American medicine's understanding of professionalism. For slightly over a century, the prohibition on advertising was deemed a hallmark of medicine, law, and other "true professions." In 1975, however, the U.S. Federal Trade Commission (FTC) applied the Sherman Anti-Trust Act first to the legal profession[82] and, in 1982, to the AMA's prohibition on physician advertising. The FTC argued, reiterating arguments first aired by Homberger, that the AMA prohibition against medical advertising was an illegal constraint of free trade and that consumers of medical services should have the same rights to information enjoyed by other consumers of commercial services.[83] The decision terminated the prohibition on advertising that for more than a century had been considered a hallmark of the American professions, essential to their very definition. Yet even though law firms, hospitals, and medical practices advertised, they retained their status as the prototypes of everything professional. Homberger was right: the prohibition against advertising was a historical accident, an intrusion of older ideals of gentlemanly honor into the new concept of a professional—and it was ultimately found inessential to medicine's status as a profession.

THE EXCLUSION OF FEMALE PHYSICIANS

Gentlemen are male by definition and white by historical precedent. Were professionals also to be defined as male and white as well? This issue was raised at the AMA's 1866 national meeting, when the question was raised as to whether consulting with regularly educated female practitioners violated the consultation clause. Henry Ingersoll Bowditch, who was chairing the committee on ethics, defended consultation with female medical practitioners as consonant with the *Code of Medical of Ethics*. "Every member of this Association," Bowditch argued, "has the right to consult with any regularly and thoroughly educated practitioner of medicine, whether male or female."

> In our code the masculine gender is indeed used in the article relating to the consultations of physicians, but this is always so used in all statute laws passed by legislative bodies; yet they embrace, of course, alike men and women in their rules and penalties.... This being admitted, the [Code

> states] the following, "A regular medical education furnishes the only presumptive evidence of professional abilities and acquirements; and ought to be the only acknowledged right of an individual to the exercise and honors of his profession." Bearing in mind the previous remarks upon the proper interpretation of the use of the masculine gender in alluding to medical practitioners [and]... according to the rules of reason unbiased by prejudice... [a member of this Association] has no right to refuse a consultation simply on the ground of sex. If the Association does not adopt this view, it ought, for consistency's sake forthwith to publish an explanatory amendment to its code and to declare that its Ethics do not include mankind, but only men; in other words, the Association of learned and benevolent men should forthwith stultify itself by declaring that however learned, however skilled in our art, however virtuous a person may be, if that person be a woman and claims to practice medicine, we as a body will have nothing to do with her.... [No] body of intelligent and humane men would consent to such a result.[84]

Bowditch proposed the following resolution for adoption:

> That the question of sex has never been considered by this Association in connection with consultations among medical practitioners, and that, in the opinion of this meeting, every member of this body has a perfect right to consult with anyone who presents "the only presumptive evidence of professional abilities and acquirements" required by this Association, "a regular medical education."[85]

After "much debate," a special session was devoted to the issue at which three founding members of the AMA debated Bowditch's resolution: gynecologist Washington Atlee of Pennsylvania (1808–1878) spoke in favor, D. Francis Condie (1796–1875) and Davis spoke against. Atlee' offered a "vigorous... advocati[ion] of the recognition of female practitioners" describing the "difficulties which had been thrown in the way of women making progress in their studies; but now they had a college of their own [The Women's Medical College of Pennsylvania founded in 1850, now Drexel College of Medicine], which was free of all reasonable objections. In other countries women had achieved the highest honors as medical practitioners."[86] Condie responded that women "would achieve higher honors in following the line of duty which had been marked out for them in the order of nature [i.e., bearing and raising children], and would do more good than in turning out physicians."[87] After this remark "was greeted with enthusiastic applause," Condie went on suggested that "the question [of] whether a male physician would consult with them ought to be left to individual judgment; let every member decide for himself.... [T]he resolution [sh]ould be...table[d], and the course to be followed left entirely to individual discretion."[88]

Davis opened his presentation with a reaffirmation of Bowditch's finding that the AMA "had never taken action upon any matter which distinguished practitioners either on account of sex or color." Having linked issues of a practitioner's sex to questions about a practitioner's "color" (i.e., race), Davis called for a "local" rather than a national interpretation of *membership*—thus switching the issue from "consultation" to "membership." "If any local association saw fit to enact a law restricting its members," Davis stated, "that was a matter for such societies to determine; but those so interfered with should not claim the legislative power of this Association to pass *ex post facto* laws for their especial benefit."[89] Having stipulated that local societies should have a right to enact segregationist rules excluding African Americans and women, Davis concludes that

> the law of the Creator has assigned [to woman] her sphere of duties; but if there was one who conscientiously believed that she could be of greater service as a physician, why should we be opposed. He was in favor of the broadest equality. If she was equal in the profession, let her be equal on the farm and in the ditch [as a laborer]. Let the members consult with whom they please if they are professionally qualified. He moved that the whole matter be indefinitely postponed.[90]

The motion carried. Davis thereby helped to defeat Bowditch's motion by linking the issue of *consultation* with female practitioners to *membership* for African-American practitioners. He also argued that local medical societies had the prerogative of adopting segregationist rules to deny membership to African-American and female physicians and that the national society, the AMA, did not have the right to prevent such discriminatory membership rules. Having supported the legitimacy of segregation and exclusion by local societies, Davis declared, sarcastically, that he did not oppose female physicians—even though they defied the Creator in rejecting the role of bearing and rearing children that He had designed for them. Davis would elaborate on his views on female physicians eighteen years later, in an editorial in the *Journal of the American Medical Association*, in which he argues that a "professional education...is an enormous outlay of physiological force; much more than a woman can afford if she is to produce her proper functions as a producer of men."[91]

National events at the time of the AMA's national conference, in May 1868, provide the context against which Davis's remarks should be read. The nation was debating the Fourteenth Amendment to the U.S. Constitution, which would be ratified two months later, on July 9, 1868.[92] Among other things, the amendment supported the controversial civil rights act of 1866 (passed over the veto of President Andrew Johnson [1808–1875]) according civil rights to newly freed African Americans. The amendment and the earlier civil rights laws outlawed racially discriminatory laws, known as Black Codes, that had been enacted by former Confederate states to deprive African Americans of their civil rights. It specifically prevents a state from denying "to any person within its jurisdiction the equal protection of the laws" or depriving them of "life, liberty or property without due process of law."

Read in the context of this debate, Davis's proposal—that "[i]f any local association saw fit to enact a law restricting its members, that was a matter for such societies to determine; but those so interfered with should not claim the legislative power of this Association to pass *ex post facto* laws for their especial benefit"[93]—would accord to state medical societies a right to use a Black Code, or Jim Crow admission criteria, thereby denying African Americans and women equal protection under the AMA's constitution or its *Code of Medical Ethics*. Davis would later advocate for such "local" treatment of African Americans, and the AMA adopted this policy—tolerating racial segregation in Southern medical societies and hospitals until forced to abandon it by the civil rights acts of the 1960s.

The defeat of Bowditch's proposal set a pattern for debates in 1870[94] and 1871, when proposals to prohibit discrimination against delegates from colleges or hospitals that taught or employed women medical students or physicians were also defeated. The high point of these debates occurred in 1871, when the AMA delegates defeated, by a vote of 83 to 26, a constitutional amendment permitting representatives of women's medical colleges and hospitals employing women physicians to serve as AMA delegates.[95] At the same national meeting, the delegates also defeated, on a vote of 45 to 41, a proposal acknowledging AMA members' individual right "to meet in consultation the graduates and teachers of Women's Medical Colleges."[96]

Underlying all of these debates was an inherited ethos of male chauvinism—the notion that females' God-given role was bearing and rearing children—entrenched in older ideals of gentlemanly honor. Gentlemen were males, as Alfred Stillé (1813–1900) informed the assembled delegates to the AMA's 1871 national meeting in a rambling Presidential Address, and it is unnatural for women to assume a male role. Stillé's address opens with the recognition that, strictly speaking, Bowditch's analysis is correct: the graduates of regular female medical colleges had received "appropriate training" and, given the wording of the AMA code, it would be "illogical... to refuse to recognize their professional standing." Nonetheless, Stillé remarks, "many laws [are] founded in error and... we are entitled to criticize them, and even to protest against them" by invoking natural law.[98]

> The laws of nature are eternal and immutable. The law which makes the man the father and woman the mother of children impresses upon both of them

> characters which are inseparable from their functions and their relative positions in the world; gives government to the one and subordination to the other; to the one intellect, to the other heart.... The transposition of functions in the moral or in the social world produces an unnatural being that is a satire on its proper sex.... In every department of active life man excels woman....
>
> Women may possibly become persuasive preachers, or even safe practitioners of domestic medicine; but learned and subtle divines, great lawyers, scientific physicians—never.... On the whole, then, we believe that all experience teaches that woman is characterized by a combination of distinctive qualities, of which the most striking are uncertainty of rational judgment, capriciousness of sentiment, fickleness of purpose, and indecision of action, which totally unfit her for professional pursuits.... If, then, woman is unfitted by nature to become a physician, we should, when we oppose her pretensions, be acquitted of any malicious or unkindly spirit [because]...in the practice of a scientific art...she usually displays a strange ignorance of the logic of reason, and a profound contempt for the logic of facts.[99]

The profession of medicine, in short, remains a gentlemanly prerogative because women are unfitted for it by their very nature. Of course "male representatives of female colleges" are undeniably male, but Stillé dismisses that issue because it is "not yet ripe for decision on its merits alone"[99]—a position that effectively denies females even the prospect of representation by (presumable logical and rational) males.

Having justified the exclusion of women from medicine, Stillé turns to "[a] subject kindred in some of its aspects to the one that has just been partially discussed, [that] convulsed the last annual meeting of the Association" in 1870—that is, the admission and representation of African-American physicians—which Stillé had supported.[101] Noting "the impossibility of harmonizing opinions so radically antagonistic," Stillé now commended "the...wisdom to await the soothing influences of time, and to exclude from our midst discussions which engender hostility and bitterness, instead of those feelings of brotherhood in a common family which it was one of the objects of this Association."[101]

The Exclusion of African-American Physicians

As Stillé remarked, the tranquility of the AMA—and his own—had been rattled the previous year, 1870, when three regularly educated, licensed, African-American physicians, Alexander Thomas Augusta (1825–1890), Charles Burleigh Purvis (1842–1929), and Alpheus W. Tucker, sought recognition as delegates at the

AMA's national meeting in Washington, D.C. Two medical societies represented Washington's regular practitioners: the all-white Medical Society of the District of Columbia (MSDC, founded in 1817 and still functioning) and a racially integrated society formed in 1869, the National Medical Society (NMS). The NMS had been founded, according to a congressional investigating committee, after the all-white MSDC refused to admit these same three African-American physicians, denying them membership "solely on account of color"[102]—a finding that prompted an unsuccessful attempt by Republican Senator Charles Sumner (1811–1874) to seek revocation of the MSDC's charter.

In this year charged with racial tension—the civil rights law had been passed over a presidential veto, the Fourteenth and Fifteenth Amendments were being debated, and a federal grand jury had just declared the Ku Klux Klan a terrorist organization—each of the two DC delegations challenged the credentials of the other. The MSDC's credentials were challenged on various grounds but mainly because, as the U.S. Congress and District of Columbia courts confirmed, they practiced racial discrimination against regularly educated African-American physicians. The NMS delegation was challenged primarily because it had been formed "in contempt of the organized Medical Society and has attempted, through legislative influence, to break down" the MSDC by appealing the MSDC's discriminatory practices to the U.S. Congress, thereby threatening the MSDC's charter.[103]

The matter was referred to the Committee on Ethics, thereby defining the matter of racial discrimination as an issue of medical ethics. At this time, the Committee was also considering a challenge to the credentials of an all-white Massachusetts delegation whose society was accused of harboring homeopaths. The Committee on Ethics had not yet been formed, so the AMA president appointed Stillé as chair, with Davis and delegates from Delaware, Kentucky (which had enacted a segregationist Black Code), and the U. S. Army (i.e., the Union Army) as members. On the next day, the committee ruled unanimously that "[t]he charge of tolerating in the Massachusetts Medical Society, men acknowledged to have become Homeopaths and Eclectics, is fully proved, and is plainly in violation of the Code of Ethics."[104] Following standard restorative justice practices, since members of the delegation admitted the charge, the committee ruled that the delegation would be admitted with full privileges, with the proviso that "unless said Society takes the necessary steps to purge itself of irregular practitioners, it ought not to be entitled to future representation."[105] After this announcement, similar treatment was requested for the D.C. medical societies; that is, that "all delegates from the District of Columbia be admitted." This motion "lost, ayes 107, nays 142"[106]—the first indication that African-American physicians would not be accorded the gentlemanly prerogatives accorded to whites.

The Committee on Ethics issued two reports on the admissibility of the delegates from the D.C. medical societies. The majority report, by Davis and the delegates from Delaware and Kentucky, implemented Davis's policy of local control over membership. It decreed that a congressional determination that the MSDC had discriminated against admitting qualified physicians solely on account of color or race was "not of a nature to require the action of the American Medical Association" because the alleged conduct "does not come into conflict with any part of the code of ethics"[107]—note that racial discrimination was thus deemed *not* a matter of medical ethics. It also found that "the charges against the eligibility of the [NMS] have been so far sustained that we recommend that no member of that Society should be received as delegates."[108] Legal action against a fellow physician was thus considered a violation of medical ethics. Furthermore, the African Americans were to be treated differently from the white delegates from Massachusetts and from the MSDC—they were to be denied the gentlemanly prerogative of forgiveness. The issue was thus as plain as black and white: whites were to be treated as gentlemen and admitted; blacks were banned.

The minority report by Stillé and the delegate from the Union Army took the wording of the code of ethics literally. "A regular medical education furnishes the only presumptive evidence of professional abilities and acquirements... [hence] no intelligent regular practitioner, who has a license to practice from some medical board of known and acknowledged respectability... should be fastidiously excluded from fellowship." Since the African-American physicians were regularly educated and licensed, Stillé and his Union Army colleague came to the conclusion that the

> National Medical Society, the Howard Medical College, the Freedman's Hospital, and the Smallpox Hospital, are regularly organized as the constitution of the Association requires [and that since] the physicians so excluded are qualified practitioners of medicine who have complied with all the conditions of membership imposed by this Association... no sufficient ground exists for the exclusion of such institutions and physicians... [and they] are entitled to seats in the American Medical Association.[109]

Before the matter could be put to a vote, however, a delegate from Maryland raised the question about which D.C. members had voting rights. The president ruled that since the majority report found no valid objections to the members of the MSDC, and since there were no objections to this finding on the part of the minority report, the MSDC delegates could vote. Thus, with all delegates from the all-white MSDC voting, and with none from the integrated NMS voting, a vote was taken on whether to table (i.e., to reject) the minority report. On a vote of 114 to 82, the black delegates were denied admission.

Matters did not end there. A delegate from Maine demanded an explanation from Davis "on what principle the delegates of the Medical Departments of Howard University (founded 1868) were excluded from membership."[110] Davis replied that the members were *not* excluded because they taught at Howard but because they were members of the NMS, which had "used unfair and dishonorable means to procure the destruction of the [MSDC], by inducing Congress to abrogate their charter."[111] The issue was thus redefined as ungentlemanly conduct, as if it were a mere flyte rather than a petition to the U.S. Congress for relief from racial discrimination. Amid "a storm of hisses,"[112] the AMA next took up a motion from Storer Jr.'s practice partner, John L. Sullivan of Massachusetts, "[t]hat no distinction of race or color shall exclude from the Association persons claiming admission and duly accredited thereto."[113] This motion was tabled (i.e., rejected) by a vote of 106 to 60. Storer Jr. himself then sought to whitewash the defeat of this resolution by proposing

> [t]hat inasmuch as it has been distinctly stated and proved that the consideration of race and color has had nothing whatsoever to do with the decision of the question of the reception of the Washington delegates, and inasmuch as charges have been distinctly made in open session today attaching the stigma of dishonor to parties implicated, which charges have not been denied by them, though present, therefore, the report of the majority of the Committee on Ethics be declared, as to all intents and purposes, unanimously adopted by the Association.[114]

This is an odd motion since it had never been stated nor proved that considerations of race or color had nothing to do with the decision to exclude the African-American delegates, which turned, after all, on the propriety of their appeal to Congress for redress against racial discrimination. Nonetheless, the resolution passed 112 to 34.

Seldom has history been so rapidly revised to salve a guilty conscience. Everyone at that meeting knew that the real issue was race: the *New York Times* summarized the events at the AMA under the headline "The Doctors: The Question of Color";[115] the *Boston Medical and Surgical Journal* characterized it as "a muss over the question of giving the Negro doctor his rights.... The question of color is mixed up with a dozen other quarrels."[116] As Stillé remarked in his presidential speech the next year, "the colored physician, and even his white representative, [was] refused admission upon the ground that the proposal is an outrage to the Association and a personal insult to many of its members"[117]; that is, Southerners found the admission of African Americans to *their* organization, the AMA, to be "a personal insult." A white commentator reporting on these matters in the *National Medical Journal* observed that the real question facing the authors of the majority report was "how were these colored men who claimed admission to be excluded, and yet make it to appear that they were not excluded on grounds of color? Nothing less would please or satisfy the southern brethren and their sympathizers, and yet the thing was somehow monstrous, and would need a plausible excuse before others."[118] This white commentator also remarks on the hypocrisy of allowing the white Massachusetts delegation to be seated "even though charges of medical irregularity [against them] 'had been sustained'.... Here they are careful of personal rights, even in a flagrant case,... [while those of] two or three colored doctors... are most unceremoniously ignored."[119] The commentator continues:

> In all the [Civil] war I did not see a more acute attack of judicial hardening. I can conceive of how men may dispute the political status of the negro; how by reason of numbers and his ill-culture they may differ as to promiscuous citizenship, (for I myself are of that opposing element); but when a man of certified competence and character knocks at the door of a great national association, claiming to represent legitimate practice, and because of his color a body like ours goes manipulating about for some excuse to keep the man out, it is too trivial and sad to record. Why, that question was decided long ago. The equalities of science are older than that of politics.... I doubt whether in the last fifty years, a national scientific has convened anywhere that would have excluded a competent scientist on the ground of color, and least of all should a medical man take such a stand.... We degrade not him but ourselves by such breaches of the law of ethics which indwells in science.[120]

Any lingering doubts about whether race was an issue were removed in 1872, when Robert Reyburn (1833–1909), a white former Union Army officer and military surgeon, a founder of the Freedman's Hospital and of Howard University, and, at the time, dean of the Howard Medical College, presented credentials to the AMA as a delegate representing these integrated institutions. A Committee on Ethics chaired by Davis refused to recognize his credentials, contending (falsely) that in the 1870s Howard was deemed in violation of the AMA's code of ethics and stating (truly) that Howard allowed females to serve on its faculty. Reyburn replied in a short speech defending

> Howard University... [which] received all who applied for medical education, without distinction of color or of sex.... If the [American Medical] Association see fit that institutions of that class shall not be represented, of course they have the power so to act, but, at the same time, they should consider well what they were doing before taking such a step [since] every human being should be allowed the right to the very highest development that God has made him capable of.[121]

After some speeches, the AMA voted to refuse to recognize the integrated D.C. medical institutions: the Academy of Medicine, Freedman's Hospital, and Howard University.

In 1873 and 1874, Davis fully implemented a more stringent version of his "localist" strategy, deeding to local societies the prerogative of determining criteria that could include—or exclude—membership in their organizations.[122] State societies in the North would be free to recognize integrated local societies, Southern state societies (which, for this purpose would include the MSDC) could segregate if they wished—and the issue of race and sex would no longer disturb the national medical society, the AMA. For African-American physicians in the South, this meant that segregationist state societies could freely discriminate against them without violating the rules of the national society.

Excluded from the Southern state and local medical societies, within a decade, African-American medical societies were founded as an alternative.[123] In 1895, these societies banded together to form an African-American alternative to the AMA, the National Medical Association (NMA). In the words of one of its founders, the NMA was "Conceived in no spirit of racial exclusiveness, fostering no ethnic antagonism, but born of the exigencies of the [segregated] American environment.... [It] has for its object the banding together for mutual cooperation and helpfulness, the men and women of African descent who are legally and honorably engaged in the practice of the cognate professions of medicine, surgery, pharmacy and dentistry."[124]

The creation of a racially segregated medical system severely limited opportunities for African-American physicians. Nineteenth-century medical societies were more than social organizations in which physicians advanced their careers by networking with fellow professionals. They served as a conduit for liaising with municipal, county, and state governments; with licensing and regulatory bodies; and with bankers and realtors. Exclusion from these societies meant professional isolation, restricted access to information and training, and limitations on professional and business contacts. As in schools and sports, the segregation of African Americans from the mainstream of American life led to a two-tier system of medicine, separate and unequal. Tragically, to secure reunion with the well-established (white male) medical societies of the South, Davis and the AMA haggled away the civil rights of African-American physicians by sophistries that trashed the integrationist ideals of returning Union soldiers like Reyburn.

A new ending was written for the story of the AMA and African-American physicians on July 30, 2008, when, instantiating the spirit of restorative justice, another "Davis," Ronald Davis (1956–2008), Immediate Past President of the AMA, met with NMA members in Atlanta to offer an apology. "I humbly come to the physicians of today's National Medical Association, to tell you that we are sorry... [O]n behalf of the American Medical Association, I unequivocally apologize for our past behavior. We pledge to do everything in our power to right the wrongs that were done by our organization to African-American physicians and their families and their patients."[125] A formal written apology had appeared earlier in the *Journal of the American Medical Association.*[126] Both apologies were triggered by a report that the AMA had commissioned for an independent panel of scholars, the Writing Group for the History of African Americans and Organized Medicine.[127] This group was convened in 2005 and delivered its report to the AMA board in 2008.[128] President Ronald Davis summarized the Writing Group's findings as follows:

> In an article published in this issue of *JAMA*,[129] Baker and colleagues—review and analyze "the historical roots of the black-white divide in US medicine." This panel of experts, convened and supported by the AMA, found that (1) in the early years following the Civil War, the AMA declined to embrace a policy of nondiscrimination and excluded an integrated local medical society through selective enforcement of membership standards; (2) from the 1870s through the late 1960s, the AMA failed to take action against AMA-affiliated state and local medical associations that openly practiced racial exclusion in their memberships—practices that functionally excluded most African American physicians from membership in the AMA; (3) in the early decades of the 20th century, the AMA listed African American physicians as "colored" in its national physician directory and was slow to remove the designation in response to protests from the National Medical Association (NMA); and (4) the AMA was silent in debates over the Civil Rights Act of 1964 and put off repeated NMA requests to support efforts to amend the Hill-Burton Act's "separate but equal" provision, which allowed construction of segregated hospital facilities with federal funds.
>
> These dishonorable acts of omission and commission reflected the social mores and racial segregation that existed during those times throughout much of the United States. But that context does not excuse them. The medical profession, which is based on a boundless respect for human life, had an obligation to lead society away from disrespect of so many lives. The AMA failed to do so and has apologized for that failure.[130]

The NMA graciously accepted the AMA's apology, and the medical societies have since collaborated on a series of projects addressing racial disparities in American healthcare.[131]

8

THE ANTI-CODE REVOLT: LAISSEZ-FAIRE MEDICAL ETHICS, 1876–1979

Your Committee do not recommend any alteration in the present Code of Ethics.
Report of the Judicial Council, Nathan Smith Davis, 1874

The Code [of Ethics] is of necessity a dead letter...an instrument of torture and oppression [for] prosecuting a fellow member.

AMA Presidential Address, James Marion Sims, Gynecologist, 1876

Medical ethics...without...penalties...[produces] a suggestive and advisory document.

Principles of Medical Ethics, American Medical Association, 1903

These principles are intended to aid physicians.... They are not laws.

Principles of Medical Ethics, American Medical Association, 1957

The focus of this chapter is an often-ignored prequel to the bioethics revolution: the transformation of the American Medical Association's (AMA) instrument of ethical self-regulation, the 1847 *Code of Medical Ethics*, once an icon of professional pride, into a loathed instrument of inquisition. After a sampling of Nathan Smith Davis's obstructionist reading of the AMA Code (the Davis quotation that opens this chapter) and some tales of the officious, oppressive, self-satisfied regime imposed on medicine in the name of "ethics," the chapter narrates the origins of a revolt by an alliance of specialists, sanitarians, and scientists (Sims's opening quotation), who, led by the Medical Society of the State of New York (MSSNY), opted out of the AMA rather than submit to its code of ethics. Eventually, as the balance of power and prestige in medicine shifted from general practice to hospital, public health, and specialist medicine, these rebels took charge of the AMA and substituted purely advisory laissez-faire principles (see 1903 opening quotation) for the "tyranny" of the AMA's code of ethics. Consequently, laissez-faire became organized medicine's approach to non-intrapractitioner medical ethics through most of the twentieth century (the 1957 quotation). Conceptually disarmed by this permissive approach to medical ethics, the AMA could not cope with the morally disruptive technologies of the 1960s and the research scandals of the 1970s. Its ineptitude in responding to these challenges created a need and a space that would be filled by an alliance of humanist-clinicians and researchers with outsiders (bureaucrats, lawyers, legislators, philosophers, former theologians) who would invent, justify, and implement bioethics as an alternative to laissez-faire medical ethics.

DAVIS'S PHARISAICAL INTERPRETATION OF THE 1847 *CODE OF MEDICAL ETHICS*

This convoluted tale opens in the 1870s, with an analysis of Davis's "pharisaical" treatment of the AMA's 1847 *Code of Medical Ethics*. "Pharisaical" is a marvelous nineteenth-century term referencing the priests criticized by Jesus for offering an excessively narrow, hypocritically censorious reading of scripture.[1] Critics applied the term to Nathan Smith Davis because of his tendency to regard anything *not explicitly permitted* by the 1847 code of ethics as if it were expressly forbidden by the code. Davis's narrow reading of the code led to interminable, mind-numbing ethics debates at the AMA's national conventions in the 1850s and 1860s. By the 1870s, even Davis's allies were complaining loudly about the "fruitless discussion of…ethics" at conventions.[2] So Davis invented a bureaucratic mechanism to remove these debates from the convention floor: a Judicial Council that dealt with ethics issues quietly.[3] Retaining his prerogatives as ethicist-in-chief, however, Davis became the council's founding chairman.

The new Judicial Council's first order of business was to ask "thirty or forty men in different parts of the country who might be supposed to represent the general sentiment of the profession in their respective districts" whether the 1847 Code should be revised.[4] According to Davis, eleven respondents opposed the 1847 Code, contending that it should be radically revised so that it would "retain nothing except the rules governing the intercourse of physicians with each other, [or they] object[ed] to any *written* rules [whatsoever], claiming that the unwritten sense of *honor*... is sufficient to afford all needed guidance and control."[5] Nonetheless, Davis concluded, since fourteen of the twenty-five respondents favored no revision of the code whatsoever, "any important changes in the Code would be in direct opposition to the wishes of a large majority of those for whose guidance it was framed."[6]

Dismissing all calls for revision out of hand,[7] Davis focused on specialists' objections to the code's restrictions on advertising a physician's specialty training (e.g., characterizing oneself as a "gynecologist" or an "ophthalmologist" on business cards or office signs; see discussion of the Homberger dispute in Chapter 7). "Specialists," Davis contended, are really general practitioners who happen to "limit their practice to some one class of diseases." Consequently, specialists must obey the same rules as other general practitioners "for no enlightened body of men can consistently have one code of morals for one part of its members, and another code for the rest." Thus, "[i]f the one may not issue cards, hand-bills, etc., calling attention... to themselves, neither can the other."[8]

Davis's rhetorical strategy was a combination of sophistry—defining "specialist" in a manner that obscures the points under contention—and a pharisaical reading of the text, treating anything not expressly permitted in the 1847 code as if it were forbidden by the code. Thus, Davis argued that since the 1847 code "makes no mention of specialties or specialists,"[9] they are not approved by the code. This interpretation obscures the fact that when the code was written specialist training was nonexistent in the United States. Two of the code's primary authors, Emerson and Hays, for example, were pioneering specialists—Emerson in epidemiology and Hays in ophthalmology[10]—yet they received the same training as their co-author, Bell, a general practitioner. A quarter of a century later, however, specialty medicine had evolved, and no one could competently practice gynecology or ophthalmology without additional training. In Europe, specialized training was indicated in medical directories and on physicians' business cards and office signs.[11] American gynecologists, ophthalmologists, and other specialists sought the same treatment—but Davis's sophistries and pharisaical readings thwarted their initiatives.

Davis extended a (poisoned) olive branch to the specialists in an apparent compromise: "those who wish to pursue a special practice [can] make known their position to their brethren and the public... not by special... titles, such as *oculist, gynecologist*, but by a simple honest notice appended to the ordinary card of the general practitioner, saying, 'Practice limited to diseases of the eye and ear,' or 'to diseases peculiar to women.'" "Such a simple notice of limitation," Davis suggested, would not be "regarded as a claim to special or superior qualifications," or "give the specialist any privileges" or "invest him with a special advantage inconsistent with the equality of rights and duties pertaining to the profession."[12] Thus, in the name of "honesty," physicians who had invested additional time and money to undergo specialty training should inform the public that their practice was *more limited* than that of general practitioners, who had not received such training. Adding insult to sophistry, Davis denied "gynecologists" and "ophthalmologists" use of their names. "What's in a name?" Juliet protested, "That which we call a rose by any other name would smell as sweet." Except that Davis thought "gynecologist" sounded sweeter to the public's ear than "practice limited to diseases peculiar to women." Davis's pharisaical reading of the code would drive specialty medicine out of the AMA, forcing it to evolve separately from the national society, rather than as branches of it, which is how it evolved in Britain.

Davis also focused his conservative gaze on contract practice. Medical contracts had been in use in the Americas from the colonial period onward. Individuals and municipalities contracted for cures; that is, they paid physicians a fee only if cured by a certain time,[13] or they contracted with physicians, like Emerson, to serve as a quarantine officer for a specific time period. Medical societies favored a different form of payment: fee for service. Thus, societies would publish fee ranges for specific services: home visits, office visits, night visits, delivering a baby, protracted delivery of a baby, minor surgery, major or difficult surgery, consultations, and so forth. Contract practice, in contrast, paid physicians not for specific services but either for outcomes (contract for cures) or for service for a specified time period. Contracts were becoming commonplace as mining and railroad companies, residential schools and colleges explored contracting with physicians to be on call to attend to their employees or students on an annual basis.

Contract practice was a hotly debated issue in the late 1860s and 1870s. In 1869, the AMA even voted to classify all "contract physicians" as "irregulars,"[14] relegating them to the same status as homeopaths and Thomsonians: it later retracted this classification in 1877, after local societies protested.[15] Some respondents to Davis's survey had urged that the code of ethics be revised to legitimate contract practice. Davis, however, found no reason for revision, opining that the code as written was "inconsistent with all contracts or, agreements to attend individuals, families, companies, corporations, or any associations or institutions...for a specified sum per month or year."[16] Hinting at his motive, Davis remarks further that the very "idea of asking members of the profession to bid against each other...is repugnant to every feeling of professional honor."[17] He observes, moreover, that "[i]t is...very desirable to so manage all our pecuniary relations...that we avoid creating the impression on the public mind that the profession...[is] little better than mere trades-unions, having for their chief object mutual pecuniary protection."[18] In Davis's mind the medical profession inhabited an elevated social space: gentlemanly, noncommercial, charitable, honorable, serving the public as neither a business nor a trade union, and above such ungentlemanly practices as advertising, competing with peers by claiming special expertise, or bidding for contracts.

ENDING EXCLUSION AND CHALLENGING THE CODE: SIMS'S PRESIDENTIAL ADDRESS, 1876

In 1876, South Carolina-born New Yorker James Marion Sims, honored in his own time as "the father of modern gynecology,"[19] became the first eminent specialist to publicly challenge the legitimacy of the AMA's *Code of Medical Ethics*. Sims had no love for codes of medical ethics, having been censured and expelled from the New York Academy of Medicine (NYAM) just five years earlier for breaching patient confidentiality and for self-promotional advertising, having revealed medical information about one of his patients in the pages of the *New York Times* (see discussion in Chapter 5). Presiding as AMA president, Sims may have felt that he held the moral high ground since he had just made institutional history by resolving "the woman question and the Negro question" (see discussion in Chapter 7). Welcoming Sarah Ann Hackett Stevenson of Illinois (1841–1909) as a delegate to the AMA's national meeting, Sims opened the organization's doors by presidential fiat to any other "woman entering the medical profession" and to "any colored man [who] should rise to the dignity of representing a State or County Medical Society." "Thus," he proclaimed, "these knotty questions are settled forever."[20] From this point forward, African-American and female delegates would no longer be excluded from national meetings of the AMA—although local societies retained the prerogative of excluding African Americans and women from membership.

Having officially ended the ignominy of gender and racial discrimination, Sims turned to the instrument that had been used to exclude African-American and female physicians from the AMA, its *Code of Medical Ethics*.

> I would not shock the moral sense of this august body by speaking of [the *Code of Medical Ethics*] in irreverent terms; for I know that there are many, indeed a large majority, of this Association who believe it to be as perfect as the Decalogue, and as incapable of improvement. It is looked upon by some of its High Priests as the Holy of Holies, and not to be desecrated by the touch of vulgar hands. It is only by observing the practical operation of laws that we can judge of their fitness and usefulness. Let us measure our Code by this universal standard.[21]

Measuring the code by this utilitarian standard, Sims found it wanting. Why, he asked, may French physicians advertise their names and specialties in directories while American physicians "wishing to change [their] place of residence [struggle to] notify the world...without violating the Code of Ethics."[22] "These are honest and honorable men and would not willfully do anything wrong. But they feel...hampered by rules that are unjust and oppressive. Pardon me if I ask you, 'Is the Code of Ethics up to the requirements of the times, when it compels honorable men to do dishonorable things to promote an honest action?'"[23] Probing the prohibition on patents (see discussion in Chapter 7), Sims observes, "[a]ccording to our Code, [an inventor] dare not, take out a patent...simply because he is a practicing physician.... Does the profession at large, or does the public, derive any benefit by thus depriving him of his invention? None whatever. We simply compel him to give his invention, his time and labor, to enrich the instrument maker."[24] "Indeed," Sims concludes, "When we speak of violating the spirit of the Code, we may all as one man cry out, 'He that is without sin among you, let him first cast a stone.'"[25]

Sims was pointing out that by condemning as unethical such morally innocent practices as informing patients of a change in address, the AMA's code of ethics was at variance with practitioners' understanding of the morality of medicine. Alluding, perhaps, to his own censure by the NYAM, Sims remarks that because Davis's reading of the code makes ethics the enemy of the innocent, it can be used as "an engine of torture and oppression—that men, jealously, maliciously intent upon persecuting a fellow member, may distort...to suit their malign purposes, thus entering into a regular conspiracy to blacken character."[26] Sims continues:

> This is the first time that the validity, the constitutionality, of the Code has been openly called in question. But every honest thinking man here, with a particle of self-respect and self-reliance, has at times felt an inward protest against its unequal operation.... The time will come (but not yet) when your organic laws, like the constitution of our country, will require modifications and amendments to suit a higher intelligence, a broader education, and a greater destiny. Remember, that when our Code was adopted, we had no telegraph...and but few railroads; the profession was not educated up to its present level, medicine was more of a mystery than it is now.... Modern thought and modern progress...will never be content with the slow uncertain movement of olden times.[27]

Nonetheless, except for repeal of the ruling condemning contract practitioners as "irregulars,"[28] Sims's recommendations for revising the code of ethics came to naught.

NEW YORKERS REBEL, OPTING FOR A NEW CODE OF ETHICS

As gynecological, ophthalmological, and other specialty societies began to form from the 1860s onward, they did so outside of the AMA, mindful of the association's hostility to advertising and its rejection of the very concept of specialization. Yet specialists themselves were still members in good standing of county medical societies and were often delegates to AMA conventions—even, as in Sims's case, serving as its president. By the 1880s, specialists' schizophrenic relationship with the AMA broke down in a conflict that would ultimately split the MSSNY into two rival societies and that would lead, in 1881, to a congress of the specialist societies that had formed outside of the AMA, the Congress of American Physicians and Surgeons. By 1886, such luminaries as Sir William Osler (1849–1919) and Francis Delafield (1841–1915) transformed the congress into a national medical society that served as a rival to the AMA, the Association of American Physicians (AAP, founded in 1886 and still functioning). In his inaugural address as president of the AAP, Delafield proudly proclaimed that this was "an association in which there will be no medical politics and no medical ethics."[29]

How had the AMA's *Code of Medical Ethics*, once the pride of the profession, become so anathema that it led to the formation of a rival national medical society whose president denounced the very idea of medical ethics? The precipitating incident occurred in New York State. Two physicians, one a graduate of a homeopathic college,[30] the other a graduate of a women's college,[31] applied for membership to two different county medical societies. Mindful of New York State's new licensing law,[32] both applicants submitted signed affidavits affirming that they would not engage in irregular medical practices and would abide by their society's ethics codes and bylaws. Seeking to sustain their purity (see discussion of the Warner-Wolpe purity hypothesis in Chapter 6), the *comita* of these two county societies were inclined to reject these applications. Yet, because the applicants held valid licenses to practice in New York State and because the *comita* were uncertain of the legal significance of the applicants' affidavits, they sought legal counsel. Both of the law firms consulted proffered precisely the same advice—admit the applicants! So a graduate of a homeopathic college and of a women's medical college were admitted to two different county medical societies in New York State. Contesting this decision, physicians from these societies appealed to the national society, filing complaints with the AMA's Judicial Council. The Judicial Council then censured the offending county societies for violating the AMA's *Code of Medical Ethics* and excluded their delegates from the national convention. In retaliation, a *comita* from an excluded county society censured the physician who had complained to the AMA.

This messy mix of censure and retaliatory censure was dumped into the lap of the MSSNY, which appointed a two-person *comita* to resolve the issue. The two persons were Cornelius Agnew (1830–1888), of the College of Physicians and Surgeons, and Thomas Hun (1808–1896), of Albany Medical College.[33] They ruled in favor of the local medical societies on the grounds that "in their applications for membership" the licensed female and homeopathic physician had "declared their allegiance to the codes of Ethics."[34] In justifying their ruling, Agnew and Hun expressly reject the impurity-stigma conception of homeopathy, construing homeopathy as an "error" rather than a sin.

> It seems eminently desirable and proper, that all homeopaths and irregular practitioners should be advised and encouraged to renounce their errors and qualify themselves for admission to what we esteem the regular profession. It would be a singular position for the profession to take, that a person who had once entered on an erroneous system of medicine, should be considered as having committed a sin against the profession, for which no subsequent repentance could atone.[35]

Commenting on these issues in his presidential address to the MSSNY, William Bailey (1825–1898) mused that "[w]e have perhaps, reached a time, when it may be well to drop the word 'ethics,' with its present and past meaning, and adopt some new term which will express or suggest a different idea... when we may assume that only gentlemen occupy the profession, and need no code for civil treatment of each other."[36] After all, Bailey remarked, codes of ethics are "but an appendix to [the] real work and scope" of a medical society whose primary function is "educational and intellectual."[37] To implement these ideas, a committee was formed to revise the MSSNY's code of ethics.

In February 1882, this committee recommended a new code. The opening twenty-six lines of the new code reaffirm traditional prohibitions against advertising and patents, repeating, virtually word for word, the statement of these prohibitions in the AMA's Code. This near verbatim reproduction of text underlines that the MSSNY was not challenging the AMA over these issues. In the next forty-eight lines of the code, however, absences speak louder than words. Notably absent was the AMA's prohibition against consulting with homeopaths; missing from the code as well was any discussion of the ethics of the physician–patient relationship. Bailey had suggested that if the MSSNY could "not drop its written law of ethics entirely," it should "at least, limit it to a much narrower field of regulation."[38] He had also remarked that "constant association with the sick and afflicted naturally develops [the physician's] sympathetic nature.... He inevitably becomes the confidential friend of the family, and being true to the trust placed in his discretion and honor, carefully guards their secrets and honors their confidence."[39] Consequently, since living the medical life naturally inspires one to become sympathetic, formal codes of ethics for the physician–patient relations seem redundant. Thus, no rules for confidentiality were needed because confidentiality was naturally implicit in the physician–patient relationship. Instantiating Bailey's theory, the MSSNY's new code lacks any statement on physicians' duties with respect to confidentiality.

Some MSSNY members, soon labeled "Old Coders," objected to the new code; others, soon labeled "New Coders," advocated for the new code; and yet a third group, "No Coders," backed an even more radical notion: that no code of medical ethics was necessary. A verbal donnybrook broke out between the Coders: Old, New, and No. Two former Union Army surgeons took the lead in a formal debate: Truman Squire (1823–1889) from Elmira, New York, championed the Old Code; Daniel Bennett St. John Roosa (1838–1908) otologist, ophthalmologist, and City University of New York (NYU) professor became the voice of No Coders. Roosa urged abolishing the "sentimental code of our forefathers, which tells us how our patients should behave towards us and which enters into such innumerable details, as to the relations we sustain to our fellow-men, that it is impossible to believe that the authors of it thought the medical profession was entitled to any discretion in the management of its own professional affairs." "The sentiment of the profession," Roosa proclaimed on behalf of fellow specialists, is to "wipe out the code of ethics from its beginning to its end…[leaving] such matters to be settled by the individual discretion and wisdom and good faith of each man in affiliation with this Society."[40]

Speaking for Old Coders, who tended to be general practitioners, Squire protested that the "report of the Committee comes far short of what we should have as a code of ethics…it cannot properly be called a code; for a code should be a system—should be a whole; this is only fragmentary, it does not contain any declaration of the moral principles, the more important of which should govern us as a profession if we are to have a code." "It does not," for example, "require physicians to say that there is any dividing line between the practice of medicine and the practice of quackery," and "nothing is said in regard to confidential communications."[41]

"The spirit which governed us in making up this code," replied New Coder Samuel Oakley Vanderpoel (1824–1886), chair of pathology and clinical medicine at Albany Medical College and former president of the MSSNY, "was that it would be impossible to affect…gentlemanly conduct between man and man. We cannot make a man a gentleman unless he is made so by nature; it is utterly impossible to bind men in these relations by a code of medical ethics." Consequently, "we left [discussion of the physician–patient relationship] out of our report….We believe that no written restrictions can affect the moral character of the man….We made a code as liberal as we can."[42]

The MSSNY's new president, Abraham Jacobi (1830–1919), professor at the College of Physicians and Surgeons, voiced more practical concerns. A German-Jewish political refugee who had fled to New York City after being imprisoned for participating in the revolution of 1848, Jacobi had established the first hospital-based department of pediatrics in the United States at the Jews Hospital (founded in 1852, now the Mount Sinai Medical Center). Mindful of the assistance that homeopaths were rendering him in public health campaigns for boiled (i.e., pasteurized) milk, pure drinking water, and in defeating antivivisectionist legislation,[43] Jacobi endorsed the new code, arguing that it was good medical politics to cement an alliance with the homeopaths.

> The homeopaths claim that they do not differ from us, as formerly they did and proudly claimed to do.... A crowd of men facing the profession with the battle cry of "*similia similibus*" and "no quarter," exclude themselves and cannot expect kind treatment at our hands. When the ranks, however, are dissolved, and... men come into your camp for reconciliation, and a parley, the case is different.
>
> [Moreover] it is more than expedient, it is absolutely necessary, that in many steps to be taken before the Legislature of the State we should be in full concord with those who share with us the honor of being called lawful practitioners.... In that hope, I am quite prepared to submit to the reports and recommendations of your committees... on the revision of the code of ethics.[44]

Jacobi also noted that the current generation of homeopaths was taking cognizance of the (Forbes-Holmes) scientific critique of their therapeutics and was working with regulars to adopt common educational standards. Thus, as Jacobi put it diplomatically, "imbued with that spirit of logic and experimental science, characteristic of modern medicine, we may overlook our differences, and meet with a spirit of reconciliation."[45]

After the speeches ended, parliamentary skirmishes began: the MSSNY adopted the new code by a vote of 52 to 18. In the same year, 1882, the AMA Judicial Council censured the MSSNY, excluding its delegates from the national convention.[46] This led to a motion at the next MSSNY meeting to rescind the new code and return to the old code: that motion was defeated by a vote of 105 (for retaining the new code) to 99 (for returning to the old code). These votes culminated in a walkout in which Old Coders split from the MSSNY to form the New York State Medical Association. The upshot was that regular medical societies in New York split into two statewide medical societies: one, consisting primarily of general practitioners, adhered to the Old Code and was recognized by the AMA; and the other, led by Agnew, Jacobi, and Roosa, was comprised mainly of specialists, scientists, and sanitarians. It subscribed to the New Code and was excluded from the AMA. Adding fuel to an already combustible conflict, the AMA vindictively barred Jacobi and other New Coders from the International Congress of Medicine that it hosted in 1887—even though these men were largely responsible for bringing this prestigious European event to America. As Surgeon General John Shaw Billings wrote to a fellow organizer, "All New Code men were dropped [from the International Conference. The other organizers] and myself have resigned from the committee. It is a bad piece of business."[47] America's regular medical profession was engaging in fratricide.

The Battle of the Ethics Books: 1882–1884

On a more cerebral level, the conflict was played out in a battle of ethics books. Firing the opening salvo was Austin Flint (1812–1886), distinguished long-standing NYAM president (from 1872–1885), who was about to become president of the AMA (1884).[48] Seeking to persuade New and No Coders of the value of the AMA's *Code of Medical Ethics*, Flint published the code with an elaborate commentary in which he defended the need to formulate a special ethics for physician–patient interactions. Medical practice, Flint contended, creates "peculiar responsibilities." For, unlike ordinary people, physicians become "intimately acquainted" with "the private character of…patients" whose "weaknesses, faults, vices, cannot be concealed" and so physicians may not gossip about people in the manner of laypersons. Physicians also deal intimately with patients' bodies and so are "exposed to peculiar temptations" that require an ethics of constraint. Moreover, physicians are required to offer "opinions concerning the nature…and the termination of diseases to patients and their friends" and are called upon to offer "testimony…in courts of law."[49] The rules of moral conduct formulated in the AMA code offer a guide to proper courses of action in these extraordinary contexts and also serve to constrain those whose "moral perceptions may be defective."[50]

Flint also argued that it is important to formally state a physician's duty of confidentiality,[51] if only to note that it does not imply the "absurd…view…that nothing is to be communicated to friends, acquaintances or the public respecting…the condition of a patient in respect of danger.…[Information] may properly be made known to those who are interested in the patient's welfare."[52] The patient's right of confidentiality is otherwise absolute and extends even to criminals. "No matter how heinous the crime, the wretched criminal has a right to medical services in sickness [and]…the duty of the doctor…relates exclusively to the patient [and not to the state]. He would be debarred from medical services were it understood that physicians are to play the role of…informers.…The ethical rule is without exceptions."[53] Flint recognizes that this may put a physician at odds with courts of law, but the conscientious physician refuses to testify, whatever the personal consequences.[54]

In 1882, Jacobi and other New Coders formed a Society for the Prevention of the Re-enactment of the Present Code of Ethics of the American Medical Association. The society replied to Flint with a collection of essays.[55] Roosa, the only essayist to discuss confidentiality, stakes out a position strikingly different from Flint's. Dismissing the idea that gentlemen need a code to inform them of the proprieties of the physician–patient relationship as "*unnecessary and positively puerile*," Roosa remarks, "[a]s to the obligation of secrecy in professional matters . . . the law determines just how far information obtained by physicians may be made a matter of evidence."[56] Although New York State law in the 1880s privileged patients' communications to their physicians, nonetheless, as Flint notes in his response, there were exceptions: a "female's name," for example, "is not privileged" if she consults a physician about an illegal abortion.[57] Flint contended that physicians' moral obligations of "professional confidence" were applicable even in these contexts. Consequently, if the courts demand disclosure of the names of women seeking illegal abortions, physicians should brave "penalties incident to . . . the requirement [that] professional confidence should be inviolable."[58] For Flint, the morality of professional conduct superseded the obligation to obey the law; for Roosa, personal conscience was limited by the strictures of law.

Alfred Charles Post (1806–1886), Delafield's colleague at the College of Physicians and Surgeons, epitomized No Coder libertarianism in his slogan, "Why is my liberty judged by another conscience?"[59] Post proclaimed it "the natural right of every practitioner of the healing art to act, according to the dictates of his own conscience . . . . This is a right of which he ought not to be deprived by the action of a bare majority of his colleagues in the profession, or even by that of a very large and decided majority."[60] Worse still, Post protested, was the "bitter and persecuting spirit . . . exhibited by some of the advocates of the old code" in imposing their moral views on others.[61] Reiterating these libertarian themes, Lewis Pilcher (1845–1934), founding editor of the *Annals of Surgery* (from 1885 to 1934) and future president of the American Surgical Association (1918), issued a searing indictment of the AMA's *Code of Medical Ethics*. The code, Pilcher charged, "has tended to foster the creation of . . . a class of men who think much of the strict letter of the code . . . medical Pharisees . . . who . . . feel at liberty to coolly ride rough-shod over the rights of others when such rights are not protected by any distinct provision of the code."[62]

The AMA code thus "fostered . . . a spirit of censoriousness in the profession. It tends to make every man a spy upon his neighbor, and has made persecutions of the most petty nature possible. . . . It has created a multitude of star-chambers all over the land, in which men have assumed the right to sit in judgment upon . . . their peers as to the motives and methods of their professional conduct."[63] Pilcher was proposing as an alternative what might be called laissez-faire libertarian ethics—the ethics of letting physicians use their own individual conscience as a guide to their professional conduct.

> A physician is not a member of a guild or corporation, the rules of which he must comply with in order to retain his membership therein, and to enjoy its benefits, but a member of a liberal profession, the rules of which are the unwritten law of humanity. . . . The approval of his own conscience, the respect and good-will of his colleagues, and the confidence of the people will always be the marks that will indicate the perfection with which he complies with the ethics of his profession, while their loss is the worst of penalties that can follow his dereliction.[64]

"There is but one logical outcome to my reasoning," Pilcher contended—laissez-faire ethics, "the rejection of the present code of the American Medical Association, or of any like set of definite ethical rules . . . as of any authority to control my professional acts."[65]

THE AMERICAN MEDICAL ASSOCIATION DEBATES REFORMING ITS *CODE OF MEDICAL ETHICS*

The *JAMA* Debates, 1892–1895

Ongoing arguments over the code of ethics led to formation of a committee in 1892 that proposed a new code for the AMA itself. The pages of the *Journal of the American Medical Association* (*JAMA*) were soon filled with letters debating this proposal, which, however, became entangled with an ethics debate about *JAMA*'s advertising policies. Davis was at the center of both debates. In 1883, he had consolidated his power base by transforming the AMA's *Transactions* into the *Journal of the American Medical Association*, and he had assumed editorship of the new journal. Previously, Davis had edited the *Chicago Medical Examiner* from 1860 to 1875, where he held himself up as a paragon of rectitude on the proprieties of advertising. In one editorial, "Give an Inch and an Ell is Taken," he argued that any liberality given with respect to endorsements will be abused, so a conscientious editor should accept none whatsoever. Since an "ell" is a measurement once used by tailors—about the length of a man's arm from shoulder to wrist—the sense of the article is "give an advertiser an inch and they will take a mile." As proof of the wisdom of never permitting the use of practitioner's names as endorsements, Davis cited an advertisement in a rival journal in which physicians who had allowed their names to be used on the business cards of a group of syphologists found their names published as endorsing the syphologists. "Our own rule,"

Davis pontificated, "has been . . . to allow no use of our name for any *special* purpose whatever."[66, 67]

Censorious though he was of others, as a practical matter, Davis needed revenue for his journal's upkeep. So, from time to time, Davis allowed himself an inch or two to raise revenue, publishing advertisements that included physicians' endorsements. The following advertisement from Storer Jr. is typical of those that he sometimes published.

> TO PHYSICIANS.—His attempts to extend a more advanced knowledge of his specialty to physicians already in practice having been so favorably commented upon by those of the profession who have attended the previous courses, and by the medical press, PROF. HORATIO R. STORER, Will deliver his third private course of twelve lectures upon the
>
> TREATMENT OF THE SURGICAL DISEASES OF WOMEN
>
> . . . Fee $50 and Diploma required to be shown. Certificates of attendance upon the course already completed have been issued to the following gentleman:
>
> Drs. J. B. Walker, Union, Me.; Alexander J. Stone, Augusta, Me. [seventeen other names with degrees and states are listed] Money receipts to Feb. 24th Drs. V. L. Halburt $3, [eighteen names follow].[68]

Forty physicians are mentioned by name in this advertisement, all effectively endorsing Storer Jr.'s lectures and thus seeming to flaunt Davis's antiendorsement policy. Yet, asserting the self-entitlement of the holier-than-thou, Davis breached his own rules, confident in his virtuousness and purity—and of his ability to silence any critics.

Davis brought the same mix of high-minded ethical pomposity and pragmatic expediency to *JAMA*, allowing himself occasional transgressions to sustain *JAMA*'s revenue stream. In 1893, Professor Solomon Solis-Cohen (1857–1948) of Jefferson Medical College introduced a motion at the AMA's national meeting censuring *JAMA* for advertising patent medicines without publishing their ingredients, thereby violating the age-old prohibition against endorsing secret nostrums.[69] In a signed letter to *JAMA*, "As to 'Nostrum' Advertisements in the Journal"[70] Solis-Cohen called out the emperor of ethics on his unclothed hypocrisy: advertising secret nostrums—an act prohibited by every major code of ethics from Percival's through the AMA's 1847 code of ethics. A flood of letters followed: some chided *JAMA*, others condemned Solis-Cohen.

Because Davis was at the center of both the *JAMA* advertising issue and of the debate over a new code, the two became entangled in a protracted serial correspondence ensued under such pen names as "A Conservative Member,"[71] "Inquirer,"[72] and the like. The use of pen names brought forth name-calling, including anti-Semitic jibes at Solis-Cohen. One correspondent, writing under the pen name "Medicus," challenged the motives of "these people," the "Hebriacs," "the Hebrew children of Philadelphia,"[73] who dared to challenge *JAMA*'s need for advertising revenue. In response, "[a] member of the [AMA] and a Jew...[protested] dragging questions of race and religion into the discussion."[74] The issue of pen names was resolved the next year when *JAMA* established a policy "that anonymous publications...will not...be published."[75] The secret nostrum issue was resolved in 1893, when John Hamilton (1847–1898), *JAMA*'s second editor (1893–1898),[76] instituted a policy that *JAMA* would "accept no advertisements of medicinal preparations [without] a formula containing the official or chemical name of each composing ingredient."[77]

A New Code for the AMA Proposed and Rejected, 1894

In 1894, the committee for revising the AMA's code of ethics presented two reports to the AMA's national meeting: the majority report proposed a new code of medical ethics; the minority report defended the old code. Speaking for the majority, committee chair Henry D. Holton (1838–1917), a Vermont gynecologist and future president of the American Public Health Association (APHA; founded in 1872; Holton became president in 1902) reported that "[t]hree-fourths of all letters received...desired some change in the Code,"[78] including, omitting "all sections of the Code that describe the obligations of the patients to their physicians, and of the public to physicians" because "the Code is not designed either for patients or the public."[79] So the new version of the AMA code omitted these sections. Moreover, since the committee could "find no good reason why [the code] should say anything respecting the patenting of medical devices,"[80] the new code did not prohibit patents. More controversially, in language carefully crafted to rebut Davis's 1874 speech denying specialists the right to advertise, the new code also declared that since "the field of medical knowledge is now so vast, no one mind can compass it in all its details. Nor can any one hand obtain the dexterity essential for the performance of all the delicate and daring operations of modern surgery. Specialists should not be something less than general practitioners, but general practitioners and something more."[81]

More radically still, the new code recognized as a legitimate colleague *any* "practitioner who has a license to practice from some medical board of known and acknowledged legal authority...and who is in good moral and professional standing in the place in which he resides"[82]; that is, the proposed new code recognized legally licensed homeopaths as legitimate peers—thereby permitting the readmission of the MSSNY. Holton also announced with pride that the code was written in gender-neutral language because "there are so many women practitioners of acknowledged learning, reputation and skill, the language of the revision omits all reference to sex."[83] Finally, to end the cycle of expulsions and to reunite the profession, the new code was to be purely advisory, without "any system of penal enactments."[84]

Holton was well aware that these revisions were controversial and remarked that although the delegates "may vote [the new code] down, as had been the cry of some," yet, "it will not down! For twenty years it has haunted us." Quoting Sims's 1876 speech, Holton reiterated the prediction that "[t]he time will come when your organic laws... will require modifications... to suit a broader education and a greater destiny." Holton asked the delegates, "Has not the time arrived for the fulfillment of that prophecy?"[85] Responding for the minority was Henry Didama (1823–1905) of the Medical College of Syracuse University, former president of the New York State Medical Association (which was loyal to the AMA's Old Code). "It cannot have escaped your notice, that certain varieties of [specialist] advertising condemned by the present standard Code are commended in the [proposed] revision and that the patenting of surgical instruments... forbidden by the standard [code] are intentionally ignored by the revisers."[86] What irked Didama most was the issue that prompted Old Coders to bolt the MSSNY, the recognition of "any possessor of a *license*," including homeopaths, as acceptable peers.[87]

In one fell swoop, the reformers were asking the delegates to accept a new code legitimizing specialist advertising and surgeons' patents, as well as female physicians and homeopaths. Any one of these revisions would have been a radical challenge, but to ask delegates to enact them all in a single package was too much for them to swallow. As a first step, it was a step too far. The proposal was voted down 135 votes against to 30 in favor.[88] The next year an exasperated eighty-eight-year-old Nathan Smith Davis observed that "[a]lmost every year somebody... is continually finding something to find fault with [in the code]. (Applause.)... I have arisen... to move that all of the amendments to the Constitution... be indefinitely postponed."[89] Acting on Davis's suggestion the delegates voted

> [t]hat the American Medical Association renews and hereby confirms its long-standing allegiance to and defense of the letter and spirit of the unamended *Code of Ethics* and etiquette of the American Medical Association.... [and that] any revision of the code... should be rejected by every regular practitioner of medicine as being inimical to the honor of the medical profession.[90]

The AMA's 1847 code would remain unamended and unrevised into the twentieth century.

THE AMERICAN MEDICAL ASSOCIATION ADOPTS LAISSEZ-FAIRE LIBERTARIANISM

The AMA's Principles of Medical Ethics, 1903

A natural reaction to autocrats who dictate in the name of centralized authority is to push the pendulum in the opposite direction. Not unnaturally, therefore, libertarianism became the central theme of a new laissez-faire version of medical ethics proposed to the AMA in 1903. Leading the reform movement was Manhattan physician E. Eliot Harris (fl. 1900) and his eminent ally, New York surgeon Joseph D. Bryant (1845–1914), former president of the NYAM (1897) and, in 1902, president of the AMA. Working together, the two strove to heal the breach between specialists and generalists and between Old, New, and No Coders. They started at the point where the breach first occurred, in New York, reuniting New York's medical societies under a single compromise code of medical ethics.[91]

Harris then suggested that the AMA adopt the compromise New York code as "the ethical…laws of the [AMA]."[92] To review this proposal, a committee was formed comprised of Harris (chair), Bryant, AMA trustee Thomas Happel of Tennessee (1847–1909), and William Henry Welch (1850–1934), a future AMA president (1910) who was, in 1902, dean of the Johns Hopkins school of medicine, founding editor of the *Journal of Experimental Medicine* (founded in 1894), and immediate past president of the AMA's rival, the AAP. The committee immediately rejected the idea of substituting the compromise New York code for the AMA's 1847 code of ethics and proposed instead a code similar in substance to the one that the AMA rejected in 1894 but very different in style.[93]

Conscious that a factor in the failure of the 1894 code reforms was the displacement of resonant Percivalean prose with plodding bureaucratic verbiage that rendered the ethics of physician–patient relationship with all the eloquence of a lease agreement, the 1902 reformers preserved Percivalean cadences wherever possible. Thus, whereas the unsuccessful 1894 reformers opened their section on the physician–patient relationship with the line "Being possessed of the requisite knowledge and skill for the treatment of disease, and also of the sanction of government for their employment, physicians should consider these acquisitions as sacred talents committed to their trust, and should use them diligently, honestly and solely for the benefit of their patients,"[94] the 1902 reformers opened with a familiar sounding line: "Physicians should not only be ever ready to obey the calls of the sick and the injured but should be mindful of the high character of their mission and of the responsibilities they must incur in the discharge of momentous duties."[95]

Absences spoke as loudly as words in the proposed new code. Absent, unremarked, unmissed, and unmourned was any mention of patients' obligations to their physicians or the public's obligations to the profession. Also unremarked, but nonetheless remarkable, the pronouns in the updated *Principles* were gender neutral. Thus, the statement "mindful of the high character of *their* mission" eliminates masculine pronouns used in this line in the 1847 Code, which reads "*his* mind ought to be imbued with the greatness of *his* mission." Calling no notice whatsoever to these changes, the committee reassured the AMA that it "retained, to a large extent, the phraseology of the existing [1847] code, while aiming at condensation of expression and a better understanding of some of its statements." The 1902 reformers also added the soothing comment that, insofar they revised the code's text, the revisions had been accepted "unanimously, without dissension or distrust on the part of its members . . . and without regard to any past or present disagreements or misunderstandings whatsoever."[96]

By conserving traditional language, by diplomatically declining to emphasize potentially controversial changes, and by underlining their unanimity, the 1902 reformers made palatable a text that, from its title, "*Principles*," to its prefatory comments, to its deletion of the sections on the patient's and the public's obligations to their physicians and to the profession of medicine, to its gender-neutral pronouns was just as radical as—and in many respects identical to—the code overwhelmingly rejected in 1894. Yet, to the casual reader, and no doubt to ordinary AMA delegates, the repetition of familiar cadences allowed the *Principles* to be read as restatements of familiar precepts updated for a new century. Percivalean-sounding prose reaffirmed physicians' virtues of attention and humanity. Physicians' obligations of confidentiality and delicacy were also preserved, as were their duties of serving as a "minister of hope and comfort to the sick" and of never abandoning a patient. Even the paternalistic imperative of rehabilitating "patients suffering under the counsels of evil conduct" was retained.[97]

It also helped that the 1902 report coincided with broader efforts to update the AMA's constitution and bylaws and that the past presidents of both the AMA and AAP, Bryant and Welch, were on the committee that endorsed these proposals. The AMA convention accepted the code with remarkably little debate. Manuscript versions of the code, however, tell a more turbulent tale. Following precedents set by their 1894 predecessors, the 1902 committee had deleted those sections of the code's text that stipulate patients' and the public's obligations to their physicians and to the profession. In doing, so they inadvertently destroyed conceptual foundations of the AMA's code of ethics as a statement of the *reciprocal* duties and obligations of physicians, patients, the profession, and the public *to each other*. For if patients and the public have no obligations to their physicians or to the profession, the notion of reciprocity becomes meaningless.

Recognition that their new code needed a different conceptual foundation seems to have dawned somewhat belatedly on the 1902 committee. Early drafts of the 1902 *Principles* initially included sections on patients' and the publics' responsibilities to physicians and to the profession. On later drafts, these sections are crossed out.[98] and a typescript appended to the galley proofs states that the word "'code' has been eliminated from the text and replaced by the expression 'Principles of Medical Ethics.'"[99] This new title, the explanation continues, was "adopted as adequately descriptive" because "[i]t is wiser to formulate the principles of medical ethics, without definite reference to 'code' or penalties," leaving to "the respective states, to form such a code, and establish such rules as they may regard fitting and proper, for regulating the professional conduct of their members, provided of course, that in doing so there shall be no infringement on the established ethical principles of this Association."[100] This change, the committee explained, is "intended to facilitate the business of the parent organization and promote its harmony by leaving to the state association large discretionary powers concerning membership and other admittedly state affairs."[101]

Thus, forced by the logic of their revisions to reconsider the foundations of professional medical ethics and acutely aware of the discord sowed by the authoritarianism of the earlier contractarian version of the AMA *Code of Medical Ethics*, the committee sought harmony at the national level by embracing "principles" in the abstract while devolving actual ethical decision making and enforcement to local societies. A natural concomitant of this strategy of harmony through devolution was the decision to offer "principles of medical ethics, without definite reference to 'code' or penalties." A letter from the chair of the 1910 AMA Judicial Council to the editor of *JAMA* explains this devolutionist approach:

> This country is so large and custom, as well as conditions of life, vary so widely with the character of communities, states and groups of states which comprise the country, that the committee believe it to be an impossible task for the American Medical Association to cover the whole ground and provide anything like the variety of [ethical] questions which arise and are bound to arise. The Association sets forth general principles of ethics and it seems to your committee far better to allow the individual state societies to provide the details in such a way and as far as they deem wise.[102]

Devolution was a natural reaction to a half-century of officious moralizing by Davis and the "medical Pharisees" at national meetings of the AMA. To use Pilcher's turn of phrase, from their seats of centralized authority they had been "at liberty to coolly ride rough-shod over the rights of others,"[103] creating a "spirit of censoriousness in the profession" that "has made persecutions of the most petty nature possible."[104] In reaction, as Pilcher predicted, AMA members rejected not only "the [1847] code," but also "any like set of definite ethical rules of any authority to control [their] professional acts."[105] Making precisely this point, the preamble to the 1903 *Principles* expressly declares, "[t]he American Medical Association promulgates [its *Principles*] as a suggestive and advisory document." Some similar statement of the laissez-faire status of the AMA's ethics principles would be reaffirmed in AMA ethics documents through the 1970s.

Devolutionist Laissez-Faire Ethical Libertarianism, 1912–1976

In 1903, the reign of the Pharisees ended and the era of laissez-faire devolutionist medical ethics commenced. Yet, in less than a decade, the pendulum began to swing away from devolved laissez-faire ethics. A devolutionist system of ethics can be effective only if it is enforced at the local level. Yet the jurispathic impact of Davis's policies, in combination with the atrophy of traditions of restorative justice predicated on ideals of gentlemanly honor and the increasing financial attractiveness of such commercial practices as advertising and fee splitting, foredoomed the devolutionist laissez-faire experiment. By 1911, the Judicial Council was complaining that, as a consequence of the policies enacted in 1903, "[e]xcepting in one or two states, there is no control of membership by either the state or the American Medical Association. It is left absolutely with the component county society." This, in turn, led to unresolved "questions of secret division of fees, contract practice, advertising, etc. [which] should be met and given careful, judicious and deliberate consideration."[106] So the Council recommended that a national ethics council be "re-created as a permanent body; that its functions should be made much broader than they have been in the past"[107]; that is, it recommended that the AMA reassert central authority to police the ethical conduct of practitioners.

The issue that most vexed the Judicial Council was the "parasitic practices that…should be called by their proper names and printed in letters of burning condemnation so that…the guilty may be easily recognized and properly sequestered from the great mass of honest, conscientious, and supremely trustworthy medical men…who should not have their good work tarnished by a questionable few."[108] The name of this outrageous practice was "fee splitting"—the secret division of fees between referring practitioners and specialists. The issue had been raised in 1900, when delegates rejected a resolution condemning "commissions or a division of fees under whatever guise it may be made," on the grounds that "it would be impossible for this Association to get at the truth…on all such questions."[109] In 1902, county medical societies were empowered to expel members "guilty of division of fees, either the giving or receiving of part of a fee without the full knowledge of the patient."[110] This position is reflected in the 1903 *Principles of Medical Ethics*, which state that "it is derogatory to professional character for physicians to pay or to offer to pay commissions to any person whatsoever who may recommend to them patients…[or] for physicians to solicit or to receive such commissions."[111] Yet, as the Judicial Council observed, even though the local societies were authorized to expel members for fee splitting, the practice was becoming increasingly widespread, in part because local societies were not expelling miscreant members—the AMA's laissez-faire devolutionist approach to ethics left the organization impotent to address its members' manifestly immoral conduct.

The Typhoid Mary Case and the American Public Health Association's Proposal

Coincidently, at the same 1911 meeting, the AMA's Preventive Medicine and Public Health Committee forwarded from the APHA's Committee on Reporting Typhoid Fever[112] a request that the traditional statement, "when pestilence prevails, it is [physicians'] duty to face the danger, and to continue their labors for the alleviation of suffering people, even at the risk of their own lives," be amended so that it continues, "not omitting the foremost duty at any and all times of notifying the properly constituted health authorities of every case of infectious or contagious disease of which they become aware."[113] Because the 1903 Code states that the "obligation of secrecy" is so strong that "no infirmity... observed during medical attendance should ever be divulged by physicians, except when imperatively required by the laws, "the APHA's request seemed straightforwardly incompatible with the AMA's 1903 *Principles of Medical Ethics*."[114]

Prompting the APHA's request was an incident involving a nonphysician, George Soper (1870–1948), an engineer who would later become Director of the American Society for the Control of Cancer (founded in 1913, now the American Cancer Society). Soper had discovered the identity of an asymptomatic typhoid carrier, Mary Mallon (1869–1938), more popularly referred to as "Typhoid Mary." As a nonphysician, Soper was not bound by confidentiality and, as he wrote in *JAMA* in 1907,

> Believing that sufficient had been learned concerning [Mary Mallon's] history to show that the cook was a... cause of typhoid and a menace to the public health, I laid the facts concerning the four principal [typhoid] epidemics [attributable to Mallon] before Dr. Herman M. Biggs, medical officer of health of the New York City Department of Health on March 11, 1907, with the suggestion that the woman be taken into custody by the department and her excretions made the subject of careful bacteriological examination. I had been unable to obtain her consent to any examination. The department acted favorably on the suggestion and caused the cook to be removed to the Detention Hospital. She reached there March 19, 1907, after a severe struggle in which she showed remarkable bodily strength and agility.[115]

Mallon was later released on the understanding that she never work as a cook. In 1911–12, however, it became evident that she had again found employment as a cook and was the source of a typhoid outbreak that resulted in dozens of illnesses and at least one death. Mallon was subsequently incarcerated for the rest of her life, becoming the heroine of an iconic tale of the conflict between civil liberties and public health, and—more to the point of this discussion—the center of a debate over the limits of a physician's duty of confidentiality.[116] The Soper article and the Mallon case raised the question of whether the 1903 AMA *Principles of Medical Ethics* should be revised to permit—or even to require—physicians to report to public health authorities the occurrence of typhoid and other contagious diseases in their patients and/or the identity of contagious disease carrier like Mary Mallon.

Revising the *Principles of Medical Ethics*, 1912

As it happened, Frank Billings (1854–1932), dean of Chicago's Rush Medical College (1900–1920), AMA president during the 1903 code revisions, and, more recently, president of the AAP (1906), chaired the AMA's Judicial Council in 1911–1912. Under his leadership, the Council drafted and circulated a revised version of the *Principles* that asserted some claim to moral authority with respect to professionalism—but still stopped short of according the Judicial Council power to investigate ethics abuses or to penalize miscreants.[117] These principles were adopted at the AMA's 1912 meeting.[118] In contrast to the 1903 code, with its libertarian declaration that "the American Medical Association promulgates [its *Principles*] as suggestive and advisory," the 1912 *Principles* reassert a measure of ethical authority, claiming that physicians are obligated to adhere to the professional obligations stipulated in the *Principles* by virtue of their choice of medicine as a vocation. In choosing medicine as a vocation, one becomes bound by the ethics implicit in the role of a physician (as the intern N case in Chapter 1 illustrates). The conceptual parameters of this claim are spelled out in the following passage.

> *The Physician's Responsibility*
> Section 1.—A profession has for its prime object the service it can render to humanity; reward or financial remuneration should be a subordinate consideration. The practice of medicine is a profession. In choosing this profession an individual assumes an obligation to conduct himself according to its ideals.[119]

This conception of the moral requisites of accepting medicine as a profession provides a justification for a new, more powerful, condemnation of fee splitting.

> *Chapter II. Article VI.—Compensation... Secret Division of Fees Condemned*
> Sec. 3. It is detrimental to the public good and degrading to the profession, and therefore unprofessional, to give or receive a commission. It is also unprofessional to divide a fee for medical advice or surgical treatment, unless the patient or his next friend is fully informed as to the terms of the transaction.[120]

The logic of this condemnation is straightforward: since by definition "a profession has for its prime object the service it can render to humanity," rather than aiming at "reward or financial remuneration," and since secret fee splitting places financial remuneration above patients' interests, it is inherently "unprofessional."[121] The 1912 *Principles* is the first AMA medical code to explicitly assert that medical ethics is a form of professional ethics in the sense of an ethics justified primarily because one has chosen to become a member of a *profession*.[122] It is also the first to use "unprofessional" as a term of moral condemnation. Perhaps unintentionally, the AMA had begun to conceive of professionalism—its mission of service to humanity—as the foundation of its moral claims on its members. Professionalism was thus no longer a form of gentlemanly honor in modern guise. It was now a concept in its own right that generated an internal logic that dictated appropriate conduct for members of the profession. Notably, insofar as the physician's professional mission is characterized as "service to humanity" rather than "exclusively to the patient... without exception,"[123] the 1912 concept of professionalism created conceptual space for a professional duty to report infectious disease to health authorities and even to identify carriers by name.

How had this radical conceptual shift, this broad redefinition of the profession's objectives, become possible? One important factor was a generational shift in concepts of health and disease. The Davis- Flint generation was no longer commanding the AMA in 1911–1912. President Billings had come of age at a time when Bernard, Koch, and Pasteur offered a new approach to bacteriology and physiology that reinvigorated communal and environmental approaches to health and that emphasized such public health measures as pasteurized milk, sanitary water supplies, sewage disposal, and vaccination.[124] President Billings himself was a researcher on the germ theory of disease, and, during his presidency, he deployed the AMA's clout with Congress to lobby for a U.S. Public Health (and Marine Hospital) Service (founded in 1902) and to help enact the Pure Food and Drug Act (1906).

In 1912, a fellow public health reformer, Abraham Jacobi, became president of the AMA—a turn of events that surprised Jacobi, who joked, "I never expected this distinguished honor of presiding over this body... [since] I had to say a sharp word or two [about the AMA] now and then."[125] As a committed public health and environmental reformer (he championed the reforestation of the Mississippi flood plain),[126] Jacobi enthusiastically endorsed the APHA's request for an amendment. With the backing of Billings and Jacobi, the amendment was enacted and the 1912 *Principles* made it "the duty of a physician to notify... public health authorities of every case of communicable disease under his care."[127] Given their conception of disease and the causes they embraced, it was natural for these leaders to endorse a broad communal conception of the goals of the medical profession; that is, "service to humanity," rather than "exclusively to the patient."

Nonetheless, the professionalism of the 1912 *Principles* was tempered by a laissez-faire conception of ethical decisionmaking. For example, after reiterating that the professional obligation of confidentiality as "a trust [that] should never be revealed except when imperatively required by the laws of the state," the 1912 *Principles* make a laissez-faire pivot on the issue of identifying individual disease carriers.

> There are occasions... when a physician must determine whether or not his duty to society requires him to take definite action to protect a healthy individual from becoming infected because the physician has knowledge, obtained through the confidences entrusted to him as a physician of a communicable disease to which the healthy individual is about to be exposed. *In such a case the physician should act as he would desire another to act toward one of his own family under like circumstances.* Before he determines his course, the physician should know the civil law of his commonwealth concerning privileged communications.[128]

So, in resolving the conflict between the physician's duties to patients and to society, the *Principles* offer procedural guidance in the form of a recommendation for reflection in terms of the Golden Rule—and then, in true laissez-faire fashion, permits each physician to decide the issue according to the dictates of his or her individual personal conscience.

The 1912 *Principles* also take a devolutionist approach to the issue of specialists' business cards, office signs, and directories, stating that these are issues to be resolved by local customs. So, although "solicitation of patients by circulars or advertisements or by personal communications or interviews" was condemned as "unprofessional,"[129] nonetheless, "publication or circulation of ordinary simple business cards, being a matter of personal taste or custom, and sometimes of convenience," is not per se improper"; but, "it is unprofessional to disregard local customs or offend recognized ideals in publishing or circulating such cards."[130] Much the same devolutionist approach is taken toward contract practice: "it is unprofessional for a physician to dispose of his services under conditions that make it impossible to render adequate service to his patient or which interfere with reasonable competition among the physicians of a community."[131] Yet the interpretation of "adequate service" and "reasonable competition" is the prerogative of the local societies, devolving the issue for them to decide. Moreover, the prohibition against holding patents was eased somewhat: although it was still unprofessional to hold a patent, in which one personally "receive[d] remuneration from patents or medicines," the institution to which one was affiliated, could hold a patent on them.[132] Here again, the bounds of propriety in these matters were to be determined by the sensibilities of the local medical society.

With respect to patient emergencies and nonabandonment, the 1912 *Principles* is also sensitive to local sentiment: "a physician... should... respond to any request for his assistance in any emergency" and should provide services "whenever temperate public opinion expects the service." Moreover, the physician "should not abandon or neglect a patient because the disease is deemed incurable; nor should he withdraw from a case... until a sufficient notice of a desire to be released has been given the patient or his friends." Nonetheless, to give physicians leverage in contract negotiations, these statements are prefaced by the laissez-faire assertion that, "[a] physician is free to choose whom he will serve."[133] Thus, a physician is free to choose *not* to accept contracts to serve colleges, factories, mines, and schools—and physicians in the Jim Crow South are free not to accept African Americans as patients. Note, moreover, that as the return of the masculine pronoun in the quoted sentence indicates, the quietly reformist preference for gender neutral pronouns in the 1903 *Principles* was discarded in the 1912 version—the grammatical presumption is that all physicians are male.

Taking Action Against Fee Splitting

The primary motive for the 1912 reforms had been to address the growth of fee splitting. Consequently, the 1912 *Principles* state unequivocally that "[i]t is detrimental to the public good and degrading to the profession, and therefore unprofessional, to give or receive a commission. It is also unprofessional to divide a fee for medical advice or surgical treatment, unless the patient or his next friend is fully informed as to the terms of the transaction"[134] Yet the prerogative of enforcing the principle prohibiting fee splitting remained with the county societies—who were reluctant to pursue the issue.

Concerned that devolving enforcement to the local societies might not curtail the practice of fee splitting, the AMA authorized a member of the Judicial Council, Alexander Lambert (1861–1938), professor of medicine at Cornell Medical College and a future AMA president (1919–1920), to investigate "the secret division of fees, taking of commissions, and contract practice."[135] The Committee reported at the 1913 AMA national meeting that it had sent to every county medical society and their members an "anonymous" questionnaire."[136] About half responded. On the basis of this data, the committee found that "the prevalence [of fee splitting and "kick backs" or commissions] varies in different sections of the United States."[137] It was higher in large cities, like "New York City," where, "among certain groups of men, it is without a doubt the rule rather than the exception."[138]

The underlying reason for fee splitting was that "hardly more than 10 per cent of physicians in the United States are able to earn a comfortable income."[139] Nonetheless 77.3 percent of respondents held that fee splitting was not "justifiable;" only 9.3 percent believe the practice justifiable, and 13.4 percent were unclear or "doubtful" about its moral status.[140]

> [Common] reasons given for this secret fee splitting…is that it is justifiable because of the disproportionate fee between the amount paid the surgeon and the amount paid the physician.…Another reason is that it is nobody's business what a surgeon does with his fee after he earns it.…Other answers are more frankly truthful, such as "purely on the grounds of good business," and "because everyone else is doing it," and "unless you do some other man will." These frankly but tacitly admit the low standard of commercialism on which these men have put their profession.[141]

The Committee concluded that, "If through secret fee splitting and commissions the standards are changed from giving to patients the best service possible to squeezing them for the best attainable fees, then will the medical profession be weighed and found wanting. The confidence and respect now given to it by the public will be destroyed."[142]

The Committee's proposed three remedies: ethics education, expulsion, and transparency. Medical colleges should formally teach medical ethics so that "young men [will] not be turned loose on the world ignorant of the high ideals and standards [the profession] has always and will always stand for."[143] Unfortunately, these recommendations came at the very moment when the Carnegie Foundation's 1910 Flexner Report on medical education led to a major drive to focus medical school curriculum entirely on the physical sciences and practical clinical skills,[144] thus purging from the medical school curriculum any subject matter not focused on medical science and its application to clinical practice.[145] Out of sync with the major direction of medical education reform, the recommendation to include more medical ethics in the medical school curriculum had no impact—quite the reverse; the impact of the Flexner reforms led to the neglect of medical ethics education, which was given, at best, a perfunctory nod.

Worse yet, the Lambert committee was unwilling to challenge the laissez-faire stance of the *Principles* by requesting investigatory or punitive authority—instead, it accommodated its proposals to the devolution of enforcement to local societies and, to reiterate, local societies were reluctant to reprimand their own members.

Thus, its recommendations that practitioners who fee split should be expelled from medical societies also had little impact.[146] The AMA did, however, initiate a century-long campaign against fee splitting and related practices. In 1924, the Judicial Council tried to swim against the devolutionist tide by requesting and receiving the power to recommend the expulsion of any "county society found to enroll so many fee-splitting, or otherwise unethical, members as to render it impossible for that society to enforce the ethical standards of the medical profession."[147] Few county societies, however, were actually investigated or expelled. From this point forward, the AMA undertook "bully pulpit" campaigns against patient referrals to facilities in which physicians held a financial interest, including diagnostic laboratories,[148] healthcare appliance outlets,[149] pharmacies,[150] and hospitals.[151] It also campaigned against traditional fee splitting[152] and commissions for "steering" patients to commercial organizations or laboratories.[153]

The Continuity of Laissez-Faire Medical Ethics: The *Principles* of 1949 and 1957

The mix of professionalism tempered by devolutionist laissez-faire attitude toward ethics formulated in the 1912 *Principles* governed the AMA through the interwar period. In the post-World War II period, the rapid spread of "voluntary prepayment health insurance plans [and the] formation of medical [practice] groups" compelled the Judicial Council to consider changes.[154] Influenced by the opening salvos of the Cold War—the American airlift of food and medical supplies to besieged Western Berlin, the formation of the North Atlantic Treaty Alliance (NATO) to defend the "Free World" against communism—an interim version of the *Principles*, issued in 1949, proclaimed ideals of freedom and internationalism. It also condemned the "war crimes of a medical nature committed by the Germans during the past war"[155] and opened with a statement on "The Physician's Responsibility" by Sir Thomas Watson (1792–1882), long-serving president of the Royal College of Physicians:

> The profession of Medicine, having for its end the common good of mankind, knows nothing of national enmities, of political strife, of sectarian dissensions. Disease and pain the conditions of its ministry, it is disquieted by no misgivings concerning the justice and honesty of its client's cause; but dispenses its peculiar benefits, without stint or scruple, to men of every country, and party and rank, and religion, and to men of no religion at all.[156]

Having affirmed medicine's global nature and its national, religious, and sectarian neutrality, the interim 1949 version of the *Principles* nonetheless valorized laissez-faire ethics with a prefatory misquotation from James Percival, misidentified as the author of *Medical Ethics*: "These principles are not laws to govern but are principles to guide correct conduct."[157]

As every student of medical ethics should have known, but evidently did not, the first name of the Percival who wrote *Medical Ethics*, was "Thomas." James was one of Thomas Percival's sons who predeceased his father in 1793, depressing Thomas so profoundly that he ceased work on the manuscript that would be published a decade later, in 1803, as *Medical Ethics*—which, ironically, is a very law-like code of professional duties. Curiously, the misquotation invokes Percival's book to herald its opposite: a non–law-like, non–duty-based set of libertarian principles. Finding little to support laissez-faire ethics in the actual text of *Medical Ethics*, the 1949 *Principles* invoke instead the spirit of Hippocrates to valorize its description of the "Character of the Physician" as "pure…diligent…conscientious in caring for the sick [and] as was said by Hippocrates 'modest, sober, patient, prompt to do his duty without anxiety; pious without superstition, conducting himself with propriety in his profession.'"[158] Thus, despite the internationalism of its prefatory quotation, the 1949 *Principles* were substantially similar to precursors.

From 1949 to 1956, the Judicial Council tweaked and amended statements of the AMA *Principles* until, in 1957, it undertook a radical revision of the text: forty-seven sections of Judicial Council reports were assembled "under appropriate titles to serve as a practical, useable reference document for the guidance of the profession."[159] The titles took the form of ethical principles. Principle I, for example, states that "THE PRINCIPAL objective of the medical profession is to render service to humanity with full respect for the dignity of man. Physicians should merit the confidence of patients entrusted to their care, rendering to each a full measure of service and devotion."[160] The body of the text that follows consists of relevant Judicial Council commentaries. The original eighty-two-page typescript was literally a cut-and-paste affair in a nonmetaphorical sense: judicial commentaries were cut from earlier documents and pasted under typewritten principles.[161] A more cohesive version of this assemblage was published with a useable index in a special June 7, 1958 edition of *JAMA*.

In this new format, ten principles of AMA ethics were placed cheek-by-jowl with a half-century of materials assembled from Judicial Council Opinions and Reports and earlier statements of the *Principles*. Principle 9, for example, reiterates a standard statement on confidentiality, more or less as it appears in the 1912, 1949, and 1955 versions of the *Principles*. Specifying the application of this principle to communicable disease carriers, physicians are held to have a responsibility to report the occurrence of these cases to authorities, although they need not report the name of the actual carrier. The issue of naming carriers (like Mary Mallon) should be resolved in terms of the Golden Rule: the physician should act as "the physician…would desire another to act towards one of his own family in like circumstances."[162] On another information-sharing question, a physician is advised that *he* "should assure himself that the patients, his relatives or his responsible friends have such knowledge of the patient's condition as will serve the best interests of the patient and the family."[163] Thus, physicians *may* inform patients' friends and families of a patient's condition, as long as they act in the patient's interest. Patients' access to their own medical records, however, is considered inadvisable, but here, too, the Golden Rule applies: a "physician... must always act as he would wish to be treated were he in a like situation."[164]

The permissive language of this advice is encapsulated in the laissez-faire declaration that prefaces the 1957–58 *Principles*: "These principles are intended to aid physicians individually and collectively in maintaining a high level of ethical conduct. They are not laws but standards by which a physician may determine the propriety of his conduct in his relations with patients, with colleagues, with members of allied professions, and the public."[165] Note the permissive term "may." The 1957 format would be followed with minor modifications in later editions of the AMA *Principles*, which would also perpetuate the practice of prefacing the *Principles* with a laissez-faire declaration that these principles were not "laws" but "standards" meant to guide rather than dictate—many versions of the *Principles* also invoke the libertarian ethical standard of the Golden Rule.

THE INSULARITY OF THE AMERICAN MEDICAL ASSOCIATION'S MEDICAL ETHICS, 1913–1970

The 1957 version of the *Principles* also cemented a tendency toward insularity that scholars often remark when commenting on professional medical ethics as propounded by the AMA: its inward-turning gaze and seeming blindness or indifference to ethical and social issues impacting and surrounding medicine.[166] The professional medical ethics of the AMA had divorced itself from issues of social justice after the divisive debates over the status of African-American and female physicians that roiled the organization in the 1870s; nonetheless, Davis and many others in the AMA remained sensitive to ethical and social issues in society at large. Thus, the pages of Davis's *JAMA* reflected the rich array of social and ethical issues swirling around the regular American medical profession in the 1880s and 1890s. These include, as one would expect, professional concerns about advertising,[167] contract practice,[168] female physicians (education of),[169] laissez-faire medical ethics (i.e., "the guide of each man must be his own conscience"),[170] medical ethics education,[171] patent medicines,[172] sects (e.g., homeopathy),[173] specialty medicine,[174] the New Code–No code controversy,[175] the view that medical societies "should exclude all... ethical... discussions,"[176] and the AMA's code of ethics and its revision.[177] Beyond these professional concerns, however, were lively discussions of capital punishment (humanism in),[178] casuistry versus principlism,[179] experimentation (animal[180] and human[181]), experimentation (honesty in),[182] falsification of death certificates,[183] the Hippocratic oath,[184] self-expurgation of medical texts,[185] vivisection and antivivisection,[186] as well as the ethics of the beginning and end of life: abortion,[187] birth control,[188] craniotomy/feticide/partial birth abortion,[189] and, at the other end of the lifecycle, euthanasia (in the sense of mercy killing)[190] and the value of human life.[191]

Prior to the advent of laissez-faire professional ethics, the full range of ethical and social issues impacting medicine and its practitioners was discussed in *JAMA*, or by some AMA committee, or at AMA conventions. In striking contrast, after laissez-faire medical ethics was proclaimed in the 1903 and 1912 *Principles*, the AMA ignored major national debates on ethical issues, even those directly impacting medicine. Debates over eugenic sterilization and euthanasia illustrate this insularity. Eugenicist arguments for the compulsory sterilization of persons deemed unfit to reproduce because of such presumed genetic defects as "feeble mindedness" or habitual criminality took legislative form in the United States in 1907, when Indiana became the first state to legalize compulsory sterilization on eugenic grounds. Other states soon passed similar laws, including Virginia, which passed a compulsory sterilization bill in 1925. Two years later, in 1927, Carrie Buck, an inmate of Virginia's State Colony for Epileptics and the Feeble Minded (founded in 1910, now the Central Virginia Training Center), appealed to the courts to reverse a decision by the Virginia eugenics board to have her sterilized. The case went to the U.S. Supreme Court. Oliver Wendell Holmes Jr. (1841–1935) wrote the Court's decision. Son of the physician of the same name, Oliver Holmes Jr. was a Union Army Civil War veteran who had been wounded in the battles at Antietam and Fredericksburg and whose firsthand experience of the carnage of war appears to have influenced his decision. He found against Carrie Buck and in favor of a states' rights to sterilize the "feeble minded" for eugenic reasons.

> We have seen more than once that the public welfare may call upon the best citizens for their lives [i.e., during the Civil War]. It would be strange if it could not call upon those who already sap the strength of the State for these lesser sacrifices, often not felt to be such by those concerned, in order to prevent our being swamped with incompetence. It is better for all the world if, instead of waiting to execute degenerate offspring for crime or to let them starve for their imbecility, society can prevent those who are manifestly unfit from continuing their kind. The principle that sustains compulsory vaccination is broad enough to cover cutting the Fallopian tubes. *Jacobson v. Massachusetts*, 197 U.S. 11. Three generations of imbeciles are enough.[192]

Conscious of decades of national debate over eugenic sterilization, the AMA considered studying eugenic sterilization—but it never did.[193] A 1933 report mentioned the subject in passing, but without comment.[194] In 1936, a Committee to Study Contraceptive Practices commented that "our present knowledge of heredity is so limited that there appears to be very little scientific basis to justify limitation of conception for eugenic reasons."[195] If publicized, this finding might have made a major impact on the national debate over eugenic sterilization. Seventy years earlier, a similar report by Horatio Storer Jr. had culminated in the criminalization of prequickening abortion. The AMA of Storer's era, however, operated under a code of ethics conceptualized as a social contract in which the profession and the public had reciprocal duties toward each other. The laissez-faire principles of the twentieth century were conceived as advice to individual members and did not presuppose any organizational obligation to society: so the AMA said and did nothing with respect to eugenic sterilization—it did not even publicize its findings. Most, but not all, medical societies were equally quiescent. The singular contrast is the American Neurological Association (ANA, founded in 1874–1875, still functioning), which publicly proclaimed that the compulsory sterilization of criminals had no scientific foundation.[196]

A similar pattern emerges with respect to euthanasia and end-of-life care. In 1906, bills were introduced in Iowa and Ohio to legalize euthanasia, in the sense of mercy killing. Although neither bill was enacted into law, it is noteworthy that the AMA—which enacted its laissez-faire *Principles* three years earlier, in 1903—took no stand in the debate.[197] A related debate raged in the AMA's hometown, Chicago, a decade later in 1915. Dr. Harry Haiselden (1817–1919), chief surgeon at the German-American Hospital, systematically declined to perform life-saving surgery on children born with severe birth defects, allowing them to die. Haiselden was transparent about his practices, permitting the press to interview parents and to photograph the infants he was allowing to die. A feature silent film dramatizing Haiselden's practices and starring Haiselden himself, *The Black Stork*, played in theaters from 1917 to 1942.[198] According to the leading authority on Haiselden, historian Martin Pernick, newspapers from Ann Arbor, Baltimore, Boston, Detroit, New York, Philadelphia, St. Louis, Washington D.C., and, of course, Chicago, covered the story.[199] Some 333 people took a public stand on Haiselden's practices, but the AMA uttered not one word. Before 1903, the organization would have spoken out on the subject. In the 1870s, it had launched a national campaign to save prequickened fetal life, and, in the 1880s, Davis had editorialized about the value of saving human life and specifically denounced euthanasia in the sense of mercy killing.[200]

The AMA first took official notice of euthanasia, in the sense of mercy killing, in 1973, when it addressed issues raised by Bjorn Ibsen's morally disruptive technology, the ventilator. State medical societies were recommending the implementation of formal advance directives; that is, instructions to physicians written *in advance* of a person's loss of decision-making capacity stating, while the person is still capacitated, her or his preferences with respect to end-of-life care, including whether to discontinue ventilator support. Pushed to address these issues by state medical societies, the AMA declined to endorse advance directives; it simply remarked "that individuals have the right to express [end-of-life care] wishes." The AMA observed further that physicians "may, and indeed should, feel free to question those wishes with patient's... representatives or by appropriate judicial proceedings when the circumstances of a particular situation seem to require it."[201] In other words, patients are free express their "wishes" for end-of-life-care, but, after they became incapacitated, physicians should feel free to challenge these "wishes," thereby overriding a patient's express wishes with respect to end-of-life care.

Having declined to lend its imprimatur to advance directives, and having given physicians permission to challenge advance directives, the AMA denounced "[t]he intentional termination of the life of one human being by another—mercy killing—[as] contrary to that for which the medical profession stands and is contrary to the policy of the American Medical Association." However, the statement continues, "[t]he cessation of the employment of extraordinary means to prolong the life of the body when there is irrefutable evidence that biological death is imminent is the decision of the patient and/or his immediate family. The advice and judgment of the physician should be freely available to the patient and/or his family."[202] In other words, insofar as an end-of-life intervention can be considered "extraordinary means," patients or their family members may decline the intervention. The term "extraordinary means" was drawn from a policy statement by the MSSNY,[203] which, in turn, borrowed it from a 1957 statement on end-of-life care by Roman Catholic Pope Pius XII (1876–1958; pope 1939–1958).[204]

This first attempt by the AMA to offer official guidance on the cessation of treatment in end-of-life care flopped. Whatever the extraordinary–ordinary distinction means in Catholic moral theology—a complex issue still vexing theologians[205]—it was meaningless in the context of the critical care technologies of the 1960s and 1970s (artificial nutrition and hydration, ventilators, etc.). Worse yet non-Catholic medical practitioners, families, and patients (i.e., the majority of Americans) were naturally ignorant of the theological tradition that made the distinction meaningful, and they would have no reason to accept the pronouncements of a Roman Catholic pope as authoritative. More strikingly, the AMA's appeal to the moral authority of a Roman Catholic Pope, rather than to its own Ethical and Judicial Council, raised issues about the AMA's competency to respond to the moral disruptions of emerging medical technologies: Ibsen's ventilator, Scribner's hemodialysis machine, Edward's and Steptoe's in vitro fertilization, and so forth. After a half-century adrift in the rhetoric of laissez-faire medical ethics, the AMA seemed to have lost its moral moorings. The ethical guidance that would ultimately be recognized as authoritative would come from a surprising source: a hodge-podge alliance of humanistic clinicians and scientists with *lumpen intelligentsia* from law, philosophy, and theology who created a new field that came to be called "bioethics."

9

AMERICAN RESEARCH ETHICS, 1800–1946

We have no right to use patients entrusted to our care for the purposes of experimentation unless direct benefit to the individual is likely to follow. Once this limit is transgressed, the sacred cord which binds physician and patient snaps instantly. Risk to the individual may be taken with his consent and full knowledge of the circumstances [as was done in] the yellow fever experiments in Cuba under the direction of [Walter] Reed and [James] Carroll.

Sir William Osler, 1907[1]

Very many college professors . . . have been . . . educated abroad . . . in the great centers of Europe, where patients have no other aspect than as "clinical material," without very much regard for the life or health of that material. . . . The humanitarian view is dominant in [America], and even in the eleemosynary institutions, supported wholly by charity, there is a unanimous demand on the part of the public that the inmates be treated with something like the recognition of the Golden Rule [which] demand[s] good care of the patient first and abstract benefits to science as an after consideration. . . . It should be well understood . . . that no patient need be subjected to a clinical examination or clinical treatment without his consent, whether he be a private or a charity patient.

The Modern Hospital, Hornsby and Schmidt, 1913[2]

> The patient, and the patient only, must say whether he or she is to be operated upon .... [P]ermit for operation is signed by the patient in any language that he or she can write, and the signature is witnessed by at least two persons.... The form of this permit is given forthwith.
>
> I, the undersigned ____ a patient at the____ Hospital, hereby certify that I have full knowledge of the operation to be performed upon me and do hereby give my express consent thereto, and in consideration of the performance of the said operation by said Dr. ____and the said Hospital___ from any and all claim of any kind that I may have against them at any time hereafter as the result of the said operation, or because of the same or of anything arising in the connection therewith.
>
> *The Modern Hospital*, Hornsby and Schmidt, 1913[3]

> Every human being of adult years and sound mind has a right to determine what shall be done with his own body; and a surgeon who performs an operation without his patient's consent commits an assault for which he is liable in damages.
>
> Justice Benjamin Cardozo (1870–1938), *Schloendorff v. Society of New York Hospital*, 211 N.Y. 125, 105 N.E. 92 (1914)

SOME MISCONCEPTIONS ABOUT THE HISTORY OF INFORMED CONSENT

Every field has foundation myths, "just-so" stories of its origins that sound good in the telling but that do not bear up under historical scrutiny. One of the just-so stories that bioethicists tell their students, the public, and the press is that they introduced the practice of requiring medical practitioners and researchers to obtain "informed consent" from patients and research subjects. To quote one of the founders of the field, law school professor Jay Katz (1922–2008), before the rise of bioethics "[d]octors felt that...they were obligated to attend to their patients...without consulting with their patients about the decisions that needed to be made.... The legal doctrine of informed consent is only 25 years old [i.e., it arose in the 1960s]."[4] Another of the field's founders, John C. Fletcher (1932–2004), wrote that as late as "1952 the norm of voluntary informed consent...was not part of the ethos of American researchers."[5]

Yet legal recognition of consent as a prerequisite to experimentation arose well before the 1960s. It dates to the very first law regulating health professionals in the British colonies, the Duke of York's Law of 1665. This law states that "no person or persons employed...as chirugeons, midwives, physicians, or others [may] presume to set forth or exercise any act contrary to the known approved rule of art"—that is to say, no one may engage in experimental surgery or medicine—"upon or towards the body of any...without the...consent of the patient or patients if they be *mentis compotes*, much less contrary to such consent."[6] Bioethicists revolutionized our conception of consent and of the patient–physician and subject–researcher relationships. Yet they did not invent the practice of consenting patients or research subjects; rather, they created a new understanding of the moral basis of consent and new enforcement mechanisms,[7] thereby—or so I shall argue in the next chapter—launching an ethics revolution.

Still, the bioethicists' just-so story seems intuitively correct. As every schoolchild ought to know, social class, gender, racial, and religious divisions visibly stratified American society until the 1960s, when these strata were shaken by egalitarian ethical, moral, and legal ideals enacted in such measures as the Civil Rights and Voting Rights Acts. Similarly, before the enactment of Medicare and Medicaid in the 1960s, American hospitals and other medical institutions mirrored the stratifications of American society. Private hospitals divided according to religious denominations (Catholic, Episcopalian, Jewish, Methodist, Presbyterian, etc.) and served the affluent in private wards and the deserving poor in charity wards; public hospitals served everyone else—and, in the South, the races were treated apart. So it might seem self-evident, given the gap in prestige, power, social status, and civil and human rights between white male researchers and the disenfranchised, servile, indigent, and colored people who served as subjects, that researchers could exploit subjects at will—without seeking their consent. Yet, fact being stranger than just-so stories, it was in just these inegalitarian contexts that practices of consent seeking became the expected standard of conduct in American medical research.

As a practical matter, researchers of yesteryear, much like researchers today, needed to recruit subjects, retain their services through the course of an experiment, and ensure their subjects' cooperation. These mundane practical considerations—recruitment, retention, and cooperation—prompted researchers to offer their subjects monetary and nonmonetary compensation and to seek their consensual cooperation. The law also moderated researchers' conduct: Anglo-American law has consistently held that, to reiterate the wording of the Duke of York's law, no medical practitioner may "presume to" experiment "upon or towards the body of any...without the...consent of the patient or patients if they be *mentis compotes*, much less contrary to such consent."[8] So said Anglo-American law in the seventeenth century, and so it would reaffirm in every subsequent century—albeit with greater emphasis on knowledgeable and appreciative consent from the mid-twentieth century onward.[9] So, since neither a license to practice medicine nor a medical diploma accords its holder the right to assault or batter anyone, consent was sought to mitigate the likelihood of lawsuits, irrespective of whether the patient or subject was female or male, in service or bound, or even enslaved—since masters could sue if researchers damaged their "property." Subjects' voluntary consent, especially if documented by consent forms or contracts, provided protection against prosecution for assault or battery—and, by the end of the nineteenth century, it also provided some protection against a rising tide of medical malpractice lawsuits.[10]

Another factor encouraging researchers to seek consent from their subjects was the public nature of the research enterprise itself. To contribute to the progress of medical science, to bring honor and prestige to researchers and to advance their careers, experimenters needed to disseminate accounts of their experiments to their peers, their funders, and often to the public as well. Insofar as research was a public enterprise subject to professional and communal scrutiny, researchers had reason to treat their subjects in ways that would be perceived as morally and politically acceptable. Peer acceptance of experiments confirming the mosquito transmission theory of yellow fever, for example, was facilitated by opinion makers like Johns Hopkins professor Sir William Osler. Thus, in the 1898 edition of his textbook, *The Principles and Practice of Medicine*, the standard medical text of its day, Osler condemned the research practices of Italian bacteriologist Giuseppe Sanarelli (1864–1900) as "marred by a series of unjustifiable experiments upon men which should receive the unqualified condemnation of the profession."[11] By contrast, in the 1901 edition, Osler praised experiments directed by the Yellow Fever Commission of the United States Army—Aristides Agramonte (1868–1931), James Carroll (1854–1907), Jesse W. Lazear (1866–1900), and Walter Reed (1851–1902)—as "remarkable," "conducted in the most rigid and scientific manner."[12] Significantly, Osler declared the sacrifice of human life in this experiment morally justifiable because "young soldiers [served] voluntarily, without any compensation, and purely in the interests of humanity."[13]

No matter how impressive their scientific achievements, American researchers risked condemnation by peers like Osler and faced possible loss of funding, public censure, and legal consequences if they transgressed professional ethics or public moral sensibilities. Volunteerism and consent—supplemented, in risky nontherapeutic experiments by the Golden Rule requirement of serving as a subject one's self—served to reconcile risks to human subjects with medical ethics and public morality. At a deeper level, as self-justifying and/or soul-searching statements in researchers' diaries, letters, and publications indicate, volunteerism, consent, and contracts preserved researchers' sense of moral and psychological well-being by assuaging feelings of guilt associated with any indignities, discomforts, disabilities, or deaths they might inflict on their subjects.

Nontherapeutic experiments, in particular, were morally problematic on their face because, instead of holding out the promise of making sick patients better, they risked making healthy people sick, and sick people even sicker—an inversion of the primary objectives of healthcare. To quote, John Hornsby M.D. (1861–circa 1924), secretary of the American Medical Association's (AMA) Hospital Section and founding member of the American Hospital Association (AHA; founded in 1906, still functioning), such experiments seem to violate the "Golden Rule [of healthcare which] demand[s] good care of the patient first and abstract benefits to science as an after consideration."[14] Voluntarism, consent, and above all else, the researchers' willingness to follow the Golden Rule by doing unto themselves what they would ask of others, elevated the moral status of nontherapeutic experiments by demonstrating the researcher's belief that the risks they asked of others were worth undertaking.

The Role of Total Institutions and Pet Keeping

Two social factors exacerbated ethical issues surrounding medical research in post-Civil War America: the rising population of Americans in total institutions and the newly fashionable practice of pet keeping. *Total institutions*, as classically defined by sociologist Erving Goffman (1922–1982), are those whose members are cut off from the rest of society and whose activities are regulated from dawn to dusk and often through the night.[15] Armies, asylums, hospitals, orphanages, prisons, and schools are total institutions in this sense. The highly regulated nature of these settings makes them methodologically ideal for conducting controlled trials. Yet the same highly controlling environment also undermines the likelihood that soldiers, inmates, patients, or students in these institutions have a real choice about participating in an experiment. Compounding the problem, institutionalization can strip one of the personal prerogatives and legal rights that a noninstitutionalized person normally enjoys. So, paradoxically, the highly regulated environment that makes total institutions methodologically attractive to researchers also renders them morally problematic.

Animal laboratories are total institutions with none of these disadvantages; yet they have limitations because nonhuman animals are not ideal models for human physiology since they may not be susceptible to human diseases (e.g., yellow fever). Despite these limitations, demonstrations and experiments on living animals had been integral to Scottish and American medicine ever since Monro *primus* opened the doors of his anatomy class in eighteenth-century Edinburgh. Yet, ironically, just as animal experimentation was beginning to yield results in the emerging sciences of bacteriology and physiology, the morality of experimenting on animals was being called into question.

Urban Americans had begun to perceive some animals not as food sources and labor extenders but as family members and child substitutes: that is, around the time of the Civil War, they began keeping some domesticated animals as "pets."[16] Prior to this, keeping animals for emotional satisfaction rather than for utilitarian reasons (i.e., pet keeping) was unusual. Cats and dogs, for example, were regarded as utilitarian creatures, as mousers and hunters, not as pets. Thus, Noah Webster's dictionaries of 1828 and 1841 did not define the noun "pet" in the twenty-first-century sense of "a domesticated animal kept for pleasure rather than utility"; instead these dictionaries define the noun "pet" as "any person or animal especially cherished and indulged; a fondling; a darling; often, a favorite child." By 1866, however, the emotional relationships previously reserved for favorite children began to be projected onto birds and other caged or domesticated animals. Pet keeping became commonplace enough to warrant publication of the first American book on the subject, *The Book of Household Pets* in 1866. The first American humane society, the American Society for the Prevention of Cruelty to Animals (ASPCA), was founded in the same year.[16] As some animals were transubstantiated into pets, experimenting on them came to be seen as "inhumane." So, from the end of the Civil War to the outbreak of World War I (which the United States entered in 1917), a strident antivivisectionist movement lobbied for legislation to restrict or prohibit animal experimentation. This agitation eventually morphed into an anti–human vivisectionist movement that lobbied against human as well as animal experimentation, demanding legislative oversight of both.

THREE SIGNIFICANT CASES IN RESEARCH ETHICS: BEAUMONT, SIMS, AND REED

Three cases and some controversies are analyzed in this chapter to flesh out these abstruse observations. They illustrate how moral, ethical, and legal ideals, together with practical and political considerations and changing social norms, combine to support consent practices in the pre-bioethics era. The first case involves nontherapeutic experiments and a signed notarized consent contract between a research subject, a French-Canadian (Quebecoise), Alexis Bidagan dit St. Martin, and a U.S. military surgeon known as the Father of Gastric Physiology, William Beaumont. The second case involves a controversial physician introduced in the previous chapter, J. Marion Sims; and the third involves the yellow fever experiments conducted by Walter Reed and his team.

Alexis St. Martin, William Beaumont, and the First American Consent Form

The Beaumont-St. Martin saga has two protagonists, one an illiterate French-speaking research subject, Alexis St. Martin, about whose thoughts we know little; the other, a literate researcher, William Beaumont, who, throughout his life, kept journals in which he jotted down random thoughts, drafts of aphorisms, and passages from books and newspapers along with his case notes.[17] Some early entries in these journals indicate that, like most American physicians of his day, Beaumont embraced an Edinburgh-style medical ethics based on a physician's virtues of beneficence, sympathy, and hopefulness. Beaumont embraced the view that his patients' health ought to be his first concern, that he was to act gently, sympathetically, and humanely towards his patients, and that he was to use his medical skill to instill hope, preserve health, and prevent his patients' death. As Beaumont wrote in his journal,

> Physicians when tending their patients should make their health their first object. So gentle and sympathizing should be their disposition in the apartment of the sick that pain and distress should seem suspended in their presence. So exhilarating ought their visits to be that hope should follow in their footsteps, so salutatory their prescriptions that death should drop his commission in combat with his skill.[18]

Later entries in the journal indicate that after Beaumont became a military surgeon during the War of 1812–1815, he also embraced an ethics of gentlemanly and military honor, flyting with an artillery officer whom he posted[19] as a "contemptible *liar*, a base villain, and a poltroon" (i.e., a craven coward).[20] After his adversary declined to duel, the officers of the regiment condemned the adversary for "conduct unbecoming an officer and a gentleman," and commended Dr. Beaumont for acting on "principles... which honor and justice should dictate to every gentleman in a similar situation."[21]

The journal also records Beaumont's adoption of yet another set of values. While "looking over an old newspaper [Beaumont] came across Doc. [Benjamin] Franklin's 'project for attaining moral perfection.'"[22] Impressed by the self-improvement project, Beaumont copied Franklin's list of virtues in its entirety and resolved to master them. Among the virtues Beaumont sought to cultivate were those of

> (4) Resolution—Resolve to perform without fail what you resolve. (5) Frugality—Make no expense but to do good to others or yourself; waste nothing.... (7) Sincerity—Use no hurtful deceit; think innocently and justly, and, if you speak, speak accordingly. (8) Justice—Wrong none by doing injuries, or omitting the benefits that are your duty.[23]

These virtues—*resolve, frugality, sincerity,* and *justice*—structured Beaumont's dealings with St. Martin. Beaumont was resolute in recruiting St. Martin as a subject and in continuing his series of experiments, despite being stationed in frontier outposts. Yet, in part because he paid St. Martin out of his own pocket,

Beaumont was always extremely frugal in his negotiations with St. Martin; but he was also sincere in the sense of never having recourse to deception. Finally, Beaumont subscribed to ideals of personal justice in the sense of avoiding wrongdoing and treating others as duty demands. Beaumont's sense of justice, however, was not the egalitarian sense of justice that shaped the bioethics movement; it was a sense of personal justice—an ideal of fair dealings between persons of different classes, including persons of lower social classes.

Some apparently original moral precepts that Beaumont penned in his journal at the time that he was working with St. Martin shed light on their relationship.

> (1) He that disgraces his character by degrading unprincipled conduct should be shunned and despised by all decent classes of the community....
>
> (2) Dread of the future, & fear of consequences are not the natural attributes of virtue and innocence but rather the offspring of guilt and cowardice.
>
> (3) Know God from universal creation, read his words in the *Book of Nature*, study his *laws* in the *various* Systems of the Universe, and *learn* his wisdom in the phenomena of *animal life*.
>
> (4) He that voluntarily stands as the champion of a false and falling system or a worthless & unworthy character is either a *knave* or a *fool* and ought to be [despised? disproved?] and avoided by the present and future generations.[24]

The expression, used in item 1, "all decent classes of the community," reflects Beaumont's view that communities consist of persons of different social classes. His was a class-conscious era in which ethical precepts were also class conscious. Acts of gentlemanly honor—flyting, dueling, and the like—apply only within the gentlemanly class: a gentlemen would never flyte or duel with someone from the serving classes. Nonetheless, Beaumont recognized many "decent classes" in a community. Proposition (3) characterizes scientific inquiry as learning God's wisdom by studying the book of nature as revealed in life—and so by peering into St. Martin's stomach, Beaumont likely thought of himself as reading God's book of revelation. From his perspective, moreover, it would be foolish, unworthy (as indicated in 4), and despicable in the eyes of future generations to fail to take such an opportunity to remove false understandings or systems of physiology. As historian Ronald Numbers remarks, American physicians of Beaumont's generation believed that they "had a 'moral duty' to take every opportunity to observe and experiment. In this climate, failing to experiment became unethical."[25]

Beaumont's first journal entry about Saint Martin describes him as "[a] Canadian lad about 19 years old, hardy, robust & healthy, [who] was accidentally shot by the unlucky discharge of a gun on the 6th of June 1822."[26] Despite the apparent hopelessness of the case, Beaumont resolutely did everything in his power to heal his patient and to alleviate his suffering. After seven months of treatment, on

December 2, 1822, Beaumont noted in his journal that even though "the orifice within the stomach is still visible," St. Martin's "health [is] daily improving—his spirits good…and all the functions of his system natural and healthy." Beaumont then posed a key therapeutic question: "Can the puncture of the stomach be successfully closed by mechanical means?"[27] To test the possibility of closure, Beaumont explored several innovative interventions, but he characterized none of them as "experimental," apparently because his intent was therapeutic.

On May 30, 1823, when St. Martin "complained of a pain in the head, nausea, and some irregularity of the bowels," Beaumont decided on an intervention to treat St. Martin's constipation in a manner that appears experimental. He gave St. Martin a

> Cathartic [to accelerate defecation]…*administered*, it is presumed as never medicine was before administered to man since the creation of the world!—to wit,—by pouring it in through the ribs at the puncture into the stomach—!!—I administered it in the form of a dry powder. It occasioned a slight nausea in less than 10 minutes and operated briskly as a cathartic in less than two hours.
>
> 31st 1823: [Patient] feels relieved by the operation of the medicine given yesterday—administered in the same manner today.[28]

The cathartic "administered…as never medicine was before" was clearly innovative yet, since Beaumont's intent was therapeutic, he did not characterize it as an "experiment." Historian Ronald Numbers suggests that the innovative nature of this intervention gave Beaumont the notion of performing deliberate, nontherapeutic experiments on St. Martin.[29] Beaumont himself offered an account of this transition in a January 1834 memo soliciting funds from the U.S. Congress. Here, Beaumont portrays himself as a resolute savior, a caring physician seeking justice for an abandoned patient.

> In [June 1823 St. Martin's] wound was partially healed; but he was still abject, altogether miserable and helpless.—In this situation he was declared a "common pauper" by the civic authorizes of the County and was resolved by them, that they were not able to support, and declined taking care of him—and in pursuance of what they probably believed to be their duty, were about to transport him to the place of his nativity [a hamlet outside Montreal] a distance of nearly fifteen hundred miles.
>
> Knowing the life of St. Martin must inevitably be sacrificed, if such attempt to remove him should be carried into execution at that time, your memorialist…*resolved*, as the only way to rescue St. Martin from impending misery and death, to assume the responsibility of arresting the process of

transportation by taking him into his own private family, where all the care and attention were bestowed that his condition required....

In this situation Your Memorialist received, kept, nursed, medically treated & sustained St. Martin, at great inconvenience and expense for nearly two years—dressed his wounds *daily* ... nursed him, fed him, clothed him, lodged him and furnished him with such necessaries and comforts as his condition and suffering required.

At the end of these two years he had become able to walk, and help himself a little, though wholly unable to provide for his own necessities. In this situation Your Memorialist maintained St. Martin in his family for the considerable time for the *special* purpose of Physiological experiments, after he should have sufficiently recovered, to admit of the process being commenced.

The peculiar condition of St. Martin's stomach, Your Memorialist verily believes, afforded the greatest facilities for improving an important branch of Medical Science, that *ever* had, or *ever would*, probably be presented—the wound, in healing, having left an open aperture, of considerable size, directly into the stomach, thro which food, drink and other substances, could be passed into, and from, any part of its cavity, and by means of which Experiments and observations of the highest importance to Physiological investigation have been and may continue to be made, with the most useful and satisfactory results.[30]

The memo—in effect, a grant proposal—continues with a request for funding. One point to notice here is that Beaumont seems to recognize a transformation in his relationship to St. Martin. Initially, he was St. Martin's physician, playing the role he had learned as an apprentice in Vermont: placing his patient's interests first, while gently, sympathetically, humanely—and resolutely—using innovative treatments to save his patient's life and restore his health. Nonetheless, the case fascinated Beaumont because a fistula (permanent opening) around the wound allowed him to insert and remove small pieces of food from St. Martin's stomach, tracking the digestive process and thus observing the physiology of digestion—God's laws as revealed in the Book of Nature. So, fearing that both St. Martin's life and his own studies were endangered by the plan to repatriate St. Martin to Montreal, in June 1823, Beaumont took St. Martin into his own household and provided him with medical treatment *gratis*.

A letter that Beaumont's wife, Deborah (1787–1871) wrote to her parents in December 1823 reflects St. Martin's initial status in the Beaumont household. He was, she wrote, a "creature... an invalid boy [who would] do a thing for me, [since her hands were full with] two babies and [she was expecting] a third [baby] and [had to] do all [her] own serving, milking, baking, [and] make [her] own butter."[31] In her eyes, this thirty-year-old "invalid boy"[32] was a mere "creature"—a dependent with a lower status than a proper servant—who could help with some household chores: he was neither a patient nor a research subject. At some point in the next year, however, this invalid-boy-creature-who-helped-out assumed a different role as Beaumont initiated a series of deliberate physiological experiments using St. Martin as his subject. Only then does Beaumont use the term "experiment" in his journal, in such headings as "Experiment 1st," a study of the digestion of corned beef.[33] "Experiment," as Beaumont used the term in his journals and publications, refers exclusively to nontherapeutic interventions for scientific purposes.

At no time during the 1820s, neither before these experiments had commenced nor in any letters or publications about the experiments, does Beaumont use the term "consent" or "contract." The situation is thus precisely as envisioned in bioethicists' just-so version of the history of research ethics: an empowered physician-benefactor takes advantage of a patient's gratitude and dependence to exploit him as a research subject without the patient-subjects' consent—and, as it turned out, against the patient's wishes. For, in August 1825, when Beaumont and his extended family, including St. Martin, were traveling near the Canadian border, St. Martin left them without notice. St. Martin's sudden departure changed the dynamics of his relationship with Beaumont. Having voiced his dissatisfaction with his arrangement with Beaumont with his feet, so to speak, St. Martin deprived Beaumont of his research subject at the very moment when Beaumont was coming into prominence as a researcher.

Seeking to regain his research subject, Beaumont commissioned the American Fur Company to locate St. Martin and persuade him to return to service. In a letter of August 1827, an agent of the Fur Company informed Beaumont that he "[s]ucceeded in finding your ungrateful Boy Alexis St. Martin. He is *Married* … he is poor and miserable beyond Description and his wound is worse than when he left you.… I did all I could to bring him up but could not succeed."[34] A second letter informed Beaumont that

> there will be no difficulty in getting [St. Martin] Back at any reasonable Price Providing you will employ his Wife!!!—also—he is miserably Poor and will remain So while he lives unless he comes back to you. I think you had better write to me in New York requesting me to engage Alexis & his Wife to come up and remain with you one or two years.[35]

In 1829, the American Fur Company secured St. Martin's "service" to Beaumont by adopting a standard contract used to employ trappers. Ironically, the first consent document in the history of American medical research was not motivated by medical ethical ideals or by fear of public or peer censure; the motive was eminently practical: the need to recruit a research subject. Thus, as it turns out, the American Fur Company of New York was the first American contract research organization (CRO).

After the fur company contract expired St. Martin left Beaumont's service and returned to Canada. In 1832, and again in 1834, Beaumont and St. Martin negotiated contracts without using the fur company as an intermediary—although, as historian Alexa Green has observed, these contracts were also modeled on those used by the fur company.[36] In the 1832 contract, St. Martin agrees to "go, or travel, or reside in any part of the world [as Beaumont's] covenant Servant" for one year and "during said term" to "submit to, assist and promote by all means in his power... [such] Philosophical or Medical experiments" as Beaumont "shall direct or cause to be made on or in [his] Stomach... either through or by the means of the aperture or opening in the side... and will obey, suffer and comply with all reasonable and proper orders or experiments." These experiments, however, "shall be reasonably and properly used... for the purposes of science and scientific improvements, the furtherance of knowledge in regard to the power, properties and capacity of the human Stomach." Beaumont, in turn was to provide St. Martin with "good, suitable and sufficient subsistence, washing, lodging and wearing apparel and in sickness good proper & suitable medicine & medical attendance & nursing."[37] Beaumont was also to pay St. Martin $150—a payment that would be valued at $37,500 in 2010 dollars (i.e., a full year's salary for an unskilled laborer). St. Martin was paid more in the two-year 1833 contract, $200 per year, or an annual salary of $48,700 in 2010 dollars.[38] Supplemental agreements guaranteed St. Martin's wife paid employment.

Writing in 1912, Beaumont's first biographer, Jesse Meyer, M.D. (1873–1913) observed of this contract that its "like... has never been duplicated in human history."[39] What Meyer probably had in mind was that, in contrast to early twentieth-century consent forms, the Beaumont-St. Martin agreement is not an agreement to forego suing the researcher (i.e., to "hold the researcher harmless"); it is an employment contract, adopted from the format used by the American Fur Company to recruit and retain someone as a "covenant Servant." It was the sort of contract one might make with a live-in housemaid or a groundskeeper. As any other contract for employment would, it stipulates the expected duration of employment (one year), and it contains a job description: serving as a subject in the experiments to be conducted. In addition, the contract offers St. Martin a health benefit guaranteeing him good medical care in the event of "sickness." In return, the employee, St. Martin, is obligated to "obey, suffer and comply with all reasonable and proper orders or experiments." Thus, St. Martin seems to have a right to decline any unreasonable or improper experiment.

For a variety of reasons, such a contract for employment would never pass muster as a twenty-first-century informed consent form. It is vague about the details of the experiments, noting only that they are to be performed through the existing aperture (fistula) into St. Martin's stomach; it says nothing about risks to the subject; and it lacks any discussion of privacy or confidentiality. Contemporary institutional research boards (IRBs) would also question whether the illiterate French-speaking subject actually understood the complex English-language contract to which he had affixed his mark or whether he knew the extent of the risks involved in the experiments or appreciated their possible impact on him. More striking, because contemporary consent documents are designed to formalize a research subject's rights, a conscientious IRB would also challenge whether anyone as vulnerable as St. Martin could give truly "voluntary" consent. An IRB today would also probe whether the prospect of a full year's salary plus room, board, clothing, and healthcare for himself and employment for his wife might not "unduly induce" or "unduly influence" (to use bioethical terms) St. Martin's decision making—concepts that make no sense whatsoever in the context of labor negotiations, where financial inducements are never "unduly" inducing or influential.

Although the Beaumont-St. Martin contract would be unacceptable by standards of twenty-first-century bioethicists, historian Ronald Numbers concludes that "Beaumont appears to have been no more insensitive or less concerned about the welfare of his subject than other nineteenth-century physiologists. Indeed, his paternal interest in St. Martin may place him a cut above his contemporaries."[40] Numbers' observation attests to the changes in research ethics, underlining the fact that the humanitarian and legal concerns of the 1900s and later bioethical concerns about research subjects' rights were unconceived and unimaginable in the America of the 1830s. Prior to the bioethics revolution, American commentators characterized Beaumont's experiments on St. Martin as praiseworthy, morally unproblematic contributions to medical science and accepted the validity of St. Martin's consent to serve as a human subject without question.[41]

The Beaumont-St. Martin relationship came to a sad end. Although Beaumont was ingenious in finding alternative funding sources through the Army and the U.S. Congress, his limited salary as a military surgeon forced him to cultivate the virtue of frugality—which led to a series of failed contract negotiations. In the end, Beaumont could not provide the sums requested by St. Martin and his wife, so his experiments ceased. After Beaumont's death, St. Martin made a living exhibiting his fistula to physicians and even to gawking bystanders. When St. Martin died, his relatives allowed his body to decompose and then buried it at a secret site so that no physician or medical student could "resurrect" the stomach with the famous fistula.[42]

Fittingly, in June 1962, the Canadian Physiological Society erected a bilingual plaque commemorating St. Martin's contributions to their science. The English reads,

> In memory of
> Alexis Bidagan St. Martin

Born April 18, 1794 at Berthier
Died, June 28, 1880 at St Thomas
Buried June 28, 1880 in an unmarked grave close by this tablet.

Grievously wounded by the accidental discharge of a shotgun on June 6, 1822…he made a miraculous recovery under the care of Dr. William Beaumont.…After his wounds had healed, he was left with an opening into the stomach and became the subject of Dr. Beaumont's pioneering work on the physiology of digestion.

Through his work he served all humanity.[43]

Anarcha, Betsy, Lucy, and J. Marion Sims: Consent to Surgical Experiments

Anarcha, Betsy, and Lucy were three African-American slave women in Alabama whose protracted deliveries left them persistently incontinent. The trio was, in all likelihood, illiterate, and what little we know about them must be gleaned from the speeches, letters, publications, and unfinished autobiography of pioneering gynecologist J. Marion Sims. Sims first mentioned this trio in 1854, when he acknowledged that, but for the "heroic fortitude of [these] patients," he would have failed to develop the first effective repair of obstetric fistulas[44]—a hole between the bladder and vagina that rendered these women continuously incontinent of urine and often of feces as well. According to the World Health Organization (WHO), each year 50,000–100,000 women who give birth without the aid of modern medicine develop such fistulas as a result of obstructed labor. These women "suffer constant incontinence, shame, social segregation and health problems. It is estimated that more than 2 million women live with untreated obstetric fistula in Asia and sub-Saharan Africa."[45]

Unusually for medical researchers even today, Sims consistently shared credit for developing the first effective repair for such fistulas with his research subjects. Thus, in an 1857 address to the New York Academy of Medicine Sims credited

> The indomitable courage of these long-suffering women, more than to any one other single circumstance, is the world indebted for the results of these persevering efforts. Had they faltered, then would woman have continued to suffer from the dreadful injuries produced by parturition, and then should the broad domain of surgery not known one of the most useful improvements that shall forever grace its annals.[46]

As Sims recounts the tale,[47] his quest to invent a surgical repair for obstetric fistulas began when he was a twenty-seven-year-old Alabama country doctor earning a living attending to the medical needs of plantation owners, their families, and their slaves. An older physician had called on Sims to assist him in treating Anarcha,

> a young colored woman about seventeen years of age...who had been in labor more then seventy-two hours. The child's head was so impacted in the pelvis that the labor pains had almost entirely ceased...the [stillborn] child was brought away with forceps. [Unfortunately] there was an extensive sloughing of the soft parts the mother having lost control of both the bladder and the rectum. Of course, aside from death this was about the worst accident that could have happened to the poor young girl....The case was hopelessly incurable.[48]

A month later, another plantation owner consulted Sims about "[h]is negro girl, Lucy, about eighteen years old, [who] had given birth to a child two months ago and since that time...had been unable to hold any water." Sims replied: "She has a fistula in the bladder—a hole in it [so] the urine runs all the time....I don't want to see her....It is absolutely incurable." According to Sims' autobiography, the plantation owner replied, "You are putting on airs. When you were my family doctor and used to see my family or my niggers, you never objected to an investigation of their cases....I am going to send Lucy in."[49] Sims recounts that Lucy showed up at his office the following day.

> I had a little hospital of eight beds built in the corner of my yard for taking care of my negro patients and for negro surgical cases; and so when Lucy came I gave her a bed....I examined her case very minutely. I told her that I was unable to do anything for her, and I said, "Tomorrow afternoon I have to send you home." She was very disappointed, for her condition was loathsome and she was in hope that she would be cured.[50]

Chance favoring the prepared mind, Sims had an "aha" moment while attending a white woman, Mrs. Merrill, "the wife of a dissipated old man...a respectable woman who obtained a living by washing and taking in sewing, and was much appreciated and respected among her neighbors."[51] Placing Mrs. Merrill in an odd position to correct her inverted uterus, Sims discovered what later came to be known as the "Sims position," which offered a clear view of a woman's internal organs.

> [Sims] said to [him]self...why can I not take the incurable case of vesico-vaginal [obstetric] fistula which seems now to be so incomprehensible and put the girl in this position and see exactly what are the relations of the surrounding tissues. Fired with this idea...I jumped into my buggy and drove

> hurriedly home.... Arriving there, I said [to another patient with obstetric fistula], "Betsey... I want to make one more examination of your case." She willingly consented. I got a table about three feet long and put a coverlet upon it and mounted her on the table on her knees with her head resting on the palms of her hands. I placed two [medical] students one on each side of the pelvis and they laid hold of the nates, and pulled them open.... Introducing the bent handle of the spoon I saw everything, as no man had ever seen before. The fistula was as plain as the nose on a man's face. The edges were clear and well defined, and distinct, and the opening could be measured as accurately as if it had been cut out of a piece of plain paper.... I said at once, "Why can not these things be cured? It seems to me that there is nothing to do but to pare the edges of the fistula and bring it together nicely, introduce a catheter in the neck of the bladder and drain the urine off continually and the case will be cured."[52]

It took Sims almost four years of experiments—from 1845 to 1849—to learn how to close an obstetric fistula with sutures that did not become infected in the pre-asepsis, pre-antiseptics, pre-antibiotic, and pre-anesthesia era of the 1840s. Ironically, the AMA would first approve ether as a safe and effective anesthetic in May 1849,[53] the same month in which Sims managed his first successful postoperative recovery from fistula repair surgery. Even after the AMA's announcement, however, Sims and many other physicians trained in the pre-anesthesia era considered ether anesthesia too risky to use for anything except major surgery.[54]

Anarcha was the first of Sims's patients to enjoy a successful postoperative recovery from a fistula repair;[55] successful repairs of Betsy and Lucy's fistulas soon followed. Yet, since Sims had to earn a living, he did not pen an article on repairing obstetric fistulas until two years later. At the time, he was suffering from persistent diarrhea and believed that he would soon "die... in bed [so he] wrote out the history of [his] operations... and sent the article to Dr. Isaac Hays the editor of *The American Journal of the Medical Sciences*. It was published in... 1852,"[56] as, or so Sims believed at the time, his "last... offering to the medical profession before I should quit this world."[57]

Deeply in debt and struggling to regain his health, Sims decided to leave the South for healthier Northern climes. Since funds from the sale of his house and property were insufficient to repay his debts, Sims contemplated raising additional funds by selling his house slaves. When they protested, however, he freed them, remarking in his autobiography that he "would not put any of them in slavery against their will."[58] Sims "left Montgomery [Alabama] for New York [City] about the first of May (1853), so near dead that no one thought that [he] would ever get to New York. [He] had to lie down all the way on the railroad train. The diarrhea was uncontrolled."[59]

Sims regained his health in the cooler climate of New York City, where he opened a practice as a gynecological surgeon. To advertise his expertise to the physicians of his new hometown, Sims published an article on obstetric fistulas in an 1854 issue of a New York medical journal. In the article, he also praised "the heroic fortitude of [his] patients," Anarcha, Betsy, and Lucy.

> I was fortunate in having three young healthy colored girls given to me by their owners in Alabama, I agreeing to perform no operation without the full consent of the patients, and never to perform any that would, in my judgment, jeopard[ize] life, or produce greater mischief on the injured organs—the owner agreeing to let me keep them (at my own expense).[60]

Sims notes in the article that to perfect the fistula repair procedure he "operated on these three upwards of forty times...one of them [Lucy] submitted to more than twenty operations, not only cheerfully but with thanks."[61]

Sims reiterates these themes in the unfinished autobiography that he dictated about a quarter of a century later, in 1882, recalling how his brother-in-law urged him to quit his seemingly quixotic quest to develop a successful repair for obstetric fistulas:

> [M]y operations all failed [for]...four years. I kept all these negroes at my own expense all the time...this was an enormous tax for a young doctor in country practice.... [After] years of constant failure and fruitless effort...it was with difficulty that I could get any doctor to help me. But, notwithstanding the repeated failures, I had succeeded in inspiring my patients with confidence that they would be cured eventually...and at last I performed operations only with the assistance of the patients themselves.
>
> My brother-in-law...came to me one day, and he said: "I have come to have a serious talk with you.... [W]ith your young and growing family it is unjust to them to continue in this way, and carry on this series of experiments. You have no idea what it costs you to support a-half-dozen niggers, now more than three years, and my advice to you is to resign the whole subject and give it up. It is better for you and better for your family."
>
> [Sims relates replying] "I am too near the accomplishment of the work to give it up now. My patients are all perfectly satisfied with what I am doing for them. I cannot depend on the doctors, and so I have trained them to assist me in the operations. I am going on with this series of experiments to the end. It matters not what it costs, [even] if it costs me my life."[62]

These narratives reveal a great deal about Sims's conception of his relation to his subjects. He characterizes Anarcha, Betsy, Lucy as "long-suffering women,"[63] "a young colored woman...poor girl,"[64] a "servant girl...negro girl,"[65] "three young healthy colored girls given to me by their owners in Alabama,"[66] "negroes [kept] at [his] own expense,"[67] and "my patients"—this last, "patients," was the most frequent characterization.[68] In dictating his autobiography, he has his brother-in-law and the plantation owner characterize these three "negro patients" differently: they refer to them as "niggers," [69] or, "my niggers."[70] To appreciate why it was important for Sims to differentiate his speech from that of the planter and his brother-in-law, it is helpful to recall that Sims, a Southerner, was addressing Northern audiences just prior to and in the aftermath of the Civil War. His first publication on obstetric fistulas appeared in 1852—the same year that Harriet Beecher Stowe (1811–1896) sold 300,000 copies of her antislavery novel, *Uncle Tom's Cabin*, sometimes referred to as the book that started the Civil War.[71] Sims's 1857 address to the New York Academy of Medicine was delivered in the same year that the U.S. Supreme Court announced *Dred Scott* (60 US 393), a decision that infuriated Northern abolitionists by denying citizenship to freed slaves living in the North and to the descendants of freed slaves. Finally, Sims dictated his autobiography in 1883, when the memory of the quarter of a million Union soldiers' who died in a war to save the union and to end the moral blight of slavery was still part of his audience's living memory.[72]

As a Southerner practicing in New York City, Sims was well aware that slavery was an incendiary subject. So to differentiate himself linguistically from Southern bigots who denigrated Negros as "niggers," Sims portrayed his African-American subjects as "colored," or "negro," or as "girls" or "women"—but, to reiterate, most frequently he referred to them as his "patients"; that is, as women whose suffering he, as a physician, was obligated to treat. He stated unequivocally, however, that these "three young healthy colored girls were given to me by their owners"—an assertion that, without mentioning the word "slave" made evident to his audience that these young women were enslaved. Sims then reassures his audience that he did not mistreat these "colored girls," having agreed "to perform no operation without the full consent of [his] patients, and never to perform any that would, in [his] judgment, jeopard[ize] life, or produce greater mischief on the injured organs."[73] Moreover, although Sims recounts that he treated these patients in a segregated hospital for Negro patients, he also indicates that he accorded them the prerogatives of patient status—including consent. Thus, in his 1882 autobiography, Sims reports saying to "Betsy...I want to make one more examination of your case." After "she willingly consented," Sims began his examination by setting up an examination table and "[putting] *a coverlet upon* it."[74] Thus, Sims asked consent before examining his patient, the enslaved Betsy, and then covered the examination table for her comfort.

Commentators writing in the post-civil rights bioethics era have been skeptical and sometimes caustically dismissive of Sims' claims.[75] After noting that "statues of Dr. Sims can be seen in [Alabama], New York and South Carolina,"[76] one critic remarked that any knowledgeable appraisal of Sims would condemn him for "unethical experimentation with powerless Black women" and for "manipulat[ing] the social institution of slavery to perform human experimentation, which by any standard is unacceptable."[77] Other critics deplored Sims for having "failed utterly to recognize his patients as autonomous persons,"[78] and several accused Sims of addicting the slaves who served as his subjects to ensure their compliance with his experiments.[79] "It was," another critic summed up acerbically, "chattel slavery and morphine, not courage, that bound the[se] women to [Sims] surgical table."[80]

The claims about morphine addiction rest on a misunderstanding of the postoperative treatment of obstetric fistulas. According to L. Lewis Wall, a urogynecological surgeon who founded the Worldwide Fistula Fund (2003) to provide obstetric fistula repairs to women in the developing world, Sims used low doses of opiates to constipate and sedate patients postoperatively, to prevent sutures from opening before the fistula repair had healed.[81] Sims applied the same postoperative sedating-constipating regimen on all of his patients, irrespective of race or social status. Still, one might ask, how likely was it that Sims asked his slave-subjects for consent? Or, that they truly volunteered?

Studies of the nineteenth-century American medical literature have consistently found that, from the 1820s onward, consent seeking and patient refusals of treatment (i.e., refusals against medical advice) were commonly reported in published accounts of surgical cases.[82] Sims himself contrasts a case in which *he* declined to operate on a lady with a case in which a lady's guardian declined an operation. The first case involved a woman for whom "the slightest touch at the mouth of [her] vagina produced intense suffering."[83] The lady had remained a virgin through a quarter-century of marriage and was consulting Sims about the possibility of surgical treatment. Although Sims thought a surgical cure might be possible, he "declined to do anything, on the grounds that an untried process was not justifiable on one in her position in society, the hospital being the legitimate field for experimental observation.... [It was not for someone of the] high intellectual endowments of this lady, [with] her elegant culture and fine social position."[84]

Sims contrasted this case with "another similar case in which a lady had been married but two years," and " had the same instinctive dread of being touched, the same muscular agitation... on attempting to pass the finger into the vagina. As this lady's husband threatened to obtain a divorce, I looked upon her case as a proper one for experiment. Explaining to her fully our ignorance of the subject, I proposed a series of experimental incisions, which she readily assented to."[85]

After a series of innovative surgeries brought only partial relief to the patient

> [T]he mother of my patient came to the conclusion that I was experimenting on her daughter. I told her it was true, and attempted to justify the propriety of the course when a lawsuit [for] divorce was in prospect. The mother, however, was inexorable, and unfortunately removed her from my care. But [the patient's] improvement was so great that I had no doubt of her ability to fulfill the duties of a wife under some difficulties.[86]

Sims refusal to perform innovative surgery, or to perform what he considered an "experiment"[87] on a high-status "lady" of "elegant culture and fine social position"[88] is striking evidence of the influence of social status on the physician–patient relationship in the inegalitarian world in which he practiced. So too is his statement that "the hospital" (i.e., the place where the lower classes receive medical treatment) was "the legitimate field for experimental observation."[89] The practice of the time was to conduct experiments on the lower social classes to improve medicine for more effective and safer use by the higher social classes. Nonetheless, Sims was willing to abandon this accepted norm and to perform innovative surgery on a "lady" (i.e., a woman of the higher social classes) for social reasons: her husband was going to shame her by dragging her through the divorce courts, thereby announcing to the world her inability to perform her marital functions.

Sims never characterizes Anarcha, Betsy, and Lucy as "ladies." They were "three young healthy colored girls given to [Sims] by their owners." As such, they were at the bottom of the social hierarchy and so, in his view, fit subjects for experimentation. Yet Sims repeatedly stated that he would "perform no operation" on these three girls without their "full consent" as "patients"; he states further that he would never "perform any [operation] that would, in [his] judgment, jeopard[ize their] lives, or produce greater mischief on the injured organs."[90] In reading this statement, it is important to appreciate that "full consent" was understood differently in the pre-bioethics era. For bioethicists, informed consent is an exercise in rationality in which one understands, appreciates, and weighs alternatives and decides accordingly. Before bioethics, however, medical decision making was thought to be appropriately emotive. Decisions that bioethicists would dismiss as inappropriately biased or based on a "therapeutic misconception" would have been regarded as appropriately emotive from the Edinburgh moral sense perspective of nineteenth-century American medicine, which viewed physicians as appropriately "ministers of hope." Thus, Sims proudly proclaims that he "infus[ed] . . . enthusiasm [for a cure] into the hearts of the dozen sufferers who looked to me for help, and implored me to repeat operations."[91] Sims also encouraged his respectable higher status "ladies" to expect a cure from his surgical innovations.[92] Status made a difference, however, for if these ladies or their guardians lost enthusiasm for his experiments, they could simply decline and walk out of Sims office.[93]

Could Sims's enslaved African-American patients simply walk away from an experiment if they were unwilling to serve as a subject? As a practical matter, as Sims' brother-in-law pointed out, supporting African-American slave research subjects was economically burdensome, and so uncooperative subjects would likely have been sent back to their plantations. Moreover, in the pre-anesthesia era in which Sims conducted his research, it was difficult to the point of near impossibility to perform surgery on uncooperative subjects. Historian Numbers describes a case in which researchers tried to conduct Beaumont-type experiments on an uncooperative patient with a gastric fistula. In the end, the exasperated researchers stated that their research had become "impossible" because the subject lacked "the desirable good attitude.... [S]he plagued us throughout this time by her ignorance, ill-will, and insubordination.... [G]ood experiments... were impossible... because the woman... did not allow them."[94] To reiterate, without the cooperation of subjects, surgical experiments were impractical, almost impossible in the pre-anesthesia surgical era. Thus, the multiple operations that Sims reports in his publications could not have been conducted without the active collaboration of Anarcha, Betsy, Lucy, and other enslaved subjects.

The gist of Sims's account seems plausible, especially if one recalls that his patients-subjects were suffering from what one nineteenth-century physician characterized as a truly pitiful malady:

> [C]ompared with which, most of the other physical evils of life sink into utter insignificance. The urine passing into the vagina... trickles constantly down her thighs, irritates the integument with its acrid qualities, keeps her clothing constantly soaked, and exhales without cessation its peculiar odor, insupportable to herself and those all around her... [and because] neither palliative nor curable means have availed for the relief of the sufferer, [some have] been compelled to sit constantly on a chair, or stool, with a hole in the seat, through which the urine descends into a vessel beneath.[95]

The WHO offers a similar characterization of women suffering from untreated obstetric fistulas today "constant incontinence, shame, social segregation and health problems."[96] Sims gave his patients some hope of curing their incontinence, of restoring their health and thereby of delivering them from shame and social segregation. It was their only opportunity for an alternative life, and it would be natural for them to seize it. So, to reiterate, Sims's stories of thankful, cooperative, and consenting subjects seem plausible.

If one accepts the gist of Sims's account of his treatment of Anarcha, Betsy, and Lucy as generally accurate, what do Sims's experiments and post-bioethical criticisms of them tell us about medical ethics then and bioethics now? Sims remarks in his autobiography that his views on honor and dueling "were entirely changed a long long time ago."[97] His views on Negroes appear to have evolved as well. Southern medical men typically shared the views of Louisiana physician Samuel Cartwright (1793–1863), who, like Sims, was a University of Pennsylvania alumnus. Cartwright characterized "the negro [as] a slave by nature, [who] can never be happy industrious, moral or religious in any other condition than the one he was intended to fill" (i.e., slavery).[98] Sims may initially have shared this view—which would explain his surprise on discovering that his house slaves did not wish to be enslaved—yet after working closely with Anarcha, Betsy, and Lucy for four years, in 1853, Sims freed his slaves, refusing to "put any of them in slavery against their will."[99] This decision suggests that in the years that Sims worked with closely with his African-American research subjects his view had evolved away from those held by Cartwright and other Southern physicians. Thus, in his lectures and publications, Sims takes the unusual step of sharing credit for his discoveries with his research subjects, Anarcha, Betsy, and Lucy.

More definitive proof of the evolution of Sims's views on the status of African Americans is to be found about two decades later, in 1876, when Sims undertook a one-person civil rights campaign to end the exclusion of women and African Americans from national meetings of the AMA. Using his role as the AMA's president, Sims publicly welcomed into the organization a woman delegate who others were lobbying to exclude. He then gratuitously extended this welcome by stating that if "any colored man... should rise to the dignity of representing a... Medical Society we must recognize him as such. And thus these knotty questions are settled forever." Sims was overly optimistic in believing that segregation in the AMA could be ended by presidential fiat (see discussion in Chapter 8); nonetheless, his declaration attests to a significant evolution of his views on the equality and rights of African Americans.[100]

Sims' work with Anarcha, Betsy, and Lucy in the 1840s predates these events. Nonetheless, Sims appears to have exhibited toward them the ethical characteristics and obligations required by the 1847 AMA *Code of Medical Ethics*: he ministered to their medical needs and condescended to them as required by the medical ethics of that inegalitarian era. As discussed in Chapter 6, "condescension" meant that, even though his patients were his social inferiors, Sims was obligated to treat them with the same courtesy that he would extend to their social superiors and also to inspire their minds "with gratitude, respect and confidence." As he would for any "lady," he had to, and did, ask for their consent to examine and/or to experiment on them. Judged by the standards articulated in the 1847 AMA *Code*, Sims conduct toward his African-American subjects was exemplary in all respects save one—in sharing credit for his discovery with his research subjects, he publicized their names, thereby breaching his "obligation of secrecy" (AMA *Code of Medical Ethics*, 1847, chapter I, article I, section 2).

Bioethics was formed, in part, in reaction to researchers' exploitation of vulnerable populations, most notably the 399 African-American males deceived into serving as research subjects by the U.S. Public Health Service (PHS) in its Tuskegee Syphilis Study (1932–1972). To quote from one of the field's foundational documents, the Belmont Report of 1979, bioethics arose from the need to protect "racial minorities, the economically disadvantaged, the very sick, and the institutionalized [who] may continually be sought as research subjects [precisely because of] their dependent status and their frequently compromised capacity for free consent,... [or] for administrative convenience, or because they are easy to manipulate as a result of their... socioeconomic condition."[101] Viewed from this perspective, Sims' choice of research subjects, enslaved African-American women, was unconscionable. Inverting the ethical precepts and social structures under which Sims operated, a bioethics perspective would mandate that Sims restrict his experiments to white ladies who had volunteered, fully cognizant of the risks and pain involved, because, unlike the enslaved African-American women on whom Sims actually operated, these white ladies (or their guardians) could freely refuse to serve as his subjects.

Many critics condemn Sims's experiments for just these reasons, arguing that his statues should be removed from state houses and public parks to be placed in museums of researcher infamy alongside images of the Nazi doctors convicted of crimes against humanity at Nuremberg. Unlike the Nazi doctors, however, Sims openly adhered to the medical ethics of his inegalitarian era, and so he could and did publicize both his methods and the results of his experiments. To be sure, assessed by the egalitarian standards of the late twentieth-century bioethics era, his experiments are unacceptable. Yet the medical morality of nineteenth-century America, and of the AMA *Code of Medical Ethics*, asserted the moral claims of medicine in the context of an inegalitarian era of class privilege and African-American enslavement. I believe that a more balanced assessment of Sims has been offered by urogynecologist L. Lewis Wall, who, like Sims, tended to the medical needs of women suffering from obstetric fistulas:

> The operations carried out by Sims on black slave women from 1845–1849 represented his attempt to cure them of an odious and devastating condition that was then considered incurable. His operations... were performed explicitly for therapeutic purposes and, as far as we can tell from the surviving sources, were carried out with the patients' cooperation and consent. At the time Sims began his efforts to close vesicovaginal fistulas, there was no effective alternative to surgical treatment and the quality of life to which such patients were reduced by their injuries was acknowledged by all medical writers of the time as unendurable. There is no doubt that slaves in the mid-nineteenth century American South were a "vulnerable" population

who were often subjected to significant abuse by the slaveholding system. To suggest, however, that for that reason alone no attempts should have been made to cure the maladies of such enslaved women, especially when they were desperate for help and no other viable alternatives existed, seems ethically bankrupt.[102]

Contract and Consent: The Walter Reed Yellow Fever Experiments, 1900–1901

The high mortality rates associated with eighteenth- and nineteenth-century yellow fever epidemics created an environment that supported Rush's heroic model of the inspired solo researcher valiantly seeking to stem a rising onslaught of death and dismissive of pusillanimous constraints of caution. In a curious turn of history, the American experience with this same disease, yellow fever, also became paradigmatic for the more collaborative model of infectious disease research associated with the emerging sciences of bacteriology and physiology. This new empirically driven model was rigorous in its methodology, cautious in its use of human subjects, and had a propensity for Golden Rule self-experimentation and signed consent forms. The experiments most closely associated with this turn in American research ethics were conducted in 1900–1901 by the U.S. Army's Yellow Fever Commission, which was commanded by Major Walter Reed.

The commission was formed in the aftermath of the Spanish-American War of 1898, when most U.S. troops had to be hastily withdrawn from Cuba and the Philippines because of the ravages of yellow fever. Some 6,406 soldiers died during the war, 5,438 from disease.[103] Politicians, the public, and the press held U.S. Army Surgeon General George M. Sternberg (1838–1915) accountable for this tragic loss of life. The *New York Times*, for example, expressed a "lack of confidence in Sternberg…whose department's blunders are constantly occurring and who is always prepared with complete evidence that the blunder was not his fault…. Surgeon General Sternberg is unfit for the position he holds…. [T]he country has had enough of Surgeon General Sternberg."[104]

Pressured to address issues of military health, Sternberg set up a Yellow Fever Commission under Reed's command to determine how the disease was transmitted. According to the dominant theory, championed by Italian physician Giuseppe Sanarelli, yellow fever was a bacteriological disease spread by direct contact with the bacterium on an infected person's clothing, vomit, and the like. An alternative model, insect transmission, appeared in the 1890s, after a Scottish physician, Patrick Manson (1844–1922), and British military physician Ronald Ross (1857–1932) had established that insects were the vectors for transmitting malaria.[105] Cuban physician Carlos Finlay (1833–1915) believed yellow fever was transmitted in the same way, by *Aëdes aegypti* mosquitoes—but, unlike Manson and Ross, he could not corroborate his theory empirically.

Sternberg instructed Reed and his team—Agramonte, Carroll, and Lazear—to test these theories, cautioning them that no experiments involving human subjects "should . . . be made upon any individual without his full knowledge and consent."[106] Historian Susan Lederer remarks that Sternberg may have sympathized with research subjects because, as a medical student, he himself was pressured into serving as a human subject for gonorrhea experiments.[107] Sternberg was also present at the 1898 conference at which Osler publicly condemned Sanarelli's experiments as "criminal" because they had been conducted without the subject's knowledgeable consent.[108]

Sternberg must also have appreciated that restricting his researchers' experiments to consenting subjects would help to inoculate him and his researchers against politically charged public criticism. Sitting in Washington, Sternberg would have been aware that, on March 2, 1900, U.S. Senator Jacob Gallinger (1837–1918), a homeopathic physician, had introduced legislation to prohibit in the District of Columbia "the crime of human vivisection"; that is, "any scientific experiment involving pain, distress, or risk to [human] life or health."[109] Exempted from this blanket prohibition were two types of experiments on humans: experiments "having for [their] demonstrable end and object the amelioration of suffering or recovery of the patient thus treated or operated upon"[110] and Golden Rule experiments "made by medical students, physicians, surgeons, physiologists, or pathologists upon one another."[111] The constraints on researchers proposed in Gallinger's bill would unequivocally prohibit the sort of nontherapeutic experiments on nonmedical personnel that the Yellow Fever Commission planned to undertake in Cuba.

Out in the Caribbean, the yellow fever researchers also came to appreciate the political issues surrounding their experiments. In letters to their wives, Carroll and Reed describe a visit to the Spanish Consul in Cuba. As Carroll explains,

> One of the Spanish papers has taken up the matter of our experiments and accuses us of horrible cruelty in enticing Spanish emigrants out to camp by hiring them as laborers, then locking them up in a room at night and turning in a lot of infected mosquitoes to give them yellow fever, without their knowing anything about it. As a matter of fact we do take Spaniards . . . and we offer them a reward to be bitten, if they choose. No compulsion whatever is to be used, and we have American volunteers for the same work, who will be bitten and treated exactly as they are. The Consul says, that so long as the men are of age and consent fully, it is nobody's

> business. So we will go ahead. Do not speak of this to any one, because we do not want it spread any more than is necessary, until after we have finished.[112]

Reed's letter offers a similar account:

> My precious wifie:
>
> *Friday—Nov.* 23rd. I couldn't write any more, last night, but must jot down a few words this afternoon—I hope that my sweet oomsey is much better, to-day.... The days pass very rapidly here, but there is very little that I can do—my experimental station is complete except one of the buildings. I have five American non-immunes [to yellow fever], three of whom are ready to try any kind of experiment I shall propose, while the other two will try the infected bedding test [of Sanarelli's bacterial spread theory]. I have, also, 6 Spanish immigrants, recently arrived, who are working as laborer's around the camp—whether when we make the offer to them, they will be willing to accept and give their written consent, I don't know—Already some anonymous correspondent has been writing to one of the Spanish papers in Havana, telling about what we propose to do, and this paper, "La Discussion," is calling upon the authorities to stop the "*horror*," as it designates our experiments—We have thought it best to have the Spanish consul interviewed... and he very properly takes a sensible view of the matter, & sees no reason why the observations should not be made on any one who gives his full written consent, after the danger has been explained to him. So that as far as Spain's representative is concerned, we need give ourselves no bother. Of course, the newspapers here are just like those in the U.S.—anything, however false, so that a sensation is produced and the paper sold.[113]

As these letters make evident, Reed and his team understood that documenting informed consent served as an antidote to a scandal-mongering press that charged the researchers with locking the unsuspecting Spaniards "in a room at night and turning in a lot of infected mosquitoes to give them yellow fever, without their knowing anything about it."

So, for a mix of political and moral reasons in their publications and presentations, both Sternberg and Reed emphasized that their team had only experimented on people who, as Sternberg put it, "were fully informed as to the nature of the experiment and its probable results and [who] gave their full consent."[114] In a presentation at the 1901 meeting of Pan American Medical Congress, the Reed team observed that

> [T]he attack [of yellow fever] always followed within the period of incubation of the disease, and concerned only those non-immune individuals who had consented to submit themselves for experimentation. *Of*

> *a total of 16 individuals who thus* consented, *14 contracted yellow fever; whereas of 5 non-immunes, who did not* consent *and were therefore not subjected to experimentation, none acquired the disease, although* otherwise placed under exactly similar surroundings. [emphasis in the original][115]

As this truly prosaic passage makes evident, for the Reed team, the concept of a consenting individual was neither window dressing nor an afterthought: it was as integral to their methodology as their distinction between "immunes" and "non-immunes."

The Reed team had also attempted Golden Rule self-experimentation on moral grounds, to assuage their consciences, "as the best atonement they could offer for subjecting others to the risks."[116] James Carroll describes their self-experimentation agreement in a report to Sternberg:

> Early in the month of August it was decided to test the mosquito theory advanced by Dr. Finlay, and since man is the only animal known to suffer from yellow fever, there was no alternative but to make the tests upon human beings. The question arose of the tremendous responsibility of such an undertaking, which could only be justified by the enormous saving of life that would follow the establishment of the theory, even should one or several lives be sacrificed in the course of the work. The best atonement we could offer for endangering the lives of others was to take the same chances ourselves, and it was agreed by Dr. Reed, Dr. Lazear and myself that experiments should be undertaken and that we would all be bitten by contaminated mosquitoes.[117]

After Carroll and Lazear were stricken with yellow fever, however, Sternberg forbade future forays into self-experimentation, since the self-sacrificial acts of self-experimentation would deplete his staff and would not provide the sort numerical data required for scientific evidence that mosquitoes transmitted the disease. Moreover, as Carroll notes in his report, their very work as researchers unsuited them for service as subjects. Thus when "[o]n Sept. 13th Dr. Lazear himself was bitten by a stray mosquito in Las Animas Hospital; he sickened Sept. eighteenth and died Sept. 25th, 1900, a martyr to the cause."[118] Yet since a stray mosquito bite did not establish which type of mosquito caused Lazear's yellow fever—or even that mosquitoes were the vector—Lazear's death did not establish anything of scientific value about yellow fever. Martyrdom is no substitute for methodological rigor.

After Lazear's death, Sternberg also sought to have Reed supervise the experiments while sitting safely in the United States. Reed, however, insisted on returning to Cuba to oversee properly controlled scientific experiments:

> I have been so ashamed of myself for being here in a safe country, while my associates have been coming down with yellow Jack [i.e., yellow fever]. The General [Sternberg] has suggested that I do not return, but somehow I feel that, as the Senior member of a B[oar]d investigating yellow Fever, my place is in Cuba, as long as the work goes on—I shall, of course, take every precaution that I can against contracting the disease, and I certainly shall not, with the facts that we now have allow a "*loaded*" mosquito to bite me! That would be foolhardy in the extreme.[119]

On his return to Cuba, Reed had the team design a carefully controlled multi-armed experiment (with cross-over elements) that would test both the bacterial spread and mosquito-borne theories of transmission. Recruitment of volunteers commenced soon afterward. John Moran (1876–1950), an Irish-American clerk, describes how he and Private John Kissinger (1877–1946) were recruited:

> Adventure knocked at my door that October afternoon as I crossed the parade grounds of the Post Hospital. I suspect that it was by design rather than accident that Dr. Roger Post Ames [1870–1914] accosted me, with a cheery "Hello, Johnny, what's new over at Headquarters?"... In an apparently casual manner, Dr. Ames led up to the clinching point and my own major weakness of hoarding and saving money for my medical education.... Did I know that Major Reed was offering a bonus or money award of $500.00 for volunteers for a series of experiments which he was planning?... He knew that $500.00 would be a godsend to me and, furthermore, a fitting start for a young man bent on studying medicine. Neither of us gave very much thought to a possible death lurking in the background. "All right, Doc, I will sleep over it and let you know tomorrow." Repeating to myself what he told me: "Just think, Johnny, what that $500.00 will mean to you," I wended my way to my room, having already made up my mind that I would go in for the experiments....
>
> A few hours after my talk with Dr. Ames I broke the news to my roommate, Private John R. Kissinger of the Hospital Corps, informing him that I was "going in" for the experiments, but without the bonus.... When it came to moral courage, Kissinger was not found wanting. He, too, was going to volunteer and without any money reward. I tried to dissuade him, arguing that our cases were different; since I was to study medicine while he had no such ambition....
>
> True to our pact we, the two Johns, walked across the parade grounds to Officers' Quarters, next morning, headed for Major Reed's combination bedroom and private office... both of us being anxious to strike the iron while it was hot. Neither of us wanted to risk the danger of getting cold feet .... [T]he Major bade us "Good morning. What can I do for you?"... I managed to

> blurt out our mission there, having forgotten the few, but terse and to the point, words I had been memorizing for the ordeal. The Major's surprise was complete and so reflected in his countenance. He never expected such rapid-fire action as confronted him, there and then, in the persons of two human guinea pigs.... He was about to speak when Kissinger, now grown bolder, forestalled him, saying "That is not all, Sir. We are volunteering without the bonus or money award which we understand you are offering." Doubt clouded his face for a moment. "That is correct, Major," I managed to add. "We are doing it for medical science," later recorded as "humanity and science".... I was principally interested in medical science, although not unaware of the human aspect of whatever sacrifices might be in store for me.... In a quiet and modulated voice [Reed] informed us that we were gladly accepted for the experiments and that we could elect between the "Infected Clothing" and the "Infected Mosquito" tests. There and then, we both chose the mosquito test.[121]

Dr. Ames had tried to purchase Moran's services—just as Beaumont bought St. Martin's services—with a large sum of money, $500 (about $32,800 in 2010 dollars).[122] Moran, however, wanted to demonstrate his moral courage by serving "medical science," and he believed that to accept payment would rob his "adventure" of nobility. He and Kissinger displayed even greater moral courage by volunteering for what they had reason to believe was the most dangerous arm of the experiment—being bitten by loaded mosquitoes—since it was commonly believed at the army base that a mosquito bite had caused Dr. Lazear's recent death. Moran, in fact, wrote a memorial note about Dr. Lazear, who had "died... in his 34th year, a martyr to science, death cutting short a life of brilliant promise and accomplishment."[123] Moran may have envisioned that, should he die, someone would write such an epitaph about his heroic martyrdom. As it happened, both Kissinger and Moran contracted yellow fever—both survived and were awarded Congressional Medals of Honor. Kissinger, however, was disabled by his bout of yellow fever and also received a military pension. Unscathed, Moran would make a bit of a career by telling and retelling his tale of their moral courage for radio and film.

Both Kissinger and Moran signed written consent forms but since these forms appear not to have been preserved in any archive, we must assume that they were similar to those signed by such Spanish research subjects as Antonio Benino, who signed a Spanish version of the consent form below:

> The undersigned... consents to submit himself to experiments for the purpose of determining the methods of transmission of yellow fever,... and... gives his consent to undergo the said experiments for the reasons and under the conditions below stated.

> [He] understands perfectly well that in case of the development of yellow fever in him, that he endangers his life to a certain extent but it being entirely impossible for him to avoid the infection during his stay in this island, he prefers to take the chance of contracting it intentionally in the belief that he will receive from the said Commission the greatest care and the most skillful medical service.
>
> [A]t the completion of these experiments, within two months from this date [he] will receive the sum of $100 in American gold [a sum equivalent to about $ 6,560 in 2010 dollars][124] and [if he] contracts yellow fever at any time during his residence in this camp, he will receive in addition to that sum a further sum of $100 in American gold.... [I]n case of his death because of this disease... said sum (two hundred American dollars) [equivalent to about $ 13,120 in 2010, dollars will be given] to the person [he] shall designate.
>
> [He] binds himself not to leave the bounds of this camp during the period of the experiments and will forfeit all right to the benefits named in this contract if he breaks this agreement.[125]

Like the Beaumont-St. Martin contract, this is a modified employment agreement between a researcher and a foreign national in which the foreign national, Antonio Benino, is employed for a specified period of time (two months), for a specified task (serving as a research subject), for a stated purpose (determining how yellow fever is transmitted), at a specific place (the army base), in exchange for money and medical care (in the event of contracting the disease). Were the employee (Benino) to violate the agreement, he would forfeit his benefits. As any contract for employment would, these contracts document an agreement on conditions for employment and for its termination.

What distinguishes this contract from an ordinary employment contract and from the Beaumont-St. Martin contract is language reflecting "the tremendous responsibility," that the Reed team felt about "mak[ing] the tests upon human beings... should one or several lives be sacrificed in the course of the work." Their felt need to make the best "atonement we could offer for endangering the lives of others"[126] is expressed in the contract in two significant ways: an offer to pay a death benefit to the subjects' designated heirs and a discussion of risks to the subject ("he endangers his life to a certain extent"). Although vague, this disclosure of risk anticipates bioethics-era consent forms, which, like the Reed team's forms, are designed to document the subject's knowledgeable volunteerism and the researcher's respect for the subject as a person. Conversely, the large sums of money that the Reed team offered would be seen by bioethicists as "unduly influencing" a potential subject's decision making.

Intriguingly, on the moral courage conception of volunteerism financial payments were also morally objectionable since they diluted the purity of the subjects' intention to courageously volunteer to serve humanity by risking disease, disability, or death to advance science. Yet, at this early stage in the development of research ethics, these various conceptions of consent and consent forms—as a contract for a subject's services, as a means of preventing legal action for malpractice or manslaughter, as a public relations device to dampen criticism, as a testimonial to volunteerism, as a method of assuaging the responsibility or guilt of the researcher, and as recognition of service to science and humanity—were still in flux.

The courage/service to science-and-humanity conception of voluntarism also influenced the Reed team's treatment of their subjects' names. Unlike Beaumont, who would often state his subject's name, the Reed team anticipates the practices of the bioethics era by de-identifying the names of their subjects in their published reports. They usually characterized their subjects using such language as, "Case I.—W. J., American, nonimmune, aged 27." A typical case description would be written up as follows:

> Case I.—W. J., American, nonimmune, aged 27—in quarantine since December 20, 1900—with his full consent, at 11 a. m., January 4, 1901, was injected subcutaneously with 2 c. c. of blood taken from the general circulation of a case of mild yellow fever at the beginning of the second day of the disease and having a temperature of 100.8.[127]

In contrast, Moran and Kissinger's names were explicitly highlighted so that they could "reap the credit which is so justly due" them for their nobility, courage, and sacrifice.

> *Twenty-three of the men who submitted themselves for experiment by the board contracted yellow fever, beginning* with Dr. James Carroll, who was taken sick August 31, 1900, and ending with John R. Bullard, who was taken sick October 23, 1901. Conspicuous among them was *John J. Moran, a civilian clerk* . . . who was one of the earliest volunteers for the second set of experiments, and whose action was dictated by the purest motives of altruism and self-devotion. *Mr. Moran disclaimed, before submitting to the experiments, any desire for reward, and has never accepted any since, although he was offered the $200. . . .* Such was his modesty that he has made no effort, so far as known to this office, to make known his connection with these experiments and reap the credit which is so justly due him.[128]

For bioethicists, publication of subject's names without express prior consent would be anathema to their paternalistic objective—using informed consent as prophylaxis against researchers' exploitation of their subjects—for the Reed team, as for Sims, naming subjects was a way of honoring them for risks undertaken in the name of medical science.

On an immediately practical level, the Reed team's experiment yielded "the enormous saving of life" that the team believed was the only justification for deliberately risking the lives of human subjects.[129] Once the urban dwelling *Aëdes aegypti* mosquito was identified as the vector transmitting yellow fever, Major William Gorgas (1854–1920), chief sanitary officer for Havana, turned his attention from swamps to puddles, initiating a campaign to eliminate the mosquito's urban breeding grounds, ridding the city of yellow fever and demonstrating methods successfully adopted in Florida and Panama.

The impact on American research ethics was just as significant. The publicity surrounding Reed's yellow fever experiments made them a landmark moment in the history of American researcher ethics: the point at which the methodological demands of controlled clinical trials obsolesced the statistical relevance of Golden Rule self-experimentation, forcing the justificatory burden of endangering human life in nontherapeutic experiments to be carried by the notion of informed, consenting volunteers. Hereafter, the Reed team's model of documenting knowledgeable subjects' voluntary participation in experiments with consent forms became the Gold Standard for systematic nontherapeutic research, especially for research conducted in such total institutions as the military, orphanages, and prisons—or in other contexts in which the voluntary participation might be suspect or in which the experiments might prove controversial.[130]

VIVISECTIONISM: THE ETHICS OF EXPERIMENTING ON HUMAN AND NONHUMAN ANIMALS

The practice of consenting experimental subjects adopted by Sternberg and the Reed team also served to ward off antivivisectionist efforts to pass laws regulating animal and human experimentation. The American antivivisectionist movement was conceived in the aftermath of the Civil War, reached its crescendo from the 1890s through 1917, and then died out in the 1920s—but became resurgent in the bioethics era.[131] A debate among four prominent Harvard faculty members offers a sense of the early antivivisectionist movement's intellectual conception and development. The four Harvard faculty members are Henry Jacob Bigelow, the physician who censored Storer Sr.'s sexist diatribe against women seeking abortions and who was a much-quoted early voice for antivivisectionism; Henry Pickering Bowditch (1840–1911), a vivisectionist, so-to-speak, and founding member and future president of the American Physiological Society (founded in 1887, still functioning); Bowditch's friend and nonmedical protégé, the philosopher William James (1842–1910), whose opposition to antivivisectionism moderated over time;

and Bowditch's student, protégé, and successor, Walter Bradford Canon (1871–1945), who also became president of the American Physiological Society. In this early incarnation (1870s–1920s), the antivivisectionist movement had a significant impact on the ethics of research on human as well as nonhuman subjects.[132]

Henry Pickering Bowditch

Henry Pickering Bowditch was the younger cousin of the abolitionist and public health reformer, Henry Ingersoll Bowditch, mentioned in Chapter 7 as a defender of specialists' rights to advertise and of women's rights to practice medicine. Like his older cousin, Henry Pickering was an abolitionist. He served in the Union Army commanding white and—more controversially—African-American troops, and he was wounded in combat. Returning to civilian life, he completed his medical education at Harvard and then did postgraduate work in Europe. Henry Pickering then returned to Harvard where, emulating the Europeans, he set up the first American laboratory dedicated to physiological experiments.

Even before this laboratory opened its doors or conducted a single experiment, in a June 1871 address to the Massachusetts Medical Society the ever-censorious Henry Jacob Bigelow delivered a diatribe on the "horrors of Vivisection."[133] Bigelow condemned vivisection—a generic name for any form of research conducted on a living animal, nonhuman or human—as "cold-blooded cruelties... practiced under the authority of Science!"[134] Physiological research, Bigelow contended, yields only useless facts; however, even if such experiments yielded knowledge that could extend human life, it would be "[b]etter that I or my friend should die than protract existence through accumulated years of torture upon animals whose exquisite suffering we cannot fail to infer, even though they may have neither voice nor feature to express it."[135] Bigelow was particularly vexed by the repetitive infliction of pain on animals. He allowed that if a *single* experiment "though cruel, would forever settle [an important therapeutic issue] we might reluctantly admit that it is justified. But the instincts of our common humanity indignantly remonstrate against the testing of clumsy or unimportant hypotheses by prodigal experimentation, or making the torture of animals an exhibition to enlarge a medical school, or for the entertainment of students."[136]

Extending the Golden Rule to vivisectionists, Bigelow suggested that physiologists do unto themselves what they were doing to their animal subjects: "for every inch cut by... experimenter in the quivering tissues of a helpless dog or rabbit or Guinea-pig let him insert a lancet one eighth of an inch into his own skin... and he may have some faint suggestion of the atrocity he is perpetrating, when the Guinea-pig shrieks, the poor dog yells, the noble horse groans and strains."[137] In an era that identified morality with moral sentiment, the notion that physiologists were insensitive to suffering was akin, to update the reference, to accusing them of having a sociopathic personality disorder. Worse yet, Bigelow contended, instructional vivisection infects medical students with the same disorder. "Watch the students at a vivisection. It is the blood and suffering, not the science, that rivets their breathless attention . . . mak[ing] students less tender of suffering, vivisection deadens their humanity and begets indifference to it."[138]

Antivivisectionism spread rapidly. In 1880, Henry Bergh (1813–1888), founder of the ASPCA, lobbied the New York State legislature to enact laws regulating animal vivisection. By the 1890s, antivivisectionist societies were sprouting nationwide. The New England Anti-Vivisectionist Society (NEAVS founded in 1895, still functioning) had taken root in Henry Pickering's backyard and was lobbying the Massachusetts legislature for laws regulating vivisectionism. Henry Pickering denounced the proposed legislation as unnecessary because "no abuse of the right to vivisect has been shown to exist in [Massachusetts] institutions."[139]

Sidney Taber and William James

By this time, groups like the Vivisection Reform Society (VRS, founded in Chicago, in 1903, still functioning) were linking animal to human vivisection and were lobbying for legislation to regulate both. To rebut Bowditch's claim that American vivisectionism was innocent of abuse, VRS publications documented cases of abusive practices drawn from the pages of medical journals and textbooks. The VRS's secretary, Chicago lawyer Sidney Richard Taber (fl. 1862–circa 1920s) edited one of the best known of these publications, *Illustrations of Human Vivisection*. "[B]efore any reform can be hoped," Taber observed, "there must be such exposure as shall, sooner or later, awaken an effective public condemnation. Herein are delineated oppression of the weak, cruelty to the defenseless, injustice to the poor, violation of human rights."[140] Taber's volume details "the practice of subjecting human beings, men, women and children, who are patients in public charitable institutions, hospitals or asylums, to experiments involving pain, distress, mutilation, disease or danger to life, for no object connected with their individual benefit, but for scientific purposes."[141] The VRS's objective was "absolute condemnation of this hideous practice by the leading medical associations of the United States as shall stamp the human vivisector with ignominy and disrepute," by legislation regulating—but not outlawing—human and animal vivisection.[142]

Among the dozens of human rights violations that Taber found in the medical literature was the following 1870s case published in the *American Journal of the Medical Sciences*. A former military surgeon and Civil War veteran, Professor

Roberts Bartholow (1831–1904) of the Medical College of Ohio experimented on a "feeble minded" Irish domestic servant, Mary Rafferty (circa 1843–1873):

> To an institution bearing the comforting name of the Good Samaritan Hospital there came one day a poor woman by the name of Mary Rafferty. A domestic servant by occupation, strong neither in mind nor body, she had sustained an accident which made her good "material" for a dangerous experiment... an eroding ulcer had appeared which gradually had laid bare the brain substance. Apparently any cure of her trouble was seen at once to be hopeless; but she presented a chance for making scientific experiments of a kind such as had hitherto been made only upon dumb animals. We are twice told by the experimenter that she was "rather feeble-minded," and we may thus judge the value of her "consent" to experimentation—if, indeed, her consent was ever asked. She... was "cheerful in manner," and smiled "easily and frequently," with child-like confidence and perfect faith in the goodness of those about her.
>
> "It is obvious," says the experimenter at the outset, "that it is exceedingly desirable to ascertain how far the results of experiment on the brain of animals may be employed to elucidate the functions of the human brain." He commenced his vivisections... upon Mary Rafferty by inserting into the substance of the brain, thus exposed by disease, insulated needle electrodes of various lengths, and connecting them with a battery.... Let the vivisector tell the story:
>
> > When the needle entered the brain-substance, she complained of acute pain in the neck. In order to develop more decided reactions, the strength of the current was increased... her countenance exhibited great distress, and she began to cry. Very soon the left hand was extended as if in the act of taking hold of some object in front of her; the arm presently was agitated with clonic spasms; her eyes became fixed, with pupils widely dilated; lips were blue, and she frothed at the mouth; her breathing became stertorous; she lost consciousness, and was violently convulsed on the left side. The convulsion lasted five minutes, and was succeeded by coma. She returned to consciousness in twenty minutes from the beginning of the attack.[143]
>
> What had happened? Simply this: the distinguished scientist had caused in a human being precisely the same "violent epileptiform convulsion" which [others] had produced in the lower animals, and by the same method of experimentation.... Of the next experiment performed, the vivisector himself shall tell us the result:
>
> > Two days subsequent to observation... The proposed experiment was abandoned. [Mary] was pale and depressed; her lips were blue; and she had

> evident difficulty in locomotion.... She became very pale, her eyes closed, and she was about to pass into unconsciousness, when we placed her in the recumbent posture, and Dr. S... gave her, at my request, chloroform by inhalation. The day after... Mary was decidedly worse. She remained in bed, was stupid and incoherent. In the evening she had a convulsive seizure, lasting about five minutes, confined to the right side. After this attack she lapsed into profound unconsciousness, and was found to be completely paralyzed on the right side.... No movements of any kind could be excited by strong irritation of the skin of the paralyzed side.... The pupils were dilated and motionless.
>
> No coroner was called upon to make an investigation. Officially speaking, she was reported to have died of the disease from which she had been so long suffering.[144]

After noting that this case was published in a leading medical journal, Taber asks:

> What is the attitude of the eminent surgeons and physicians... of the editors of the leading medical journals, the representatives of medical opinion? Are deeds such as have been herein described regarded as laudable, if performed only upon the ignorant and poor, in the name of Science? No such creed is openly professed. Is it held in secret? Take the representative medical journals in the United States.... Possibly we may judge of their real attitude by what they have not done. During the past quarter of a century, has a single human vivisector been mentioned by name with condemnation and rebuke in the editorial columns of any medical journal of the United States.... For any such condemnation we have searched in vain. Can we imagine that the editors of medical journals throughout the United States would be so absolutely indifferent to the atrocities of human vivisection—printed and described in their own columns—unless, in reality, such deeds are regarded as excusable, if they are done "in the name of Science"?[145]

Taber thus argues that since medical societies and journals would not condemn such experiments, or rebuke those who perform them, they implicitly deemed it acceptable to abuse people with mental disability, "the feeble minded," in the name of scientific progress. Consequently, since the medical profession could not to be trusted to regulate itself, reform would require legislative action—enactment of laws regulating vivisection.

Because Taber and other reformers accepted Bigelow's contention that physicians who abused "human rights" (their terminology) had been desensitized by animal vivisection—and not by the massive slaughter, the piles of unburied dead, that researchers like Bartholow and Bowditch witnessed during their service in the Civil War—the bill proposed by the VRS also required that "Dumb Animals" be "completely anesthetized" during experiments and then killed before regaining consciousness (except when testing for poisons, vaccines, and the like). The bill also required prior review and authorization by the institution's director and written consent of human subjects. It also prohibited Mary Rafferty-type "experiment[s] upon children under fifteen years, the aged, the feeble-minded, or women during pregnancy" and required institutions to report experiments on human and nonhuman animals annually to the State Board of Health.[146]

The VRS tried to recruit to their cause one of the most famous American philosophers of the era, Henry Pickering Bowditch's friend and protégé, William James. In his previous writings, James had defended vivisection in the name of scientific progress. "To taboo vivisection," he wrote, is "the same thing as to give up seeking after a knowledge of physiology.... Vivisection, is, in other words, a painful duty."[147] When the VRS invited James to join the society, however, he declined their invitation; he noted that, although he continued to oppose governmental regulation, he now believed that

> [T]he public demand for regulation rests on a perfectly sound ethical principle, the denial of which by the scientists speaks ill for either their moral sense or their political ability. So long as the physiologists disclaim corporate responsibility, formulate no code of vivisectional ethics for laboratories to post up and enforce, propose of themselves no law, so long must the anti-vivisection agitation, with all its expensiveness, idiocy, bad temper, untruth, and vexatiousness continue, as the only possible means of bringing home to the individual experimenter the fact that the sufferings of his animals *are* somebody else's business as well as his own.[148]

As James observed, the AMA had adamantly opposed any regulation of animal vivisection since it first took note of the subject in 1884. By 1896, the threat of laws restricting vivisection was a recurrent topic of discussion at national meetings. In 1900, the AMA "earnestly protest[ed] against the passage of" Senator Gallinger's anti-vivisectionist bill on the grounds that "experimentation on animals is absolutely essential to the progress of pathology and physiology... [and] not a single instance of the practices of vivisection has been shown to have occurred."[149] It reiterated this position in more general terms in 1908,[150] when it also appointed Bowditch's protégé, Walter Cannon, to chair its Council for the Defense of Medical Research (CDMR, 1908–1926).

Two years earlier, in 1906, Cannon had succeeded Bowditch as head of Harvard's Experimental Physiology Laboratory. By accepting an appointment as chair of the CDMR, Cannon was taking on Bowditch's other role: defender of scientists' rights to experiment on living animals, nonhuman and human. Like William James, however, Cannon rejected the AMA's absolutist stance on vivisection, concluding that self-regulation was warranted both on moral grounds and to counteract the campaign to have government regulate "vivisectionism." So, Cannon had the CDMR survey laboratories and medical schools to determine their practices and to assess whether medical students were taught to treat laboratory animals humanely. He also contacted medical journal editors requesting their cooperation in reviewing publications to assure that they only published reports of humanely conducted experiments.

In the course of the survey, the CDMR discovered that newer laboratories had adopted "Rules Regarding Animals," voluntarily implementing many of the practices that the VRS had attempted to impose legislatively. These "Rules Regarding Animals" required prior approval of all experiments by the laboratory's director, anesthetization for painful experiments, painlessly killing animals to prevent suffering (except where this conflicted with an experimental design), and that laboratories hold stray or purchased animals for a period to allow repatriation to their owners.[151] Upon discovering that some laboratories had adopted these rules, the CDMR recommended that all laboratories and medical schools adopt them as well "to offset the demand of the agitators for legislation which provides for meddlesome interference by uninstructed laymen."[152] By 1910, most regular medical schools (fifty-two of the seventy-seven) had adopted "Rules Regarding Animals," as recommended by the AMA[153] and, by the 1920s, virtually all major laboratories and medical schools claimed to be compliant—many even inviting representatives of humane societies to inspect their premises.

At the same time that open laboratory polices and the "Rules Regarding Animals" were blunting much of the force of the vivisectionist critique, Bigelow's contention that it is better that humans should die than that animals be sacrificed was made concrete in a well-publicized case involving Elizabeth Gossett, née Hughes (1907–1981), the fourteen-year-old daughter of the thirty-sixth governor of New York State, former Supreme Court Justice and Republican presidential candidate, Charles Evans Hughes (1862–1948). In 1922, Elizabeth, who suffered from juvenile onset diabetes—at the time a terminal diagnosis—had her life spared by becoming one of the first patients to receive insulin, which was then manufactured from the pancreases of dogs or cows.[154] The world applauded and, in 1923, some of the discoverers of insulin received the Nobel Prize.

In 1871, Bigelow had contended that it would be "[b]etter that [he] or [a] friend should die than protract existence through accumulated years of torture upon animals."[155] Bigelow's contention was an abstract thought experiment at a time when the emerging sciences of bacteriology and physiology had yet to yield treatments that could actually save human lives. Fifty years later, faced with the choice that Bigelow had posed, forced to choose between the life of a fourteen-year-old child and the lives of dogs, the public prized those who sacrificed dogs to save the life of a human child. A choice, moreover, eased by Cannon's campaign to have laboratories adopt "Rules Regarding Animals," which required that the animals used be anesthetized. Dogs and cows might die to save a child, but, according to the Rules, they would suffer minimally.

Buoyed by the success of his campaign to protect animals used in research by professional self-regulation rather than government regulation by bureaucrats, Cannon's CDMR also recommended a series of ethical principles for research on human subjects. Foremost among these was the principle of requiring the voluntary consent of humans used as research subjects. Consent had been common practice in nontherapeutic research since the Walter Reed experiments, but Cannon was proposing that researchers seek subject consent for all experiments—as a matter of moral principle—irrespective of whether the research was considered therapeutic or nontherapeutic. The universal consent principle, moreover, was to be promulgated by the AMA and enforced through a voluntary agreement among editors, requiring them to forgo publication of any manuscript describing research on human subjects that did not declare that the subjects, or their surrogates, had expressly consented to participate in the experiment.

In an editorial arguing for a medical ethical principle of universal consent in the *Journal of the American Medical Association*, Cannon echoed Justice Cardozo's words in *Schloendorff*, proclaiming:

> There is no more primitive and fundamental right which any individual possesses that that of controlling the uses to which his own body is put .... Any hospital official or physician known to commit or to allow violation of the sacredness of the person becomes at once an object of hostility. And the law, as an expression of the public conscience, declares that deliberate injury done to the body of another is an assault, and provides severe punishment for it. Society as now constituted will obviously not countenance any operation performed for the satisfaction of the operator or... investigator... unless the consent of the person on whom the operation is performed has previously been obtained....
>
> It is clearly the duty of the physician to secure the consent of the patient or of the patient's guardian in case the patient himself is not capable of giving consent.... The medical profession is certainly not called on... to support the physician who transgresses the elementary principles of ethics.
>
> Especially are the reputation and esteem of medical men endangered by any failure on their part to stand firmly for the fundamental right of the individual to respect for his own person. For the sick commit themselves to the care of the physician and surgeon helpless and with implicit trust that their welfare alone will be considered. Any practitioner or investigator, no matter how laudable his motives, who fails in scrupulous regard for this trust is liable to do incalculable harm by rousing suspicions, fears and disrespect as to the character of medical service.[156]

Canon's point was that the practice of seeking consent from subjects should be more than a self-protective pragmatic gesture to ensure against lawsuits and bad publicity; it should be predicated on moral principle because any perceived toleration of unconsented research could undermine the trust between physician and patient essential to the very practice of medicine. Consequently, the profession must condemn as a violation of moral principle "[a]ny practitioner…who fails in scrupulous regard for this trust [since this is] liable to do incalculable harm…as to the character of medical service."[157]

Cannon's proposal was a step too far for the editors, who would not join forces to enforce the consent principles until over a half-century later, in the 1970s, after the formation of the International Committee of Medical Journal Editors (ICMJE; founded in 1978) and the World Association of Medical Editors (WAME; founded in 1995). Six decades earlier, in 1914, there was no national or international society of medical journal editors, and it must have seemed suicidal for any one journal to undertake to enforce this policy unless others were willing to enforce it as well. Journals competed for subscribers, and none could prudently forego the right to publish interesting material unless its competitors would do so. Only after medical editors agreed internationally could their journals reject publication of experiments conducted in violation of the principles of research ethics.

Cannon's initiative within the AMA was similarly abortive. The CDMR had succeeded in achieving nearly universal adoption of the "Rules Regarding Animals" because the laboratories themselves wrote the rules. Once the CDMR discovered that some laboratories and medical schools had adopted these rules, it disseminated this fact and built consensus around it. A similar effort promoting principles for the ethics of experimenting on human subjects would require the CDMR to survey hospitals about current expectations with respect to consent, establish a de facto consensus, and then turn to the AMA for authoritative validation of the consensus. Such an effort might well have succeeded since medical practitioners treated consent as a morally proper and legally prudent prerequisite to any proposed surgical procedure or nontherapeutic experimental intervention. Instead of building a consensus and then attempting to expand it, Cannon and the CDMR sought to have the AMA and journal editors impose an ethics of experimentation authoritatively from "on high," so to speak. The effort failed at the launching point because, as detailed in the previous chapter, this was an era of devolutionist laissez-faire ethics in which virtually all AMA ethics directives were advisory, and enforcement of ethical principles was left to the constituent medical societies and to individual practitioners' conscience. Moreover, as the records of the local societies indicate, by the 1920s, the medical societies' restorative justice institutions had atrophied. Censure and expulsion were replacing apologies and forgiveness, and, except in egregious cases, medical societies were reluctant to censure or to expel.

Compounding the challenge of instituting research ethics reforms was an unintended effect of the 1910 Flexner report.[158] The report precipitated a widespread reform of medical education that focused on training in medical science and its practical application in the clinic. This inadvertently denied ethics a place at the medical school lecturer's lectern or in the medical school curriculum. Formal ethics education was to be acquired *prior* to entry into medical school, as part of medical students' premedical education.[159] Once in medical school, medical students were to acquire their ethics by modeling their behavior on that of distinguished faculty and listening to their anecdotes. Formal medical ethics education, including discussion of the AMA *Principles*, was stripped out of the curriculum, and didactic discussion of medical ethics withered away.

So, curiously, as the quotations opening this chapter attest, even though during this period hospitals were promoting the practice of consenting patients and were developing forms to document patient consent, and even though a subject's consent was deemed essential for any form of nontherapeutic experimentation, Cannon and the CDMR were unable to formalize these practices as an official ethics of the AMA or of medical journalism. Consenting patients and the subjects of nontherapeutic experiments may have been the "done thing," but it would not be formally embraced by any official American medical organization until after World War II—when horror engendered by the Holocaust and fear of being tainted by the scandal of Nazi researchers would force the AMA to act. Even after the formal research ethics was officially endorsed in the 1949 internationalist version of the AMA's *Principles*, however, it slowly faded into obscurity in later (prebioethical) editions of the *Principles*.

CONCLUSION

The cases and debates in this chapter illustrate the complex tale of how medical ideals of humanitarianism and care, pressured by social agitation, law, and politics could combine with the practicalities of recruiting and retaining cooperative subjects to create a researcher morality that embraced the practice of consenting the human subjects of nontherapeutic medical experiments. Yet, although consenting subjects for some types of experiment became a moral expectation among researchers, and even as consent practices were formalized in hospital manuals, the laissez-faire devolutionist ideology embraced by the AMA and organized medicine crippled its ability to propound formal statements of research ethics and militated against efforts to officially censure persons guilty of immorally exploiting their research subjects. This disjunction between an expected morality of consent and the laissez-faire attitudes of organized medicine was bound to prove problematic. It did. As related in the next chapter, the consequent research ethics scandals became a significant factor in the empowerment of a multidisciplinary assemblage of critics whose ability to do precisely what organized medicine had been unable to do—provide, justify, and enforce principles of research ethics—would transform them from a hodge-podge of *lumpen intelligentsia* into a field that eventually came to be called "bioethics."

10

EXPLAINING THE BIRTH OF BIOETHICS, 1947–1999

I keep six honest serving-men
(They taught me all I knew);
Their names are What and Why and When
And How and Where and Who...
But different folk have different views.

Rudyard Kipling (1902)[1]

"Who was your mother?"
"Never had none!"....
"Never had any mother? What do you mean? Where were you born?"
"Never was born!" persisted Topsy.... "Never was born ... never had no father nor mother, nor nothin."[2]

Topsy, from *Uncle Tom's Cabin,* Harriet Beecher Stowe (1852)

To date, five English-language monographs have been published on the history of bioethics: David Rothman's *Strangers at the Bedside* (1991), Albert Jonsen's *The Birth of Bioethics* (1998), Tina Stevens's *Bioethics in America* (2000), Renée Fox and Judith Swazey's *Observing Bioethics* (2008), and John Evans' *The History and Future of Bioethics* (2012).[3] All five accounts are in substantial agreement about the What, When, Where, Who, and How bioethics was conceived and born; that is, they agree on the answers to the issues lyricized by Kipling—which trace back to Cicero and other Latin rhetoricians—that have traditionally served as the spine supporting good reportage. On the basic question of "what happened" and "when," they concur with Rothman's aptly titled history: what happened was that a group of strangers to medicine—bureaucrats, ex-theologians, lawyers, legislators, philosophers, and social scientists—transformed medical decision making.[4] Where and when this occurred was in America, in the 1970s. They have somewhat less agreement on how this happened, but all concur that the climate of ideas and the institutional changes that gave bioethicists entrée into the closed world of medicine occurred in the mid-1960s, well before the advent of bioethicists themselves.

As to the sixth and most intriguing question, "Why was bioethics was born?" with some exceptions, the standard account is that, like Topsy, the field just grew—although various factors are cited as facilitating its growth. Historian Rothman's answer to the "why" question is that bioethicists were invited to the bedside because new medical technologies were transforming physicians into strangers at a time when researchers were tainted by scandal. Thus, bureaucrats and the public entrusted oversight of medicine and medical research to a third party, the bioethicists. Sociologist Tina Stevens portrays bioethics as a movement emanating from a 1960s social critique of science, which reversed direction, gaining power and prominence by using the language of "ethics" to serve as an apologist for biomedicine and biomedical science. In Stevens' memorable prose, "the waxing of the social discourse of ethics tells one of the stories of the waning of the sixties. Declawed, social critique moved from protest to management."[5] Evans' explanation is framed in terms of sociologist Andrew Abbott's theory of competition over professional jurisdiction. According to Evans, bioethicists' "thin" approach to morally disruptive technologies supplanted theologians' "thick" probes into the deeper implications of emerging technologies because thin principles (act justly, do no harm) were more readily translated into bureaucrat regulations. Bureaucracies, for example, could implement bioethicists' principles by assessing whether an experiment exploits vulnerable populations or exposes them to harm. In contrast, attempts to implement theologians' "thick" concerns about the impact of technology on meaningful human relationships were stymied. Therefore, according to Evans, since bioethical approaches were more amenable to bureaucratization than were theological approaches, government bureaucrats ignored theologians and worked instead with bioethicists.

As in the ancient Asian tale of blind men trying to describe an elephant by touching only one of its parts[6]—trunk, tusk, leg, belly, tail—each historian seems to touch on a piece of the answer to the question, "why was bioethics born?" Yet none offers a comprehensive answer to the more basic question: Why did

American medicine lose jurisdiction over "medical ethics"—a subject who's very name proclaims it part of medicine's domain? To put the question using Rothman's language, why did American physicians and researchers open the doors of their fields to outsiders, to strangers?

ON THE AMERICAN ORIGINS OF BIOETHICS

Before turning to this question, it is important to appreciate than none of factors typically cited as explaining the American origins of bioethics was unique to America. Post-Hiroshima skepticism about science and technology was a worldwide phenomenon. So too were scandals involving new drugs. In the 1950s, the German *Chemie Gruenthal GmbH* developed a popular drug, thalidomide, that could reduce morning sickness in pregnant women. The drug was marketed globally and, within a decade, pediatricians worldwide—from Australia, Belgium, Brazil, Britain, Canada, Israel, Japan, Kenya, Lebanon, the Netherlands, Peru, Sweden, and Switzerland—reported an association between maternal thalidomide use and infants born with gross malformations of their arms and legs.[7] Campaigns to restrict thalidomide were launched worldwide, not just in the United States. Similarly, just as dangerous drugs and research ethics scandals were not uniquely American, neither were whistleblowing reformers—the most notable European and American reformers, Maurice Pappworth (1912–1994) of London, and Henry Beecher (1904–1976) of Boston, even corresponded with each other.[8]

Europeans, moreover, were as productive as Americans in inventing morally disruptive technologies. A Dutch physician, Willem Kolff (1911–2009), initiated the postwar surge in morally disruptive technologies by inventing a dialysis machine in 1945. American physician Belding Scribner improved on Kolff's invention a decade and a half later by inventing a shunt that made long-term kidney dialysis possible, and the consequent shortage of dialysis machines to support the needs of long-term dialysis patients was felt in Europe and in the rest of the world, not only in America. Similarly, vegetative patients were created wherever Danish physician Bjorn Ibsen's invention, the ventilator, was used, not only in America. The same pattern is evident with in vitro fertilization (IVF), which was developed by physician Patrick Steptoe (1913–1988) and physiologist Robert Edwards (1925–2013) in Britain, in 1977–1978, to assist an infertile married couple, John and Lesley Brown. The birthdate of Mrs. Brown's healthy daughter, Louise Joy, July 25, 1978, became the birthdate of alternative reproductive technologies and related ethical and legal issues worldwide, not only in America.

As this list indicates, Americans had no monopoly on morally disruptive innovations, and these innovations were as disruptive to medical morality and ethics in Europe and the rest of the world as they were in the United States. Moreover, they led to physician–humanist collaborations worldwide, not only in America. European bioethicists often challenge the notion that bioethics was born in the United States on precisely these grounds. In a review of Jonsen's *Birth of Bioethics*, published under the sarcastic title, "My country Tis of Thee—The Myopia of American Bioethics,"[9] Alistair Campbell, former president of the International Association of Bioethics (IAB, founded in 1992), condemns Jonsen for "a nationalistic arrogance surprising in so scholarly an author." Campbell contends that Jonsen's claim that bioethics should be understood within "the larger sweep of the American ethos, shows no real understanding of medicine and science in European and other non-American cultures."[10] To the contrary, Campbell accurately comments, humanist-scientist-physician collaborations and research centers and institutes arose in European and other societies around the same time that they arose in the United States.[11]

Honing his critique, Campbell caricatures Jonsen's view that bioethics was an American invention as the "Coca-Cola" analysis of bioethics. Although the cola analogy was intended derisively, it may be more apt than Campbell realized. Colas and other soft drinks (in contrast to hard liquor, wine, and beer) came to prominence in American culture as a consequence of Prohibition: a national ban on the manufacture, sale, or transportation of alcoholic beverages initiated in 1919 by the Eighteenth Amendment to the U.S. Constitution and repealed, thirteen years later, in 1933, by the Twenty-First Amendment. The intended consequence of this ban on alcoholic beverages is that, for a decade and a half, the forms of social life surrounding the consumption of alcohol were banished from the public sphere. The resulting social vacuum created space for "speakeasies" and other forms of underground social drinking, even as soda fountains replaced bars and pubs in the public sphere. For almost two decades, soft drinks became integral to social events from dances to picnics, and the generation that came of age in the 1920s and 1930s truly became the Coca-Cola and Pepsi generation. With the repeal of Prohibition, however, soft drinks again had to compete with alcoholic beverages in the public sphere, and the American market for soft drinks declined rapidly. In response, Coca-Cola and Pepsi invested resources accrued during Prohibition to develop new marketing strategies, new fountain mixers, and new bottling and distribution techniques that, in combination, transformed them into commercial powerhouses.[12] Europeans, in contrast, never enacted Prohibition and, without its aid, the European soft drink industry never evolved as robustly as the American cola industry. Consequently, when U.S. companies began marketing their beverages in Europe, their new distribution and bottling techniques and refined flavor blends gave them a competitive advantage over their rivals, and they soon dominated the European markets.[13]

To turn back to Campbell's cola analogy: something similar occurred with respect to medical ethics and bioethics. American medical societies adopted something akin to a self-imposed "prohibition" on medical ethics, creating the environment in which a robust alternative, bioethics, developed and was then exported worldwide. More specifically, as detailed in Chapters 7 and 8, the American Medical Association's (AMA) adoption of a laissez-faire approach to medical ethics from 1903 through the 1970s was, in effect, a self-imposed prohibition against making authoritative statements on medical ethics. During this entire period, the AMA characterized its *Principles of Medical Ethics* as "standards by which a physician *may* determine the propriety of his conduct," deeding the prerogative of interpreting professional standards to each individual physician's personal moral sensibilities.[14] Consequently, just as the U.S. prohibition on alcoholic beverages created a void in the marketplace that was filled by an alternative beverage industry—the colas—so, too, organized medicine's laissez-faire abandonment of medical ethics created a void in the marketplace of ideas and a vacuum of moral authority. To fill this void, legislators, bureaucrats, the courts, and American society generally sought ideas and invested moral authority elsewhere, ultimately finding it in an oddball collection of *lumpen intellentsia* who were soon valorized as ethics experts or "bioethicists."

In Europe, by contrast, organized medicine neither abandoned medical ethics nor abdicated moral authority. Consequently, just as alcoholic and caffeinated beverages retained jurisdiction over social life in European pubs and cafes, rendering soft drinks to the status of second-class beverages, so, too, organized medical and scientific societies (e.g., the British and Dutch medical societies and specialty colleges) retained jurisdiction over medical ethics—relegating aspiring European bioethicists to the status of second-tier authorities. Thus, the Royal Dutch Medical Association (founded in 1848) was able to negotiate physician-initiated euthanasia practices with Dutch legal authorities without involving "bioethicists" in any major decision.[15] Similarly, the British National Health Service (NHS, founded in 1948) was also able to initiate a covert rationing scheme limiting use of dialysis and other expensive technologies to younger patients—effectively resolving the rationing problem created by the Scribner shunt by denying access to the elderly—without annoying discussions or protests from "bioethicists."[16] Having retained jurisdiction and moral authority over medical ethics, organized medicine in Europe had the prerogative of negotiating with governments to determine the appropriate nature of end-of-life care (euthanasia) or the allocation of scarce resources (age rationing). In America, by contrast, laissez-faire ethics rendered medicine unwilling to express authoritative moral positions and thus unable to negotiate them with the U.S. government. Thus, these issues were negotiated with "outsiders" invited into the once exclusively medical jurisdiction of "medical" ethics; that is, they were negotiated with "bioethicists."

To return to Campbell's critique of Jonsen: Campbell is correct in claiming that ethics institutes were established in Britain, the Netherlands, and throughout

Europe around the same time as they were introduced in America. Moreover, moral philosophers, most notably Baroness Mary Warnock, sometimes headed committees that recommended policy on IVF and other morally disruptive technologies. The difference between Europe and America is that, to reiterate, European medical societies never abandoned their jurisdiction over medical ethics. Thus, as is documented in this chapter, to deal with American medicine's abdication from moral authority, American bureaucrats joined with government and private foundations to empower a hodgepodge of ex-theologians, lawyers, philosophers, social scientists, and humanistic nurses, physicians, and researchers to address issues raised by research ethics scandals and by morally disruptive technologies. As it turned out, this hodgepodge proved adept at providing workable resolutions to these issues. More significantly, in collaborating with each other and in communicating their views to policymakers, they created a new discourse and a new conceptual framework for approaching moral issues in biomedicine—they created the field of bioethics as an alternative to laissez-faire medical ethics.

This chapter reassembles materials that have, for the most part, been cited in standard histories of bioethics to support a vacuum-of-moral-authority explanation of why Americans invented bioethics. The account places emphasis on the dearth of "ethicists" at the early stages of "ethics regulation"; the ineffectiveness of pre-bioethical self-regulatory efforts; the role of the AMA's opposition to Medicare, Medicaid, and the racial integration of medicine as a "distraction"; and the extent to which the AMA's laissez-faire ethics constrained the AMA from responding to moral issues, including the AIDS epidemic.

THE 1960S: BUILDING A BUREAUCRATIC SCAFFOLD FOR BIOETHICS

Bureaucratic and other governmental responses to a series of scandals unfolding in the 1960s serve as a prelude to bioethics. The earliest occurred in 1962, when a bureaucrat at the U.S. Food and Drug Administration (FDA), pharmacologist Francis Oldham Kelsey was knighted in the popular press as the "Feminine Conscience of the FDA" and "Guardian of the Drug Market" for single-handedly preventing the introduction of a fetus-crippling drug, thalidomide, into America.[17] The thalidomide scare led to the 1962 Kefauver-Harris Act that reformed the process of researching and marketing new drugs. Three years later, in a well-publicized 1965 case, the New York State Division of Professional Conduct suspended the medical licenses of two physicians who had injected live cancer cells into incapacitated terminal patients without informing them or their families that the injection contained cancer cells. These physicians were found to have violated U.S. Public Health Service (PHS) rules requiring that "fully cognizant of all that is entailed, the volunteer gives his signed consent to take part in [any experiment]."[18] The next year, 1966, Harvard physician and researcher Henry Beecher cited this case as one of twenty-two cases of outrageous abuse of human subjects. Astonishingly, these cases were ripped from the pages of leading medical journals, including the journal that published Beecher's exposé, the *New England Journal of Medicine*—which had published six of the cases.[19]

As it turned out, many examples of scandalous research featured in Beecher's article had been funded by U.S. government agencies. Alarmed by Beecher's article—which has properly been deemed "the most influential single paper ever written about experimentation involving human subjects"[20]—distressed by the thalidomide scare, and prompted to action by the United States signature of the Declaration of Helsinki of Ethical Principles for Medical Research Involving Human Subjects (issued in 1964 by the World Medical Association, WMA, founded in 1947), government agencies sought to more closely monitor medical experiments involving human subjects. Completing this trifecta of governmental alarm and action, in the same year, 1966, provoked by constituent protests and stories in the popular press about a supply chain for animal experimentation that resorted to dognapping and by a graphic *Life* magazine article on doggy concentration camps, the U.S. Congress enacted the Laboratory Animal Welfare Act (AWA).[21]

One effect of these scandal-and-outrage-inspired 1960s regulations and laws was that such U.S. government agencies as the Department of Agriculture; the Department of Health, Education, and Welfare (HEW; now the Health and Human Services, HHS); the FDA; the National Institutes of Health (NIH; founded in 1930); and the office of the Surgeon General of the U.S. Public Health Service required laboratories, medical facilities, pharmaceutical companies, and other institutions receiving government support to develop institutionally based research review boards (IRBs) to monitor research on humans and institutional animal care and use committees (IACUCs) to monitor research on animals. These "satellite regulators," to use political scientist Daniel Carpenter's apt coinage,[22] applied and enforced governmental regulations to protect the welfare of research subjects, human or animal. Their impact was jurispathic; that is, institutional satellites applying governmental regulations supplanted traditional mechanisms of professional self-regulation. Thus, AWA legislation enforced by IACUCs supplanted the norms of professional self-regulation in the "Rules Regarding Animals" (see Chapter 9).

The consequent erosion of professional self-regulatory authority coincided with lobbying efforts by the AMA to forestall implementation of the 1964 Civil Rights Act in healthcare institutions[23] and to prevent the enactment of the Medicare and Medicaid federal health insurance programs for senior citizens and the poor. Taking note of the medical profession's inattention to governmental intrusions on prerogatives of professional self-regulation, in 1966, Edward Long (1908–1972) Democratic Senator from Missouri, wrote to the AMA that

> The medical profession as a whole and the [AMA] in particular have expended a great deal of . . . time and energy in an unsuccessful fight against Medicare. . . .
>
> While few were watching, and even fewer were caring, the [FDA] has vastly expanded its powers and duties.
>
> More and more it tells the physician how he is to practice his art.
>
> More and more it tells the pharmaceutical manufacturers how to run their highly complex industry in each and every detail. . . .
>
> The process whereby medical judgment is slipping from the hands of the profession into the hands of the bureaucrats is both fast and silent.[24]

The last line in the passage quoted from Senator Long's letter to the AMA presumes that physicians and pharmacists were still self-regulating their professions. The American Pharmaceutical Association (APhA, founded in 1852, now known as the American Pharmacists Association), like the AMA, had a self-regulatory professional code of ethics from 1852, the year of its founding. Yet, early in the twentieth century, around the time that AMA's code of ethics was undermined by laissez-faire ideology, the APhA code was being obsolesced as the manufacture of drugs (such as aspirin and insulin) shifted from an artisanal process in neighborhood compounding pharmacies to industrial-based mass production. As pharmaceutical manufacture industrialized, it eroded and enervated the effectiveness of professional self-regulatory oaths and codes.

RESEARCH OVERSIGHT: THE ORIGINS AND ATROPHY OF PROFESSIONAL SELF-REGULATION

Percival's Proposal for Research Ethics Committees

It is helpful to take a brief look at the history of research ethics committees to appreciate the challenges of purely professional self-regulation and some of the factors favoring their later atrophy. Although a researcher's character and conscience were traditionally regarded as the primary safeguards against abuse of research subjects, calls for an additional safeguard—peer review committees—date to the late eighteenth century. Percival issued the earliest known proposal for such a committee in his 1794 manuscript, *Medical Jurisprudence*,[25] which he reiterated in his 1803 book, *Medical Ethics:*

> Whenever cases occur, attended with circumstance not hitherto observed, or in which ordinary modes of practice have been attempted without success it is for the public good, and in an especial degree advantageous to the poor (who, being the most numerous class of society, are the greatest beneficiaries of the healing art) that *new remedies* and *new methods of chirurgical treatment* be devised. But in the accomplishment of this salutary purpose, the gentlemen of the faculty should be scrupulously and conscientiously governed by sound reason, just analogy, or well authenticated facts. And no such trials should be instituted without a previous consultation of the physicians or surgeons according to the nature of the case.[26]

Percival was proposing that ad hoc committees of physicians or surgeons be formed to review and approve proposed clinical trials at charity hospitals. Committee membership would "depend on the nature of the case"; that is, committees of physicians would review proposed experiments by fellow physicians, and committees of surgeons would review the proposals of fellow surgeons. These committees would approve a proposed clinical trial only if the trial served a "public good" by testing new therapies in situations in which the "ordinary modes of practice have been attempted without success." Thus, only potentially therapeutic innovations warranted approval, and then only if the proposed innovation could be justified by "sound reason, just analogy, or well authenticated facts"; that is, only if the review committee found that the protocol rests on a scientifically sound hypothesis. The sick poor patients in charity hospitals, moreover, should be subjected to experiments only if the resulting innovations would be "advantageous to the poor"—a constraint that rules out the view that sick poor patients should serve as clinical material to develop new therapies to be used by those enjoying superior social status. Writing in 1970, Beecher cites these lines from Percival as a precedent-setting, remarking that "echoes of all [of Percival's] points are present in the most up-to-date codes."[27]

THE FIRST AMERICAN PERCIVALEAN-STYLE RESEARCH COMMITTEE: THE NEHW-STORER CASE

Since *Medical Ethics* shaped nineteenth-century American medical societies' understanding of medical ethics, one might anticipate that Percivalean-style research ethics committees would have been common in nineteenth-century American hospitals. Yet Percival's writings on research ethics had no discernable impact on American hospitals prior to the 1860s. In part, this was because American physicians seldom conducted organized research prior to the Civil War (Beaumont and Sims being notable exceptions), and, in part, because the "clinical material" used for medical research—the hospitalized sick poor and denizens of other total institutions—were unavailable to most American physicians, who typically practiced in their own homes or in those of their patients. Hospital practice was, in fact, so irrelevant to American physicians that when Kappa Lambda societies popularized Percival's *Medical Ethics* in the 1820s, the sections on hospitals were deleted—including Percival's comments on research ethics committees.[28]

During and after the Civil War, however, hospital-based practice became more commonplace and some hospitals began to set up Percivalean-style research review committees. The earliest known example of such a committee was in the first American hospital to be run by and for women, the New England Hospital for Women (NEHW, 1862–1969).[29] The NEHW was founded and presided over by Dr. Marie Zakrzewska (1829–1902), a Berlin-Paris-educated Polish-American physician who earned an M.D. from a regular medical school, Case Reserve (founded in 1843, now Case Western Reserve University). The *sole* surgeon operating in the NEHW was the antiabortion crusader Horatio Storer Jr. A proud feminist, Storer was pleased to serve at the NEHW—a decision considered ill-advised and censurable by fellow male physicians, who neither consulted with nor recognized as legitimate female physicians. Storer also hired as his surgical associate the first American female surgeon, Dr. Anita Tyng (circa 1840–1913), a graduate of the Women's Medical College of Pennsylvania (the first degree-granting regular medical college for women, founded in 1850, now part of Allegheny University). As Storer later remarked, he hired Dr. Tyng because he "desired to do what little [he] personally could towards the real enfranchisement of women … and because [he believed in] elevating the few women … [who were] better educated."[30]

Storer's feminist proclivities, however, did little to shield him from censure when one of his patients died during an operation (a hysterectomy) that Dr. Zakrzewska considered experimental. To prevent future incidents, the NEHW hospital board drew up a plan for Percivalean-style ad hoc research ethics committees with this mandate:

> In all unusual or difficult cases in medicine, where a capital operation in surgery is proposed, the Attending and Resident Physicians and Surgeons shall hold mutual consultation, and if any one of them shall doubt as to the propriety of the proposed treatment or operation, one or more of the Consulting Physicians or Surgeons shall be invited to examine and decide upon the case.[31]

Infuriated by this proposal, Storer protested, "it is not the physician's place to judge as to necessity in surgeon's cases!"[32]

> It is not … the custom among hospital attendants … for the decision of purely surgical questions to be submitted to the medical members of the staff.… It is not the physician's place to judge as to necessity in surgeon's

> cases.... Consultations among medical men are not matters of compulsion; they are made at the request of the patient or the desire of the attendant.... I am therefore compelled to resign my connection with [this new policy].[33]

Having stated his reasons for resigning, Storer praised Dr. Tyng's skill and dedication as a surgeon, as well as the character of Dr. Zakrzewska, "the beauty and purity of whose life is already published to the world."[34] Nonetheless, he contended that, by issuing this policy on surgery, these female physicians demonstrated that women lacked the proper temperament to enter medicine "as a calling."[35]

After 1866, Storer actively opposed AMA recognition of female physicians and female medical colleges. He reconciled his deep commitment to feminism with his opposition to female physicians by contending that although he was committed to "loosing ... some of woman's present chains," he would do so solely "to increase her health, prolong her life, extend the benefits she confers on society." He would no longer "advocate for the unwomanly woman; I would not transplant them, from their proper and God-given sphere, to the pulpit, the forum, or the cares of state," nor would he "repeat the experiment, so patiently tried by [him]self. And at last so emphatically condemned—of females attempting to practice the medical profession."[36] Storer's exasperated response to his censure by physicians, and female physicians at that, documents one of the challenges of self-regulatory ethics: accountability to the judgment of those whom one accepts as one's peers, in Storer's case, fellow surgeons. Yet, precisely because peers accept a set of common values, they are typically unable, or unwilling, to challenge commonly accepted prejudices or abuses. It took physicians, female physicians in fact, to recognize the need for prior review of experimental surgery.

THE FECKLESSNESS OF PRE-BIOETHICAL PROFESSIONAL SELF-REGULATION OF RESEARCH ETHICS

Senator Long's presumption that the healthcare professions were already safeguarding the welfare of human and animal research subjects was mistaken.[37] After the NEHW-Storer incident, hospitals seldom implemented Percivalean-style prior review of proposed medical innovations or experiments. Furthermore (as discussed in Chapter 9), adhering to its laissez-faire ideology, the AMA never implemented Walter Cannon's proposal to include informed consent as an ethical principle governing human subjects research. The AMA would not endorse any research ethics principles until after 1946, when Andrew Ivy (1893–1978) shamed the organization to insulate American researchers from embarrassing comparisons with their German counterparts at the Nuremberg Medical Trials.

The AMA's first major statement on research ethics was elicited only after international pressure was brought by the WMA, which issued the 1964 Declaration of Helsinki—and even then, the AMA did not endorse the concept of prior peer review of research proposals; it endorsed research ethics in principle but, true to laissez-faire tradition, without practical enforcement mechanisms.

In the 1960s, however, the government's medical flagship, the NIH, did endorse the principle of informed consent of subjects in potentially harmful nontherapeutic experiments. Yet words were not deeds, and the NIH's official ethics statements did not become the operant morality of NIH-funded researchers. Thus, when the NIH surveyed member institutes "in 1962 [it] discovered that only nine of its fifty-two departments had any policy regarding the rights of research subjects; [and only] sixteen stated that they used written consent forms."[38] Moreover, even at the NIH's own Clinical Center (which admitted its first patient in 1953), prior peer review of risky experiments was effectively optional:

> NIH investigators ... were not required to obtain another investigator's opinion, let alone approval.... [The] NIH did have a Medical Board Committee [whose mission was to review] "any non-standard potentially hazardous procedure".... However, as one deputy director explained, "It is not necessary to present each project to any single central group." Investigators who wanted a consultation ... had the option of seeking the advice of the Medical Board Committee; but if the investigators believed that their protocols were not hazardous, they were free to proceed. The choice was the investigator's alone, and so, not surprisingly, the board was rarely consulted.[39]

Thus, even in America's leading institutions, the mechanisms of research review in the 1960s were pro forma, undermined by researchers' laissez-faire morality, their reluctance to submit to peer review, and their hesitation to pronounce judgment on each other. Consequently, satellite regulatory bodies initially did little to protect human subjects.

ENTER THE OUTSIDERS: THE IMPACT OF THE BELMONT REPORT

Resistance to Introducing Ethicists ("Outsiders") as Consultants or Reviewers

As the Storer incident illustrates, peer review is a matter for peers. Within professional communities, the concept of a peer tends to be narrowly defined: recall

Storer's outrage at the proposal that *physicians* pass judgment on his *surgical* practice. Given history's proclivity for repetition, not surprisingly, when health-care and research institutions and laboratories set up their IACUCs and IRBs in response to the regulatory mandates of the 1960s, they staffed them with fellow professionals. The very idea of incorporating ethics experts, *nonresearchers*, into the review of research was rejected as insulting. Standard histories of bioethics illustrate this reaction by citing testimony at a 1968 U.S. Senate hearing conducted by Minnesota Senator Walter Mondale (1977–1981).[39] A member of the first bioethics institute (the Hastings Center, founded in 1969 as the Institute of Society, Ethics, and the Life Sciences), Mondale discussed the idea of a national committee on ethics and medicine with various researchers, including South African cardiac surgeon Christiaan Barnard (1992–2001).

Barnard, who had just performed the first successful human-to-human heart transplant, was, at that moment, the most famous surgeon in the world. He responded to Mondale's questions about an interdisciplinary ethics oversight committee by channeling Storer's outrage:

> If we [in South Africa] could have done this [heart transplant] without a commission to give us guidance—do you feel it is necessary in this country to have some commission to guide your doctors and your scientists? I feel that if you do this, it would be an insult to your doctors and what is more it would put progress back a lot.[40]

Barnard's teacher, Owen Wangensteen (1898–1981), professor of surgery at the University of Minnesota and mentor to the generation of surgeons who would perfect cardiac transplantation, reiterated Barnard's views. Medical innovation, Wangensteen feared, could be "mangled by well-intentioned but meddlesome intruders." "I would urge you," he continued, "with all the strength I can to leave this subject to conscionable people in the profession who are struggling valiantly to advance medicine."[41] When Mondale probed whether "non-doctors, persons not in the medical profession … could bring … useful insights, or do you think it ought to be left exclusively to the medical profession?," Wangensteen replied that ethical advice should be the sole prerogative of medical professionals. "The fellow who holds the apple can peel it best.… If you are thinking of theologians, lawyers, and philosophers and others.… I cannot see how they could help. I would leave these decisions to responsible people doing the work."[42] The reaction of twentieth-century surgeons—like that of Storer, the nineteenth-century surgeon—was that one should be accountable only to peers: only researchers should review researchers. Intruding so-called ethics experts into such reviews was insulting and irresponsible.

The 1978 Belmont Report as a Watershed Moment

Historians of bioethics identify the watershed moment—the point at which the closed door of researcher self-regulation began to open to outsiders with expertise in ethics—as a set of 1970s senatorial hearings convened by Senator Edward Kennedy (1932–2009). Weeks before the assassination in 1963 of his brother, John F. Kennedy (1917–1963, U.S. president from 1961 to 1963), Senator Ted Kennedy, sent a major civil rights bill to Congress with President Kennedy's blessing. The bill would later be enacted as the 1964 Civil Rights Act. Civil rights were a Kennedy legacy. Thus, when almost a decade later, in July 26, 1972 front-page article in *The New York Times* announced that a forty-year-long study by the U.S. Public Health Service (PHS) deceived 399 African Americans into participating in a study of untreated syphilis, Senator Kennedy promptly convened hearings to investigate the so-called Tuskegee Syphilis Study and other research ethics scandals. Kennedy's hearings culminated in the National Research Act (NRA, 1974), which commissioned a National Commission for the Protection of Human Subjects of Biomedical and Behavioral Research (hereafter, the National Commission, 1974–1978) to review the protection of human subjects in U.S. government-funded research. This Commission included as part of its membership some ethics experts, including Albert Jonsen, a former Jesuit and college president, who had served on the first NIH committee to deal with a morally disruptive medical technology, the totally implantable artificial heart (1972–1973). The National Commission's staff also included such ethics experts, as Tom Beauchamp, a philosopher with a background in theology; LeRoy Walters, a professor of Christian ethics; and the eminent Anglo-American moral philosopher, Stephen Toulmin (1922–2009).

Government reports have notoriously brief half-lives. They linger for a legislative session or two and then are buried in archives and embalmed in law review articles. In the ultra-pragmatic Washington world of politics, some such fate must have seemed certain for a document drafted by a mélange of philosophers, theologians, lawyers, physicians, and social scientists bearing the odd title, "The Belmont Report."[43] Yet it was the 1978 report's philosophical tenor, its discourse of principles, that guaranteed its enduring significance. The Belmont Principles are now cited in every major document on research ethics and are taught in virtually every course or seminar on the subject offered in the United States or elsewhere. In touching deference to the power of moral principles, the U.S. bureaucracy pays tribute to the Belmont Principles on the website of the Department of Health and Human Services (HHS). The website features the full Belmont Report, complete with archives and interviews detailing the Report's history and the development of its principles.[44] This luminary status was not granted for any practical achievement, since the Report was written *after* the commission fulfilled its practical function of developing "common rules" for the various government agencies funding research on human subjects (now part of federal regulation 45 CFR 46). The Report's significance is primarily conceptual: it challenged an entrenched conception of the ethics of human subjects research that viewed the primary moral consideration in research ethics as preventing or minimizing risk of harm to human subjects.

From Osler, who had opined that "risk to the individual" is what "require[s] his consent and full knowledge,"[45] to the NIH Clinical Center, which required review of any "non-standard potentially hazardous procedure,"[46] American conceptions of a researcher's duty of obtaining informed consent had been linked to concepts of risk of bodily harm. Post-World War II codes of research ethics, as formulated in the Nuremberg Code and the 1964 Declaration of Helsinki, shared this view. Consent was viewed as mechanism for safeguarding subjects against harm. This conception was reinforced at the Nuremberg Trials because the Nazi researchers in the dock were "charged with murders, tortures, and other atrocities committed in the name of medical science."[47] Since no one volunteers to be murdered, tortured, or otherwise harmed, the informed voluntary consent rule of the Nuremberg Code was thought of as insurance against potentially harmful experiments. The 1964 Declaration of Helsinki accepted this premise, modifying the Nuremberg rules for application in clinical contexts—for example, by legitimating surrogate consent for incapacitated persons and minors—but its moral grounding was rooted in revulsion at the actions of the Nazi researchers and in notions of preventing unwanted bodily harm.

The National Commission, however, was post-Tuskegee as well as post-Holocaust: it had been mandated to "identify the basic ethical principles that should underlie the conduct of biomedical and behavioral research involving human subjects."[48] Addressing the moral outrage over the Tuskegee Syphilis experiment was unavoidable, and thus the commission needed to confront a vexing question: What moral principle was violated by an observational study of the natural course of a disease in subjects who would normally remain untreated? The challenge was that, insofar as such a study placed none of its subjects at risk of increased harm, and insofar as informed consent was thought necessary *only* in studies in which subjects were placed at additional risk of harm (the Osler and NIH position), there seemed to be no moral reason to ask subjects for informed consent. As one defender of the study commented, the PHS was not harming the Tuskegee subjects because "lack of treatment was not contrived by the USPHS but was an established fact of which they proposed to take advantage."[49] Consequently, insofar as the duty of consenting subjects was linked to risk of bodily harm, and insofar as no risk of harm was increased by a noninterventional observational study of untreated disease, no wrong was apparent in the Tuskegee study—at least not from the perspective of the then standard rationale for requiring informed consent.

The Osler-NIH harm-prevention model of informed consent was shared by a nine-member committee tasked, in 1973, by the PHS with analyzing the ethical issues raised by the Tuskegee Study. This committee concluded that the Tuskegee study was "ethically unjustified in 1932" because it broke "one fundamental ethical rule ... that a person should not be subjected to avoidable risk of *death or physical harm* unless he freely and intellectually *consents*."[50] After linking the consent requirement to risk of physical harm or death, the PHS committee concluded that, other than breaking the informed consent rule, no harm was done to the Tuskegee subjects until 1953—when penicillin became publicly available. At that point, since treatment might prevent bodily harm, "penicillin therapy should have been made available to the participants."[51]

Linking consent to harm-minimization turns the morality of the Tuskegee Study into a question of fact: Were any of the 399 African-American men studied harmed, or did they face increased risk of harm, because they participated in the study? Some commentators argue that since the "prognosis ... in patients having latent syphilis in the [Tuskegee] Study group was no better or worse than that of many hundreds of thousands of other syphilitic U.S. citizens of their generation bearing the diagnosis of latent syphilis ... [and since] the lethal complications of [the disease] have never been proven indubitably to be altered by anti-syphilitic treatment" of that era, the untreated study group was not harmed or exposed to increased risk of harm. These facts, the argument continues, "should point up [the unfounded] accusations of an irresponsible press, and the irrelevancy of certain Congressmen's emotional reaction to the Tuskegee Study."[52] In other words, since the subjects of the Tuskegee study were not harmed, the only blameworthy parties were Congress and the press; the researchers were innocent.

Writing five years after the PHS report, consultants to the National Commission came to appreciate that any conception of the ethics of informed consent grounded solely in concepts of harm prevention would fail to capture the sense of moral outrage provoked by the Tuskegee Study. Perhaps the first person to publicly express moral outrage over the study was Peter Buxton, the PHS employee who, from 1966 to 1972, peppered his superiors with memos expressing "grave moral doubts as to the propriety of [the Tuskegee Syphilis] study."[53] After his concerns were repeatedly dismissed, Buxton blew the whistle by sharing his concerns about the study with an Associated Press reporter who wrote the article in *The New York Times* that prompted Senator Kennedy's hearing.

Buxton was a star witness at the hearings, and Senator Kennedy asked him directly, "What bothered you most about the study?' Buxton did not cite out the issue of harm prevention. What bothered Buxton most was "[t]he fact that the participants really did not seem to be consulted. They were being used."[54] Nothing in the standard English-language literature on human subjects research of that era had linked the concept of informed consent with the notion of "being used."[55] "Being used" is clearly not a matter of being harmed physically, but Buxton knew intuitively that it was morally wrong.

In a deep sense, the challenge facing the National Commission was how to translate Buxton's gut feeling, his moral sensibility about the wrong of being "used," into an articulate concept. Yet, from Lady Mary Montagu's letters; to Beaumont's notebooks; to the lectures of Bard, Cullen, Gregory, Percival, Rush, Ryan, and Osler; to the initial regulations promulgated by the NIH, the primary focus of the English-language research ethics literature had been how to justify deliberately exposing people to risks of harm or death. Solutions varied from therapeutic exemptions, to Golden Rule self- and familial experimentation, to volunteerism, to labor contracts, to oral or written consent. The National Commission noted this tradition in the Belmont Report, observing that "[t]he Hippocratic maxim 'do no harm' had long been a fundamental principle of medical ethics. [French physiologist] Claude Bernard [1813–1878] extended it to the realm of research, saying that one should not injure one person regardless of the benefits that might come to others."[56] Nonetheless, to pull away from this standard conception of research ethics, the Commission asked several moral philosophers to write essays exploring the principles underlying research ethics.

The raison d'être of moral philosophy, its fundamental function, is to make articulate our often-inchoate moral sensibilities and to interrogate their rationality; that is, to make clear to ourselves and to others why that which we take to be morally praiseworthy is worthy of our praise—and why that which we condemn merits moral condemnation. As the influential Anglo-Austrian philosopher Ludwig Wittgenstein (1889–1951) once remarked, "A man will be imprisoned in a room with a door that's unlocked and opens inwards; as long as it does not occur to him to pull rather than push it."[57] The philosopher's job is to open blocked doors by suggesting alternative ways of conceiving of issues or problems—pulling rather than pushing at them.

The philosophers did their job. In a series of essays written especially for the National Commission, they fulfilled their mission of providing alternative conceptions that articulated the reasons why the Tuskegee Study was morally outrageous. As commissioner (and historian) Albert Jonsen reports, the Commission took two principles from an essay "by philosopher/physician H. Tristram Engelhardt[58] ... respect for persons as free moral agents [and] concern to support the best interests of human subjects in research" and one from "philosopher Tom Beauchamp's ... paper titled 'Distributive Justice and Morally Relevant Differences'[59] ... [reformulating] both Englehardt's and Beauchamp's principle[s as three] "crisp" principles ... respect for persons, beneficence, and justice."[60]

Engelhard developed his principles after a careful review of such major post-World War II codes of research ethics as the Nuremberg Code, the 1975 Declaration of Helsinki, various HEW regulations, and the American Psychological Association's Code of Ethics (APA; founded in 1892, first code published in 1953).[61] Without exception, all of these documents required the informed consent of human subjects as prerequisite to ethical experimentation; however, as Engelhardt put it, none "distinguish[es] … principles from procedures or guidelines employed in safeguarding principles."[62] No document had explicitly stated a moral principle justifying the consent requirement. To reiterate, they stipulated consent requirements, but they did not offer any moral basis or justification for them. Consequently, none of the established codes captured Buxton's moral insight that the Tuskegee Syphilis study was morally outrageous because subjects were being "used." Engelhardt, however, explained the moral outrage of Buxton (and the public) by observing that the researchers failed to "respect … [their subjects] as free moral agents."[63]

In its Belmont Report the National Commission refined Engelhardt's insight into the following principle:

> *Respect for Persons.*—Respect for persons [means] that individuals should be treated as autonomous agents.… An autonomous person is an individual capable of deliberation about personal goals and of acting under the direction of such deliberation. To respect autonomy is to give weight to autonomous persons' considered opinions and choices while refraining from obstructing their actions unless they are clearly detrimental to others. To show lack of respect for an autonomous agent is to repudiate that person's considered judgments, to deny an individual the freedom to act on those considered judgments, or to withhold information necessary to make a considered judgment, when there are no compelling reasons to do so.[64]

This principle captures the intuitive wrongfulness of the Tuskegee experiment. It articulates Buxton's intuition that the Tuskegee researchers wronged their subjects because they showed a "lack of respect" for their subjects by deceptively telling them that they were being treated for "bad blood" when, in fact, the researchers had no intention of treating their subjects: they were deceiving the subjects into being monitored and tested without receiving any treatment.

The Tuskegee researchers' disrespect for their subjects was persistent and pervasive. Consider the following correspondence between two researchers:

> [I]f the colored population becomes aware that accepting free hospital care [as a subject in the Tuskegee syphilis study] means a post-mortem, every darkey will leave Macon county … however, if the doctors are … requested

> to be very careful not to let the objective of the plan be known [it should work].[65]

In this communication, an official of the U.S. PHS implemented a policy of using deceptive offers of "free funerals" to secure peoples' bodies for a postmortems. Deception was the preferred policy because, had these people been informed that accepting a "free funeral" meant a postmortem, they likely would have refused the offer. The researchers wronged their subjects precisely because, to use the language of the Belmont report, they "show[ed a] lack of respect for an autonomous agent" by "repudiat[ing] that person's considered judgments." The racial pejorative "darkey," a derogatory identification of a person in terms of skin color and race that is only marginally more polite than Sims' brother's characterization of African Americans as "niggers" (see discussion in Chapter 9), reflects the researchers' racial bias. African Americans were "used," as Buxton put it, and researchers felt free to use them, to deceive them, to override their religious beliefs about postmortems because they were "darkies," second-class persons unworthy of the respect accorded to proper, presumably white, people.

The theme of injustice permeates the third Belmont principle, which, as Jonsen notes, was taken from Tom Beauchamp's essay "Distributive Justice and Morally Relevant Differences." In this essay, Beauchamp argues eloquently that no person should be denied benefits or given extra burdens on the basis of race or sex because "these are differences for which [people] have no responsibility"; that is, "these are not the sort of properties that one has a fair chance to acquire or overcome."[66] These themes of justice as fairness are reiterated throughout the Report's statement of the Principle of Justice:

> 3. *Justice*.... An injustice occurs when some benefit to which a person is entitled is denied without good reason or when some burden is imposed unduly. Another way of conceiving the principle of justice is that equals ought to be treated equally.... Until recently these questions have not generally been associated with scientific research. However [the principle was violated] ... during the nineteenth and early twentieth centuries [when] the burdens of serving as research subjects fell largely upon poor ward patients, while the benefits of improved medical care flowed primarily to private patients.... In this country, in the 1940s, the Tuskegee syphilis study used disadvantaged, rural black men to study the untreated course of a disease that is by no means confined to that population. These subjects were deprived of demonstrably effective treatment in order not to interrupt the project, long after such treatment became generally available [after 1953].
>
> ...[T]he selection of research subjects needs to be scrutinized in order to determine whether some classes (e.g., welfare patients, particular racial

> and ethnic minorities, or persons confined to institutions) are being systematically selected simply because of their easy availability, their compromised position, or their manipulability, rather than for reasons directly related to the problem being studied. Finally, whenever research supported by public funds leads to the development of therapeutic devices and procedures, justice demands both that these not provide advantages only to those who can afford them and that such research should not unduly involve persons from groups unlikely to be among the beneficiaries of subsequent applications of the research.[67]

Earlier American ideals of just treatment differ from those expounded in the Belmont Report. America inherited from its British motherland a perception of the world as naturally inegalitarian. In this world, the ineradicable poverty of the masses and the natural inequalities of class, race, and gender—recall that in 1871 the AMA's president proclaimed that "woman is unfitted by nature to become a physician"[68]—required those in the higher orders of society to favor those less fortunate with condescension, charity, and protective paternalism. Yet these inequalities were tempered by an ethics of care, stewardship, and *noblesse oblige*, grounded in ideals of gentlemanly honor and Christian charity. To quote the King James translation of the Bible, "For unto whomsoever much is given, of him shall be much required: and to whom men have committed much, of him they will ask the more" (Luke 12:48). This translated directly into the conduct of healthcare institutions for, as the Trustees of Bath hospital proclaimed, "[t]he *Rich* and *Powerful* are capable of *repelling Insults* and *Punishing Injuries*; but the *Objects* of a HOSPITAL CHARITY are *Helpless* and liable to every kind of *ill Treatment*; if they are not protected by those, to whose Care they are entrusted."[69]

America's professed ideals of egalitarianism and individualism undermined these presumptions. If everyone is equal, if everyone enjoys equal opportunities for success and earns their place in society, then the presumed superiority of those condescending or offering charity or paternalistic protection can only be viewed as insulting. Equality demands a different ethics; so, too, did the spirit of the era in which the Belmont Report was written. As historians of bioethics observe with unanimity, American bioethicists and the field they founded were conceived and born in an era of egalitarian reform that recognized no castes and asserted the civil and human rights of all persons, irrespective of class, ethnicity, gender, race, religion, social standing, status, or wealth. As one team of observers put this point:

> [B]ioethics developed in the United States [during] "a time of social protest and ferment … spearheaded by the civil rights and anti-war movements, and the beginning of the new women's movement … with their emphasis

on individual rights and choice as fundamental bases of freedom, equality, and justice."[70]

These egalitarian values are manifest in the Belmont principles: respect for persons, beneficence and, most of all, in the principle of justice. In stating the principle of justice, the commissioners expressly condemn as unjust, as a violation of the principle of the fair distribution of the burdens and benefits of research, what might be called Sims's principle (discussed in Chapter 9): the principle of imposing the "burdens of serving as research subjects largely upon poor ward patients, while the benefits of improved medical care flowed primarily to private patients." Similarly, the PHS's post-1953 refusal to provide penicillin to its Tuskegee subjects is condemned, not as a violation of the "do no harm" principle, but as an injustice, a violation of the principle of fair distribution of benefits because "these subjects were deprived of demonstrably effective treatment in order not to interrupt the project, long after such treatment became generally available."

The Belmont analysis renders the previously dominant principle of minimizing harm or increased risk of harm secondary to principles of egalitarian justice. Where trustees of the Bath hospital had paternalistically protected the weak and powerless, citing duties of care and charity, the Belmont Report offers a comparable, albeit nonpaternalist, condemnation of researchers' exploitation of "racial and ethnic minorities, or persons confined to institutions," who were "selected simply because of their easy availability, their compromised position, or their manipulability." The Report does not construe these transgressions as offenses against charity or paternalistic duty, but as an inequitable distribution of the benefits and burdens of medical innovation. Yet—*plus ça change, plus c'est la même chose!*—the Belmont conception of egalitarian justice protects the vulnerable in ways that the old order would have construed as properly paternalistic. The justifying conception may change, but the ideal of protecting the vulnerable is preserved.

The third principle in the Belmont trinity, the Principle of Beneficence, conserves the once singular norm of research ethics, the principle of harm prevention:

> *Beneficence.*—Persons are treated in an ethical manner not only by respecting their decisions and protecting them from harm, but also by making efforts to secure their well-being. Such treatment falls under the principle of beneficence.... In this document, beneficence is understood ... as an obligation: (1) do not harm and (2) maximize possible benefits and minimize possible harms.[71]

Thus, benefit maximization is not the older ideal of benefitting society by promoting medical knowledge, but rather the notion of protecting subjects participating in research from unnecessary harm and benefitting them insofar as this is possible.

One reason why the Belmont Report had such an influence on the actual practice and regulation of medical experimentation was that the Report offered practical guidance on the application of its abstract principles. Thus, the Report became relevant for HEW and its satellite regulators, the IRBs, by virtue of Part C—aptly titled "Applications."

> APPLICATIONS
>
> Applications of the general principles to the conduct of research leads to consideration of the following requirements: informed consent, risk/benefit assessment, and the selection of subjects of research.
>
> 1. *Informed Consent.*—Respect for persons requires that subjects, to the degree that they are capable, be given the opportunity to choose what shall or shall not happen to them. This opportunity is provided when adequate standards for informed consent are satisfied.... [T]he consent process can be analyzed as containing three elements: information, comprehension and voluntariness.
>
> *Information* ... generally include[s]: the research procedure, their purpose, risks and anticipated benefits, alternative procedures (where therapy is involved), and a statement offering the subject the opportunity to ask questions and to withdraw at any time from the research....
>
> A special problem of consent arises where informing subjects of some pertinent aspect of the research is likely to impair the validity of the research.... [I]ncomplete disclosure ... is justified only if it is clear that (1) [it] is truly necessary to accomplish the goals of the research, (2) there are no undisclosed risks to subjects that are more than minimal, and (3) there is an adequate plan for debriefing subjects.... Information about risks should never be withheld for the purpose of eliciting the cooperation of subjects.... Care should be taken to distinguish cases in which disclosure would destroy or invalidate the research from cases in which disclosure would simply inconvenience the investigator.[72]

The Applications section continues with carefully crafted discussions of such practical topics as research subjects comprehension of the information imparted in a consent protocol; the voluntariness of subjects' consent; how to systematically assess the balance of risks versus benefits; and just ways of selecting subjects. In practice, these discussions gave IRBs an interpretive guide and a checklist of items to be covered in approving research ethics protocols. The Belmont Report's precedent-setting blend of justification, principles, and pragmatics soon became the hallmark of bioethics.

Another important contribution of the Belmont Report (and of the National Commission) was to give IRBs and the research enterprise generally a renewed sense of moral purpose. While conserving and reinvigorating the traditional precepts of research ethics—advancing medical science to serve future patients and society; minimizing the risk of harm to experimental subjects—it embraced new ideals of respect for the people who serve as subjects and a just distribution of the benefits and burdens of research. Some of these ideals were inarticulately implicit in earlier statements of research ethics. Yet, as the philosopher Wittgenstein once wrote, "[w]hereof one cannot speak, thereof one must be silent."[73] An inarticulate gut feeling, the sort of sensibility that moved Peter Buxton to protest, is seldom persuasive to others and cannot serve to justify public policy. By making these sentiments articulate, by formulating them in terms of ethical principles, the National Commission created a new paradigm of research ethics, a nonpaternalist account of protections for the vulnerable ideally suited to an egalitarian era.

PRINCIPLES OF BIOMEDICAL ETHICS: BIOETHICS LINGUA FRANCA, FROM PIDGIN TO CREOLE

Limitations of language plagued the interdisciplinary teams of lawyers, philosophers, physicians, social and healthcare scientists, and theologians serving on, staffing, and consulting with the National Commission—and those collaborating on other projects in the emerging field of bioethics. They had to communicate with government bureaucrats and politicians, with healthcare administrators and professionals, with scientists, with the public—and with each other. Historian and witness Albert Jonsen testifies to the challenge of communicating between and across discourses:

> [When] philosophers joined the theologians as shapers of the field of bioethics, [t]he merger was not a facile one. The two disciplines had lived apart for many years and each had developed different methods and vocabulary.... They did not easily learn to converse. Dan[iel] Callahan [co-founder of the Hastings Center] recalls, "One of my toughest problems during the Hasting Center's first twenty years was persuading the philosophers to sit down with the theologians and to take them seriously. The secular philosophers did not give a damn for what the theologians were saying...." Still, a dialogue was opened, and in the [bioethics institutes and] the government Commissions and the medical school programs the theologians and philosophers began to find a common language and slowly merged into bioethicists."[74]

Sociologist-historian of bioethics John Evans cites a passage from a 1986 work by H. Tristram Engelhardt to document the same phenomenon:

> The history of bioethics over the last two decades [i.e., from 1966–1986] has been the story of a secular ethic ... that attempts to frame answers in terms of no particular tradition, but rather in ways open to rational individuals as such, has emerged.... Bioethics is developing as the lingua franca of the a world concerned with health care, but not possessing a common ethical viewpoint.[75]

Challenges of language and perspective nagged at the multidisciplinary collaborators to the new field of bioethics. Irrespective of their home discipline—whether they wrote for a government commission, a reference work, a scholarly journal, or a textbook—contributors to the early bioethics literature faced the challenge of presenting complex material of their home fields in a language accessible to colleagues from other disciplines. Responding to this challenge, the first generation of bioethicists developed a *pidgin* for cross-disciplinary communication. Curiously, the term "pidgin" is itself a pidgin evolving from a nineteenth-century Chinese-English term for a simplified language enabling people from different language and cultural spheres to communicate with each other. If a pidgin endures long enough to become a language in its own right, it typically matures into a *creole*: a complexly sophisticated language that originated as a pidgin. This progression—from communicative challenge, to various pidgins, to a common creole—characterizes the maturation of bioethics discourse.

As every schoolchild knows all too well, textbooks are a means of transmitting one generation's conception of knowledge to its successors. They are, as the philosopher and historian of science Thomas Kuhn (1922–1996) observed, the basis of "both the layman's and the practitioner's knowledge of [the field]."[76] Textbook formats, prefaces, and tables of contents reveal a great deal about a field's self-definition; they also convey to successor generations how to articulate a field's concepts and theories; that is, the proper forms of discourse. Not surprisingly, therefore, the vehicle for coalescing various bioethical pidgins into a common creole was an Oxford University Press textbook series, *Principles of Biomedical Ethics* (first edition 1979, seventh edition 2012), written by two consultants to the National Commission, Tom Beauchamp[77] and James Childress.

The two had met at Yale Divinity School in the 1960s and, a decade later, collaborated as instructors in an intensive course for graduate students and health-care professionals taught at the Kennedy Institute of Ethics (the second oldest bioethics institute, founded as The Joseph and Rose Kennedy Center for the Study of Human Reproduction and Bioethics in 1971). Their textbook grew out of this course and was based on their insight that, instead of following the standard practice of treating issues in bioethics as isolated topics, "abortion, euthanasia, behavior control, research involving human subjects, etc.," they would "concentrate on the principles that should apply to a wide range of biomedical problems—including but not limited to the aforementioned problems."[78] In the first edition of their book, they offered a quartet of principles similar to, but differing subtly from, those in the Belmont Report: the principles of autonomy, nonmaleficence (not harming), beneficence, and justice.

In the introduction to the first edition of *Principles of Biomedical Ethics*, Beauchamp and Childress explain why they had to create a pidgin language for their text:

> One major difficulty in a book of this sort is to define and then address the appropriate audience. Our intended audience includes health care professional such as physicians and nurses, research investigators, policy makers in biomedicine, and students.... For such a mixed audience, it is necessary to eliminate or at least to define technical terms for each specialty. We have tried to presume only minimal acquaintance with philosophy, theology, and medicine—merely what the average person ... on the college level could be expected to possess.[79]

An illustrative example of how Beauchamp and Childress pidginize their own field, moral philosophy, involves the concept of autonomy. The concept became prominent in the Western philosophical canon largely due to the writings of Immanuel Kant (1724–1804), a German philosopher of the Enlightenment. Kant held that "[t]he human being itself is the original creator of all its representations and concepts and ought to be the sole author of all its actions."[80] As anyone who has taken an introductory course in moral philosophy will no doubt recall, Kant's metaphysical theory of freedom of the will (autonomous agency), summarized in this statement, was expounded in series of recondite texts challenging to scholars and intimidating to laypeople. To render the Kantian concept of autonomy suitable for bioethical discourse, Beauchamp and Childress stripped it of "will" and other metaphysical accouterments, characterizing it as

> a form of liberty of action where the individual determines his or her own course of action in accordance with a plan chosen by himself or herself. The autonomous person is one who not only deliberates about and chooses such plans but who is capable of acting on the basis of such deliberations ... A person of diminished autonomy, by contrast, is highly dependent on others and in at least some respect incapable of deliberating or acting on the basis of such deliberations.[81]

This pidginized rendering of "autonomy" may not have done justice to Kant, but it effectively justified the requirement of informed consent in clinical and research contexts, rendering the concept palatable and useful for practical purposes of healthcare professionals and researchers.

Through seven editions, the pidgin in *Principles of Biomedical Ethics* became a creole that evolved into the lingua franca of bioethics. Beauchamp and Childress's primary intention, however, was not to create a creole, but rather to develop a unified, principle-based approach to the full range of issues addressed by the new field of bioethics: one that encompassed both clinical and research ethics within the same framework. In their efforts to create a broadly encompassing theory in each new edition, they integrated new ideas as the field evolved. The philosopher John Arras, a friendly critic of Beauchamp and Childress's work, likens this phenomenon to "the Borg," a collective mind-absorbing entity (from the science fiction series *Star Trek*) that absorbs all the life forms it comes in contact with into its collective self. Arras's comment aptly characterizes the development of the *Principles of Biomedical Ethics* over the course of its seven editions. The book could serve as a core text for American bioethical discourse precisely because it assimilated the wide range of concepts and discourse. To quote Wittgenstein again, "the limits of my language mean the limits of my world:"[82] through their Borg-like absorption of the ideas, concepts, and theories of others into *Principles*, Beauchamp and Childress stretched the limits of bioethics, broadening the lingua franca to reflect and facilitate the field's growth. Fittingly, in 2004, the American Society for Bioethics and Humanities (ASBH, founded in 1998) conferred on them its lifetime achievement award.

MORALLY DISRUPTIVE TECHNOLOGIES AND THE BIRTH OF BIOETHICS

Although none of the standard histories of bioethics uses the expression "morally disruptive technologies," all assign them a role in their accounts of the birth of bioethics.[83] Taking center stage in these accounts is Bjorn Ibsen's ventilator which (as discussed in Chapter 3) obsolesced cardiopulmonary criteria for death by exporting pulmonary functions onto ventilators. A key figure in this narrative is anesthesiologist Henry Beecher, who became vexed by the question of how to deal with unendingly comatose ventilator-dependent patients and by an issue raised by a Boston colleague and fellow World War II veteran, transplantation pioneer and future Nobel Laureate, James Murray (1919–2012), who sought clarification about the ethics of using permanently comatose patients as organ donors. To deal with these issues, Beecher convened an ad hoc committee of Harvard Medical School faculty whose "primary purpose [was] to define irreversible coma as a new criterion of death."[84]

In August 1968, the ad hoc Harvard committee published a special communication in the *Journal of the American Medical Association (JAMA)* arguing for a new criterion for death because

> (1) [Some ventilator patients] hearts continue to beat but [their] brain is irreversibly damaged. The burden is great on patients who suffer permanent loss of intellect, on their families, on the hospitals, and on those in need of hospital beds already occupied by these comatose patients.
> (2) Obsolete criteria for the definition of death can lead to controversy in obtaining organs for transplantation.[85]

The report offers four criteria that, in combination, indicate that a coma is irreversible: (1) unreceptivity and unresponsiveness to external stimuli, (2) absence of spontaneous movement or breathing, (3) no reflexes, and (4) a flat electroencephalogram (EEG) reading. There follows an analysis that concludes with the statement that

> if responsible medical opinion is ready to adopt [these] new criteria for pronouncing death to have occurred in an individual sustaining irreversible coma as a result of permanent brain damage… [and if] this position is adopted by the medical community, it can form the basis for change in the current legal concept of death. No statutory change in law would be necessary since the law treats this question as of fact to be determined by physicians.[86]

Having stated criteria for irreversible coma and offered a strategy for transforming these criteria into a legal definition of death, the report turns to ethics, invoking as its sole source of moral authority a 1957 papal allocution (i.e., an opinion) by Pius XII on "The Prolongation of Life."[87] Two fragments were culled from the allocution to support the claims that: (1) "it is not 'within the competence of the Church,'" to determine the moment of death and (2) "it is not obligatory to use extraordinary means indefinitely in hopeless cases." Consequently, the Committee concluded, "It is the church's view that a time comes when resuscitative efforts should stop and death be unopposed."[88] These fragments from the pronouncements of a Roman Catholic pope were the only authority or argument cited to resolve the moral issues surrounding brain death and discontinuation of life support for ventilator-dependent patients.

Serious analyses of the ad hoc committee's report expose it as a conceptual mishmash. It employs a distinction between ordinary and extraordinary means drawn from Catholic moral theology to justify cessation of resuscitation. But it never explains either this distinction or why a presumably secular American medical community should accept as authoritative a Roman Catholic pope's opinion parsed in arcane language drawn from Catholic moral theology. As Albert Jonsen remarks, the report is

> a pastiche, stitching together some medical information, a legal opinion, and a theological statement.... Its science is done without a single reference to any neurological research (indeed it has only one citation—the Pope's speech!) It mixes ... "irreversible coma" with the abolition of function at brain stem levels. Its very title confuses "irreversible coma" with "brain death."... Finally, although the title proclaims it ... the report does not "define" death.[89]

The report may have been a conceptual mishmash, but since neither medicine nor law can readily tolerate a moral vacuum with respect to activities involving issues of life and death, American law and medicine instantly valorized the ad hoc committee report. It "became authoritative soon after its publication [because] it gave physicians guidance in diagnosing [brain death] and gave transplanters access to fresh organs [and] courts could avoid indicting transplant surgeons as murders."[90] Within two years of the report's publication, Kansas, home to one of America's first intensive care units, passed a brain death act, and, by the end of the decade, over two dozen other states had passed similar acts. Thus, even though the ad hoc committee's report is unclear—even incoherent—and never actually offers a definition of brain death, the need for practical guidance on disconnecting ventilators and the desire to avoid indicting well-intending transplant surgeons on charges of homicide led to an instant valorization of it as authoritative. American law and medicine abhor a vacuum, and they will ignore incoherence, inconsistency and alien theology to resolve practical problems.

True to its laissez-faire principles, however, the AMA declined to take an authoritative stance on the definition of brain death. As late as 1977, it opined that although "[v]arious medical procedures have resulted in a hue and cry for a statutory definition of death. The [AMA's] Judicial Council is of the opinion that this is neither desirable or necessary.... [D]eath should be determined by the clinical judgment of the physician."[91] Unhampered by a tradition of laissez-faire ethics, two years previously, in 1975, the American Bar Association (ABA, founded in 1878) proposed a model death statute. Finally, in 1979, the AMA reversed course and also recommended a model statute. Yet, because these models and state laws were based on the Harvard ad hoc committee's report, which was a conceptual hodgepodge, they inherited its inconsistencies. Thus, had a hypothetical ventilator-dependent patient pronounced brain dead in Kansas been transported by ambulance to some Northeastern state, the patient's status as living or dead would change as the ambulance crossed from state to state.[92]

Inconsistency may be preferable to a vacuum, but it is still awkward and undesirable in law and medicine. Confusion over a definition of brain death was resolved by a second national bioethics commission, the President's Commission for the Study of Ethical Problems in Medicine and Biomedical and Behavioral Research (1980–1983, hereafter, President's Commission), which, in 1981, defined *death*—note, not some special concept known as "brain death" but simply "death"—as "the irreversible cessation of cardiorespiratory function or the irreversible cessation of all functions of the brain, including the brain stem."[93] The President's Commission also recommended a model Uniform Definition of Death Act (UDDA) that various states could adopt. This model act was endorsed by ABA, the AMA, and, most importantly, by the National Conference of Commissioners on Uniform State Laws (NCCUSL, founded in 1892). Acting on the NCCUSL's endorsement, most states have since adopted the UDDA, providing a uniform standard for determination of death across state lines.

The sequence of events is revealing. Acting on their own, without the imprimatur of the AMA or any other professional medical society, an informal ad hoc committee of Harvard Medical School faculty threw together a mishmash of neurology, theology, and law to propose a new criteria and definition of "brain death." In the context of a vacuum of leadership from organized medicine, and in the face of an imperative need for such a definition, American medicine and law instantly canonized the ad hoc committee's report, enacting laws and making court decisions based on it. A bioethics commission later provided the needed clarification and justification for recognizing the irreversible cessation of either cardiopulmonary or brain function as medical criteria for "death." In sum: faced with a pressing practical need and vacuum of leadership from organized medicine, a group of practitioners create a flawed "brain death" definition; the fields of medicine and law embraced this definition despite its flaws and later replaced it with a refined version created by a government bioethics commission.

What is striking about this scenario is that the problems addressed by the Harvard ad hoc committee had been around since Ibsen invented the ventilator in 1952. The papal allocution cited by the ad hoc committee as an ethical authority was issued in 1957. These issues became prominent in America after 1962, when the first American critical care units opened their doors in Kansas and Philadelphia.[94] To its credit, the AMA's Judicial Council recognized a pressing need to address these and other issues later deemed "bioethical" and convened a series of national congresses on "Medical Ethics and Professionalism" from 1965 to 1968. Among the plenary speakers at the conference was neurosurgeon William P. Williamson from the University of Kansas medical center who addressed the issue of "Life or Death—Whose Decision" at the First National Congress on Medical Ethics and Professionalism.[95] At the AMA's Second National Congress on Medical Ethics,[96] Frank Ayd (1920–2008) of the American Psychiatric Association (founded in 1844 as the Association of Medical Superintendents of American Institutions for the Insane) called on the AMA to "adopt universally acceptable criteria for diagnosing brain death . . . [specifically] that proposed by the Ad Hoc Committee of the Harvard Medical School."[97] As noted earlier, the AMA rejected this call for the next decade[99] and did not support a UDDA act until 1979. Thus, at a point when the profession was crying out for ethical guidance, the AMA, hobbled by its laissez-faire approach to ethics, refrained from taking a leadership role, stepping aside to allow an ad hoc medical committee, presidential commissions—and eventually bioethicists—to assume its discarded mantle of moral authority and leadership in a field still generally known as "medical ethics." By 1971, however, the first American bioethics institutes had been founded, the term "bioethics" had been coined, and a new field was being born.

THE PRESIDENT'S COMMISSION: BANISHING TRADITIONAL DISTINCTIONS AND SLOW CODES

The Harvard ad hoc committee seriously misjudged when they suggested that simply invoking the Catholic moral theological distinction between extraordinary and ordinary means would clarify most of the issues with respect to "patients who suffer permanent loss of intellect . . . their families . . . the hospitals, and . . . those in need of hospital beds already occupied by these comatose patients."[100] This was underscored in April 1975, when Karen Ann Quinlan (1954–1985), a comatose twenty-one-year-old Roman Catholic woman, was admitted to St. Claire's, a Roman Catholic hospital in Denville, New Jersey. The hospital placed Quinlan on an MA-1 Ventilator, an updated version of Ibsen's invention. The staff neurologist later determined that Karen was in a persistent vegetative state (a sometimes "eyes-open," seemingly wakeful, but nonetheless irreversible unconscious state indicative of severe brain damage, but not of "brain death"). After Karen Ann's parents, Joseph and Julia, consulted with their parish priest, they asked Karen's physicians to turn off Karen's MA-1 ventilator, which they considered an "extraordinary means" of treatment. The physicians refused, and the matter went to the courts. Ultimately, the courts ruled that since Karen's right to privacy would have permitted her to refuse ventilator support, Karen's father, as a duly appointed surrogate, could exercise this right on her behalf. The court also conferred legal immunity on physicians, so that disconnecting Karen's ventilator would not put them at risk of prosecution for homicide—provided that an "ethics committee" reviewed the case.[101]

The court's directive to consult an "ethics committee" had been inspired by an article in the *Baylor Law Review* by pediatrician Karen Teel.[102] The AMA's counsel objected to this directive on the grounds that ethics committees were unnecessary because "a treating physician is certainly able to determine whether a patient is in a terminal position. . . . [Moreover] most hospitals don't have 'Ethics

Committees.'"[103] The AMA counsel's observations about ethics committees were accurate: they were virtually nonexistent in 1976. As late as 1983, "A National Survey of Hospital Ethics Committees," involving more than 400 hospitals with over 200 beds found that only 4.3 percent had hospital ethics committees (HECs) and that most of these committees had been formed around 1977, the year after the Quinlan decision and the publication of a seminal article about an ethics committee at the Massachusetts General Hospital.[104] In those hospitals that had ethics committees, however, the hospital staff found them effective at "facilitating decisionmaking by clarifying important issues (73.3 percent); providing legal protection for hospital and medical staff (60 percent); shaping consistent hospital policies in regard to life support (56.3 percent); providing opportunities for professionals to air disagreements (46.7 percent)."[105]

In the absence of leadership from the AMA, which had opposed the very idea of ethics committees, only a few hospitals, mostly in large academic medical centers, had explored the use of ethics committees. Yet the empirical data indicated that committees were effective in ameliorating the moral distress caused by chaotic laissez-faire decision-making procedures. So the President's Commission encouraged other hospitals to establish HECs by publishing in its appendix "A Model Bill to Establish Hospital Ethics Committees," prepared by Mary Beth Prosnitz for the American Society of Law and Medicine (founded in 1911 as the Massachusetts Society of Examining Physicians, renamed the American Society of Law, Medicine and Ethics [ASLME] in 1972).[106] Subsequently, just two years later, in 1985, the number of hospitals with HECs had climbed to 60 percent.[107] In 1988, the Joint Commission on the Accreditation of Health Care Organizations (JCAHO, founded in 1951; now the Joint Commission) introduced a standard requiring the hospitals and healthcare institutions that it accredited to have the equivalent of HECS.[108] Today, virtually all American hospitals and healthcare institutions have HECs or their equivalent.

As Jonsen observes, "ethics committees were set an odd task," for, unlike admissions committees or pathology committees, "they had no well defined task to perform; they were ordered to think about ethics, probably the vaguest and most controversial topics," without a "touchstone beyond, perhaps, the skimpy code of the AMA."[109] Compounding the problem, organized medicine's de-emphasis of medical ethics was reflected in the American medical school curriculum. Thus, in 1972, a survey of 102 American medical schools found that *none* of the 94 schools responding required medical students to take a course in medical ethics. To reiterate, in 1972, no American medical school offered a required course on medical ethics. Fifteen medical schools openly admitted to offering no medical ethics instruction whatsoever; fifty-six responded that they touched on the subject in courses in related areas—social medicine, legal medicine, psychiatry—about one-third (thirty-three) gave students the option of taking an elective course on the medical ethics.[110] Thus, in 1972, no American medical school thought medical ethics important enough to be taught to all future physicians.

A decade later, in 1984—after the advent of bioethics—84 percent of medical schools required students to take a course in medical ethics or bioethics during their first two years of instruction. In 1998, the American Association of Medical Colleges (AAMC, founded in 1876), adopted as a learning goal for all accredited medical schools "knowledge of the theories and principles that govern ethical decisionmaking and of the major ethical dilemmas in medicine, particularly those that arise at the beginning and end of life and those that arise from the rapid expansion of knowledge of genetics."[111] A survey a decade after that, in 2008, reported that "in compliance with the [AAMC learning objectives] all 59 medical schools in the dataset required coursework in bioethics" on average "35.6 hours of instruction in bioethics."[112]

The use of the term "bioethics" rather than "medical ethics" in the 2008 survey is revealing; so, too, is AAMC's reference to "principles" and genetics in its 1998 statement of learning goals. During the era when medical schools no longer required instruction in medical ethics, no market for medical ethics textbooks existed, and so none was published. Thus, when American medical colleges began to require instruction in the subject, instructors found Beauchamp and Childress's *Principles of Biomedical Ethics* available to fill the void, and, thus, bioethical discourse and principles naturally came to occupy the space in the medical school curriculum previously taught under the rubric "medical ethics." In consequence, the founding generation of ethics committee members and successive generations of medical students learned to talk and think in terms of bioethical principles—autonomy, justice, nonmaleficence, and beneficence—rather than in the in terms of the AMA's *Principles* or other traditional discourses of medical ethics.

President's Commission's Guide to Ethical Decision Making in End-of-Life Care

Of more immediate relevance to the practice of ethics committees was the model of nonpaternalistic, shared decision making in end-of-life care articulated in the President's Commission's report, *Deciding to Forego Life-Sustaining Treatment*. The eminent lawyer and former president of Brandeis University, Morris Abram (1918–2000) chaired the commission, and fellow lawyer Alex Morgan Capron served as executive director. Daniel Brock, Allen Buchanan, and Daniel Wikler were among the philosophers on the Commission's staff. The Commission summarized its findings at the beginning of its report. Among them were:

> (1) The voluntary choice of a competent and informed patient should determine whether or not life-sustaining therapy will be undertaken, just as … [in] other decisions about medical treatment.

> (2) Health care professionals serve patients best by maintaining a presumption in favor of life, while recognizing that competent patients are entitled to forego any treatments, including those that sustain life ....
>
> *Incompetent Patients Generally*
>
> (9) To protect the interests of patients who have insufficient capacity to make particular decisions and to ensure their well-being and self-determination
>
> • An appropriate surrogate, ordinarily a family member, should be named to make decisions for such patients ....
>
> • health care institutions should explore ... administrative arrangements for review [of these decisions] such as "ethics committees" ....
>
> • State courts and legislatures should consider making provision for advance directives through which people designate others to make health care decisions on their behalf ... provid[ing] a means of preserving some self-determination for patients who may lose their decisionmaking capacity ...
>
> *Patients with Permanent Loss of Consciousness*
>
> (11) The decisions of patients' families should determine what sort of medical care permanently unconscious patients receive ....
>
> *Cardiopulmonary Resuscitation*
>
> (19) A presumption favoring resuscitation of hospitalized patients in the event of unexpected cardiac arrest is justified.
>
> (20) A competent and informed patient or an incompetent patient's surrogate is entitled to decide with the attending physician that an order not to resuscitate should be written in the chart.[113]

This prescient document offered a roadmap for the ethics of end-of-life decision making: palliative care, model natural death statutes, model legislation for health-care proxies and ethics committees, standards for determining persistent vegetative states and do not resuscitate orders. In no small part because the President's Commission lent its imprimatur and offered guidance on these matters, within two decades, its recommendations became standard practice throughout the United States.

Road building requires ground clearing. As Wittgenstein remarked, "philosophy is a battle against the bewitchment of our intelligence by means of our language."[114] So, the commission's philosophers did battle to clear the obstacles erected by the conceptual frameworks embedded in various distinctions commonly used to discuss end-of-life decision making, including the extraordinary/ordinary distinction:

> (5) Several distinctions are employed by health care professionals and others in deliberating about whether a choice that leads to an earlier death would

> be acceptable or unacceptable in a particular case. Unfortunately, people often treat these distinctions—between acts and omissions that cause death, between withholding and withdrawing care, between an intended death and one that is merely foreseeable, and between ordinary and extraordinary treatment—as though applying them decided the issue, which it does not.[115]

Having rejected the traditional ways of discussing end-of-life care, the Commission proposed an alternative:

> Good decisionmaking about life-sustaining treatments depends upon the same processes of shared decisionmaking that should be a part of shared decisionmaking that should be a part of healthcare in general. The hallmark of an ethically sound process is always that it enables competent and informed patients to reach voluntary decisions about care ... a decision to forego treatment is ethically acceptable when it has been made by suitably qualified decisionmakers who have found the risk of death to be justified in the light of all the circumstances. Neither criminal nor civil law ... forces patients to undergo procedures that will increase their suffering when they wish to avoid this by foregoing life-sustaining treatment.
>
> ... The Commission has also found no particular treatments—including such ordinary hospital interventions as parenteral nutrition or hydration, antibiotics, and transfusions—to be universally warranted and thus obligatory for a patient to accept.[116]

Seven years later, in 1990, the U.S. Supreme Court also ruled that terminal patients have a right to refuse such ordinary hospital interventions as artificial nutrition and hydration.[117]

The Commission's vision of shared end-of-life decision making left little room for such then-common practices as "slow," "show," or "no-coding" patients. In American clinical argot, "code" may be used as a verb indicating a cardiopulmonary arrest, as in, "the patient is coding"; it may also indicate the administration of cardiopulmonary resuscitation (CPR): thus "to call a code" would be to request CPR for a patients who is "coding." Code language became important in the 1970s and 1980s because critical care physicians had to make on-the-spot decisions about CPR without clear legal authority or guidance from the AMA or other professional societies. End-of-life-care discussions with patients or their families were consequently perceived as risky, and, although many ICU physicians openly discussed these issues with patients and families, others would act without any such discussion, simply designating some patients as "no-code." DNR, an acronym for "do not resuscitate," would then be written in a patient's chart. Fearing to write a DNR order, other clinicians "slow-coded" patients; that is, they administered resuscitative interventions so slowly that they were ineffective; others merely pretended to administer life support, so-called "show coding." In one case, an aggrieved family brought a hospital staff to court after discovering that a purple dot on a family member's medical record meant that the medical staff had made the patient no-code—and had done so without consulting either the patient or the patient's family.[118]

These practices arose because neither organized medicine nor the law offered clinicians official guidance on end-of-life decision making. The President's Commission sought to normalize decisions "about life-sustaining treatments" so that they involve "the same processes of shared decisionmaking that should be a part of healthcare in general."[119] The Commission thus disapproved of the charade of slow or show coding, condemning it as a "dishonest effort that needs to be justified by reasons stronger than merely providers' discomfort in discussing DNR decisions."[120] Following its standard practice, in an appendix, the Commission offered examples of the official DNR policies recommended by three state medical societies (Alabama, Minnesota, New York), six hospitals, and five federal agencies. Notably missing, however, was any guidance from the AMA, which, at this point, still offered no leadership on these pressing issues of medical ethics. In 1988, JCAHO recommended policies formalizing DNR decision making in advance of potential cardiopulmonary emergencies, and, in the 1990s, formal DNR policies and end-of-life care treatment discussions with patients and families increasingly became the accepted standard of practice in American hospitals.

THE NEW BIOETHICS AND THE OLD MEDICAL ETHICS CONFRONT AN AIDS EPIDEMIC

As an economic historian wrote in a perceptive analysis of America's response to the AIDS epidemic of the 1980s, "the American medical profession was conceptually ill prepared for an epidemic that threatened practitioners as well as patients … [because] the American Medical Association's Code allowed physicians to choose their patients."[121] Ironically, medical societies had originally organized and developed codes of ethics to support a coordinated response to epidemics. Thus, the yellow fever of epidemic of 1795 transformed a convivial meeting of medical practitioners into the Medical Society of the County of New York, and the Baltimore cholera epidemic of 1832 led to the formation of the Baltimore Medico-Chirurgical Society and to its promulgation of a system of ethics encouraging physicians to tend the sick even "when the pestilence walketh in darkness." Moreover, three physicians who tended the sick during the Philadelphia cholera epidemic of 1832—Bell, Emerson, and Hays—wrote into the AMA's code of ethics the memorable line that "when pestilence prevails, it is [physicians'] duty to face the danger, and to continue their labors for the alleviation of the suffering, even at the jeopardy of their own lives."[122]

In his 1900 presidential address to the AMA, pioneering neurosurgeon William Williams Keen (1837–1932), a Civil War veteran, encouraged his colleagues to

> Be brave men. When pestilence stalks the streets and contagion lurks in every chamber of illness, where have the doctors been found? Fleeing from danger … ? Nay … in the crowded tenements, in the hospitals … cheerfully tending to the sick, facing the disease in the midst of its victims and seeking, even in the bodies of the dead knowledge that will make them masters of the plague. Witness Rush in the yellow fever epidemic of 1797, [Samuel] Gross in the [Philadelphia] cholera epidemic of 1832, [Waldemar Mordecai] Haffkine [inventor of a vaccine against plague] and [Robert] Koch in the bubonic plague of the present time …. [P]estilence has bred its many quiet heroes who have gone about their daily duty, simply, fearlessly, devotedly … [and] the Recording Angel has dropped a tear, blotting out their faults, and writ their names high in the roll of honor.[123]

The 1912 AMA *Principles of Medical Ethics* reiterate a more prosaic expression of the physician's duty to be brave: "When an epidemic prevails, a physician must continue his labors for the alleviation of suffering people, without regard to the risk to his own health or to financial return."[124] Fulfilling this commitment, a past president of the AMA, Johns Hopkins professor William Henry Welch, rushed to points of outbreak in an effort to fight the Spanish Influenza pandemic of 1918–1919[125] (which killed an estimated 50–100 million people worldwide[126]). As late as 1976, annotations to the AMA *Principles of Ethics* state that "when an epidemic prevails, a physician must continue his labors without regard to the risk to his own health."[127]

And yet when the first American AIDS cases were reported in 1981, the AMA no longer required American physicians to tend to the epidemic-stricken! What accounted for the change? The short answer is that the 1980 version of the AMA's *Principles of Medical Ethics* still affirmed a physician's prerogative to choose whom to accept as a patient but no longer stated that physicians were responsible for caring for the epidemic-stricken. This became a practical issue in 1985, when clinical tests to detect HIV infections became available. In 1986, physicians requested a ruling from the AMA's Council on Ethical and Judicial Affairs (CEJA) on whether, in the event of a positive test for HIV/AIDS, they were obligated to breach the confidentiality of HIV/AIDS patients to protect the welfare of spouses or other sexual partners. Responding to this request for "guidelines that should help in responding to questions regarding acquired immunodeficiency syndrome (AIDS),"[128] CEJA opined that

> [P]hysicians have an obligation to assist in notifying individuals who have been exposed to the infection … [and that] a potentially or known infected individual has a duty to refrain from sexual practices or other activities that might result in further dissemination of the disease. Where testing for the HTLV-IIVHIV antibody is indicated, informed consent should be obtained.[129]

CEJA also touched on the issue of a physician's duty to treat HIV/AIDS patients:

> Physicians and other health professionals have a long tradition of tending to patients afflicted with infectious disease with compassion and courage. However, not everyone is emotionally able to care for patients with AIDS. If the health professional is unable to care for a patient with AIDS, that individual should ask to be removed from the case. Alternative arrangements for the care of the patient must be made.[130]

This odd addendum inverts Keen's admonition to "be brave," offering physicians who find themselves "not … emotionally able to care for a patient with AIDS" a right to "ask to be removed from the case [although in that event] alternative arrangements for the care of the patient must be made."[131] "Cowardice" is a noun that Keen might have used to characterize the state of being so emotionally discomforted by danger that one dodges it. Had some firefighters' organization proclaimed that since "not everyone is emotionally able to enter a burning building to save the lives of occupants, such individuals should be excused from entering burning buildings," the public would regard this as outrageous since those not emotionally able to risk their lives to save occupants of burning building were not emotionally equipped to serve as firefighters.[132] From 1847 to 1976, the official position of the AMA was that doctors, like firefighters, had a duty "when pestilence prevails" to risk their health and their lives to provide medical care for those in need. This was the heritage of Bell, Hays, Emerson, Keen, and Welch. The field's willingness to risk its members' lives during epidemics, moreover, was considered central to its status as a profession—something more than a mere money-making occupation.

The laissez-faire conception of ethics introduced in 1903, however, threatened this commitment. Consequently, subsequent statements of AMA's principles of medical ethics issued from 1912 to 1976 preserved the professions' social contractarian obligation to care for the sick as a constraint on the scope of the laissez-faire ideal. Thus, the 1912 version of its *Principles of Medical Ethics* asserts physicians' obligation to conduct themselves according to the ideals of the profession[133] and stipulates as a professional ideal that "when an epidemics prevails a physician must … alleviat[e] suffering of people, without regard to risk to his own health, or life, or financial return."[134] The 1912 *Principles*, however, rescinded the former prohibitions on contract practice[135] but stated that individual physicians had the prerogative of declining contracts they believed improper. This prerogative was formulated as, "A physician is free to choose whom he will serve. He should … always respond to any request for his assistance in an emergency."[136]

The 1957 version of the AMA's *Principles of Medical Ethics* preserved this balance between free choice and professional obligation, but with a significant difference: the statement of a physician's right to choose "whom he may serve" retained its status as a *principle* of AMA ethics;[137] by contrast, the statement of a physician's duty to care for the sick "when an epidemic prevails … without regard to the risk to his own health"[138] was downgraded to a mere *comment* on the principle of physicians "responsibilities … and the community."[139] As a mere comment, it was buried in a section that addressed a miscellany of subjects and was neither indexed nor indicated in the table of contents. Thus, unless one knew of the statement's existence, it was virtually impossible to discover it—the statement of physicians' duties during epidemics was literally buried so deeply in the commentaries that it had become indiscernable. Having been relegated to the back pages of the code, not surprisingly, in 1977, it was deleted when the AMA pruned its *Principles* of material that "did not adequately reflect current conditions of medical practice … [or that] were historical anachronisms."[140]

This deletion was not warranted by then-current conditions of American medical practice since more than 60,000 Americans had died of Asian flu during the pandemic of 1957–1958, and more than 30,000 had died during the Hong Kong flu pandemic of 1968–1969[141]—and a massive vaccination campaign had been undertaken in response to the swine flu scare of 1976.[142] Since pandemics still threatened America in the years immediately prior to the 1977 revisions, the deletion of the statement of physicians' duty to risk one's life to care for the epidemic-stricken was not a function of its irrelevance. It may have been deleted as a "historical anachronism"—which it would naturally have been considered from the perspective of laissez-faire ethics.

Yale law professor Robert Cover (1943–1986) coined the term "jurispathy," which literally means "law killing," to capture the idea that dominant normative systems have a tendency to supplant or kill alternative normative frameworks.[143] Yielding to jurispathic inclinations, in 1975, the U.S. Federal Trade Commission (founded in 1914) filed a complaint against the AMA targeting sections of its code of ethics that restricted members ability to advertise and to enter into contractual relationships (group practice, managed care organizations). After a series of negotiations, the AMA revised its *Principles*, deleting the section forbidding physicians to solicit patients through advertising. Conforming to this settlement, in 1980, the AMA issued a slimmed down seven-principled statement of ethics—and, like its

1977 precursor, it contained no statement on physicians' obligations to care for the epidemic-stricken.[144]

Consequently, when the AIDS epidemic of the 1980s broke out, the AMA's ethical principles asserted that a physician may choose whom he will serve, but it lacked any statement addressing physicians' professional obligation to care for the epidemic-stricken. Read against this background, the 1986 CEJA statement that "[p]hysicians ... have a long tradition of tending to patients afflicted with infectious disease with compassion and courage" looks like an attempt to reassert the recently deleted principle of physicians' duty to care for the epidemic-stricken. Similarly, the statement that physicians who are "not ... emotionally able to care for patients with AIDS ... should ask to be removed from the case" seems to have been intended to limit the prerogative of choosing patients to just those physicians who pleaded "emotional [in]ability." Finally, the statement "[a]lternative arrangements for the care of the patient must be made" reasserts the profession's duty to provide care for the epidemic-stricken, albeit on a collective rather than an individual basis.[145] On this reading, CEJA was not fashioning an escape clause for cowardly physicians; it was attempting the opposite: to limit physicians' options by suggesting that anyone declining to treat people suffering from HIV/AIDS was "not emotionally competent."

Whatever the intent behind the CEJA 1986 statement, it was confusing, and the AMA's House of Delegates requested a clarification. As CEJA's correspondence for this period makes clear, some physicians regarded CEJA's suggestion that physicians who declined to treat AIDS patients were emotionally incompetent as "grossly inappropriate, inflammatory, and uncalled for." Surgeons, in particular, objected to being "forced to accept any patient with any type of illness." Several surgeons reiterated the language of section VI of the 1980 AMA *Principles*, which stipulated that, except in emergencies, they had the "right to pick and choose [their] cases." Other surgeons decried as discriminatory any policy that would prohibit them from continuing to practice surgery if they had contracted HIV/AIDS. As one surgeon angrily wrote, "I do not think that [internists and family practitioners] who are not at physical risk for contracting the AIDS virus have any right, ethical, judicial or otherwise to lecture or dictate to those of us who are." Another wrote, "Your opinions are biased against [HIV infected] surgeons."[146]

This correspondence shaped the 139 lines of tightly argued prose that constitutes CEJA's four-page 1987 report, *Ethical Issues Involved in the Growing AIDS Crisis*.[147] The report opens with an assertion that HIV/AIDS patients have a right "to competent medical service with compassion and respect for human dignity and to the safeguard of their confidences within the constraints of the law." It continues:

> A physician may not ethically refuse to treat a patient whose condition is within the physician's current realm of competence solely because the patient is seropositive.... Neither those who have the disease nor those who have been infected with the virus should be subjected to discrimination based on fear or prejudice, least of all by members of the health care community....
>
> Principle VI of the 1980 Principles of Medical Ethics states that "A physician shall in the provision of appropriate patient care, except in emergencies, be free to choose whom to serve...." The Council has always interpreted this Principle as not supporting illegal or invidious discrimination. Thus, it is the view of the Council that Principle VI does not permit categorical discrimination against a patient based solely on his or her seropositivity. A physician who is not able to provide the services required by persons with AIDS should make an appropriate referral to those physicians or facilities that are equipped to provide such services.[148]

CEJA also unequivocally declared that

> [P]atients are entitled to expect that their physicians will not increase their exposure to the risk of contracting an infectious disease, even minimally .... *[I]f a risk does exist, the physician should not engage in the activity.* The Council recommends that the afflicted physician disclose his or her condition to colleagues who can assist in the individual assessment of whether the physician's medical condition or the proposed activity poses any risk to patients.... There may be an occasion when a patient who is fully informed of the physician's condition and the risks that condition presents may choose to continue his or her care with the seropositive physician. Great care must be exercised to assure that true informed consent is obtained.[149]

These statements seem to categorically constrain physicians: the first statement seems to categorically prohibit refusing to treat people suffering from HIV/AIDS because the practice is "discriminatory"—language resonant with threats of legal action. The second statement seems categorically to forbid physicians with HIV/AIDS from treating patients. Yet, on closer reading, it becomes evident that in each case CEJA allows an alternative. Thus, although physicians are categorically forbidden to discriminate against a "patient based solely on his or her seropositivity," should physicians believe they are *not competent* to provide the needed service, they "should make an appropriate referral to those physicians or facilities that are equipped to provide such services."[150] Similarly, although HIV/AIDS infected physicians are categorically prohibited from putting their patients at risk, nonetheless "a patient who is fully informed of the physician's condition and the risks ... may choose to continue his or her care with the seropositive physician."[151] It would thus appear that, although physicians may not discriminate against HIV/AIDS patients, they may legitimately refer them to AIDS clinics to minimize their own personal risk. As to HIV/AIDS-positive physicians, they are categorically prohibited from putting their patients at risk—except if they inform their patients of the risk and the patients consent to be exposed. Furthermore, "it was also clear that [AMA] officials had no plans to enforce [their 1987 AIDS statement]. The executive vice president James Sammons (1927–2001) commented that any physician with a 'psychological hang-up' about treating AIDS patients would be understood as 'not competent.'"[152] Thus, the AMA's commitment to laissez-faire ethics, reflected in the principle of patient choice, hobbled CEJA, preventing it from acting as the field's conscience during the AIDS epidemic.

This was not some academic debate of little practical significance. CEJA issued its exception and excuse-laden statements that, among other things, legitimated "turfing" patients to AIDS treatment centers at the very moment when the hospitals receiving AIDS patients, like the Mount Sinai Hospital in New York City, were having difficulty recruiting house staff precisely because they treated a disproportionately large population of AIDS patients.[153] At this very juncture, newspapers in New York and San Francisco were screaming in their headlines "What? Physicians Won't Treat Aids," and "AIDS Fears Spawns Ethics Debate as Some Doctors Withhold Care."[154]

By the 1980s, however, the AMA was no longer the sole authoritative voice in American medical ethics. Bioethicists offered an alternative voice of moral authority, as did specialty societies that, no longer ceding their moral authority to the AMA, had begun to issue their own codes of medical ethics. Thus, bioethicist-lawyer George Annas commented acerbically on the AMA's position of treating AIDS patients: "a doctor must treat an AIDS patient if the doctor wants to treat an AIDS patient."[155] Writing in a special issue of the *Hastings Center Report* on doctors' duties to treat AIDS patients, bioethicist-philosopher Benjamin Freedman (1951–1997) observed that, except for the deletion of the controversial term "emotional" from the expression "emotionally competent," the AMA's 1986 and 1987 statements on physicians competence to treat were essentially the same; that is, both were parsed to create an escape clause permitting reluctant physicians to dodge their duty to treat AIDS patients.[156]

As it happened, bioethicists were not the only parties who expressed moral positions that differed from the AMA's. In 1984, an ad hoc committee of the American College of Physicians (ACP, founded in 1915) published a full-scale manual of ethical principles that blended the older language and focus of traditional American medical ethics with the new bioethical discourse. The ACP manual addressed principles of research integrity ("The basic principle underlying all research is honesty"[157]), IRB review, patient autonomy, care for the hopelessly ill, DNR/no code orders, transplantation, and resource allocation; moreover, the writings of leading bioethicists profoundly influenced the ACP code.[158] In 1988, the ACP issued a joint position statement with the Infectious Diseases Society of America (IDSA, founded in 1964) on physicians' duties to treat AIDS patients that was incorporated into the second edition of the ACP's *Ethics Manual* (1989):[159]

> It is unethical for a physician to refuse to see a patient solely because of medical risk, or perceived risk, to the physician.... In recent decades, with better control of such risks, generations of physicians have been trained when risk has not been a prominent concern.... [W]ith the appearance of the acquired immunodeficiency syndrome (AIDS), this has changed, necessitating reaffirmation of the ethical imperative and related concerns. The College's position paper on AIDS ... emphasizes the following principles. Health professionals and institutions are obligated to provide competent and humane care to all patients, the denial of appropriate care to a class of patients is unethical; health professionals must be aware of the risks involved, how to avoid risk, and how to respond if exposed, thus minimizing danger to all.[160]

In striking contrast to the AMA's statements on AIDS, the ACP statement does not provide escape clauses or hint at alternatives to treating people with AIDS; it does not justify the obligation to treat HIV/AIDS by invoking the legal threat of prosecution for discrimination; it simply reiterates that a physician's *ethical* imperative to provide care overrides concerns about risks to the treating physician. The underlying concept here is that doctoring, like firefighting, is an inherently risky job: to accept the prestige, title, and prerogatives of "a physician" is also to accept that one must prioritize the ethical duty to save others over concerns about personal safety. After noting that physicians in recent years may not have appreciated the riskiness of practicing medicine, the ACP statement focuses on the need to minimize the risks attendant on the ethical imperative of delivering healthcare to HIV/AIDS patients. The upshot of the conflict over physicians' duties during epidemics—the tension between the AMA and ACP statements—is that

> [N]o settlement was reached on what risks might need to be borne in a future epidemic.... Writing several years after the debate has peaked ... one of the physicians ... closely involved in AIDS care ... concluded that "it seems unlikely that, given the highly individualistic nature of American medicine, we will arrive at a single standard ... for compelling treatment on the part of reluctant providers."[161]

BIOETHICS AS A RESPONSE TO A VACUUM OF MORAL AUTHORITY

This chapter posed fundamental questions: Why did organized medicine in America, and more specifically the AMA, lose jurisdiction over "medical ethics"—a subject who's very name proclaims it part of medicine's domain? Why was the AMA unable to address effectively the issues raised by morally disruptive biomedical technologies and research ethics scandals? Why had the AMA been able to lead American medicine and to rally American physicians to care for the sick during epidemics far more lethal to physicians than AIDS and yet find itself unable to do so in confronting AIDS and later epidemics? Why did the AMA allow medical colleges to abandon teaching its principles of medical ethics and abdicate from the very mission of teaching medical ethics? Why, moreover, did the AMA leave it to an ad hoc assemblage of Harvard faculty to propose a definition of brain death and resist enacting brain death legislation for more than a decade, finally abandoning the task of defining the concept of death to a bioethics commission? Why, moreover, did the AMA appropriate an irrelevant and unworkable distinction from Catholic moral theology to address issues of foregoing and discontinuing ventilator support and other critical care technologies, leaving it to a bioethics commission to develop authoritative statements on withholding and withdrawing treatment, advance directives, DNR orders, and related issues? Why, in sum, did organized medicine abdicate its moral authority, forcing the government, the courts, and society to valorize an alternative source of moral authority, the bioethicists?

The answer proposed in this chapter is that, in a rebellion against an authoritarian regime wielding power in the name of ethics in the early decades of the twentieth century, the AMA had embraced a laissez-faire conception of ethics according to which physicians should be free to follow the dictates of their personal moral sensibilities. The organization thus abdicated its role as moral conscience of the profession and promulgated nearly content-free principles of medical ethics—except with respect to issues affecting professional status (e.g., advertising) and intrapractitioner relationships. Even as organized medicine substituted personal choice for ethical policy, the Flexner Report's emphasis on science education led medical schools to substitute emulation for ethical education, creating an environment in which medical ethics failed to evolve and ethical expertise withered away in academic medicine. Thus, when organized medicine confronted the challenge of morally disruptive technologies and research ethics scandals during the 1960s and 1970s, it was so profoundly handicapped by its own laissez-faire ideology and lack of ethical expertise (either in the medical societies or in the medical academy) that it could not conceive of effective solutions—which is why it borrowed unworkable concepts from Catholic moral theology. The resulting vacuum of authoritative moral leadership created a need for action in the public sphere, as well as in critical care units, hospitals, and research centers. To meet this need, to fill that space left empty by organized medicine, as standard histories of bioethics recount in great detail, a coalition of bureaucrats, foundations, concerned humanistic physicians, and researchers joined with philosophers, lawyers, ex-theologians, and social scientists to create and valorize an alternative voice of moral authority that came to be known as "bioethics."

NOTES

ABBREVIATIONS

AMA: American Medical Association
CEJA: AMA Council on Ethical and Judicial Affairs
JAMA: *Journal of the American Medical Association*
MSCNY: Medical Society of the State of New York (County)/County of New York
MSSNY: Medical Society of the State of New York
PHD: *Proceedings of the House of Delegates* (AMA)

The American Medical Association has made the *Proceedings of the House of Delegates* from 1883 to 2011 available at the following address. The Website is regularly updated.
http://ama.nmtvault.com/jsp/browse.jsp?useDefault=true&sort_col=date&collection_filter=House+of+Delegates+Proceedings
References to the *Proceedings* are indicated as "AMA *PHD*," followed by year and page numbers, enabling access to the original document through the AMA's Website.

Transactions

The American Medical Association has digitized the complete run of its publication *Transactions* from the official record of its founding convention in New York City in 1846 through 1882, after which *Transactions* was replaced by the *Journal of the American Medical Association*. An 1883 index of the *Transactions* has been digitized. These publications are available at the following address. http://ama.nmtvault.com/jsp/browse.jsp?useDefault=true&sort_col=date&collection_filter=Transactions
The *Transactions* are numbered by the year in which a meeting was held and citations take the form "AMA *Transactions*" followed by year and page numbers. Fuller citations are given for some speeches and reports.

Endnotes.

Chapter 1: Introduction: On Medicine, Ethics, and Morality

1. Tyler 1985, 179.
2. Hooker 1849, p. xi.
3. Flint 1882; Post, Ely, Vanderpoe, et al. 1883.
4. Konold 1962.
5. Although for the most part ignored by scholars until the 1960s, physicians' moral dilemmas have been popular subjects for novels, plays, and film. For example, a 1937 novel focusing on moral dilemmas in medicine, *The Citadel,* by A. J. Cronin (1896–1981), won the National Book Award; a film version was released the following year and various television dramas were based on the book.
6. Fox and Swazey 2009, 23l; Jonsen 1993, S1.
7. Sanders and Dukeminier 1968, 366–380.
8. After 1986, the NAPH changed its name to the American Association of Kidney Patients (AAKP).
9. Pence 2008, 261.
10. Jonsen 1998, 26–27; Reich 1993, S6–S7; Reich 1994, 319–335; Reich 1995, 19–34.
11. Evans 2001; Jonsen 1998; Rothman 1991; Stevens 2000; Walter and Klein 2003.
12. Rothman 1991, Stevens 2000.
13. Kass 1990, 5–6.
14. Scholars do not accept a standard characterization of the expressions "medical ethics" or "medical morality." See Baker and McCullough 2009, 3–15.
15. Young, Sumant, Wachter, et al. 2011.
16. Cicero [44 BCE] 1921, 311.
17. Ibid., emphasis added.
18. Edelstein 1967, 342.
19. Cicero [44 BCE] 1921, 82.
20. Bosk 1981, 54.
21. Kohn, Corrigan, and Donaldson 2000; Leape and Berwick 2005.
22. Bergdolt 2008, 719–720.
23. The system of forgive-and-remember accountability described here, and in more detail by Bosk, is not limited to assessment of the conduct of physicians-in-training. It pervades academic medical centers and associated facilities.
24. The social history of medicine movement was pioneered by the Swiss-American medical historian Henry Sigerist (1891–1957), founding editor of the *Bulletin of the History of Medicine.* Social historians of medicine bring social science perspectives to bear on the history of medicine and broaden it beyond the perspective of elite practitioners. As Roy Porter (1946–2002) liked to say, it is the history of medicine written from below, from the perspective of the patient, the family, and the public, rather than only from the perspective of the practitioner

25. New Jersey Medical Society [1766] 1966, 309. This parsing of a line from the Hippocratic oath is similar to the parsing used in the Edinburgh oath discussed in Chapter 3.

26. Ibid.

27. Advertisement in the *New York Mercury*, June 27 and July 14, 1766, in Rogers and Sayer 1965, 17.

28. New Jersey Medical Society. [1766] 1966, 309.

29. Rogers and Sayer 1965, p. 27.

30. Rogers and Sayer 1965, 29.

31. Ibid.

32. American scholarship contending that medical society codes of ethics are merely propaganda traces back to Chauncey Leake (Leake 1927). Jeffrey Berlant breathed new life into this interpretation (Berlant 1975).

33. Boswell, April 7, 1775, 615.

34. Most American medical students swear a version of the Hippocratic oath shortly after entering medical school in White Coat Ceremonies at which they don their new white laboratory coats. It is also commonly repeated at graduation. On oath swearing prevalence, see Orr, Pang, Pellegrino, and Siegler 1997.

35. World Medical Association 1949.

36. "In consultations on medical cases, the junior physician present should deliver his opinion first, and then the others in the progressive order of their seniority. The same order should be observed in chirurgical cases" (Percival 1803, chapter I, article XIX, 19).

37. Percival 1803, chapter II, article XXVIII, 48–49.

38. These remarks respond to historians' criticisms of my earlier publications. See, for example, Harkness 2002.

39. Chapman 1984, 103.

Chapter 2: Midwives' Oaths of Fidelity and Diligence

1. Common Council of the City of New York 1905, 121–123.

2. Aveling [1872] 1967, 8–10; see also Forbes 1966, 145.

3. Vann Sprecher and Karras 2011, 172

4. Shorter 1991, 41; see also, Petrelli 1971, 276–292; Stock-Morton 1996, 60–95; Wiesner 2004, 70–71.

5. Bonner's was not the first English midwife's oath, but it appears to be the first to serve as a weapon in baptismal-religious conflict, and it was the progenitor of later Anglo-American midwives' oaths.

6. Witchcraft was a concern in the interrogatories of visitation and in later oaths; however, historian David Harley argues that this concern has been overemphasized. See Harley 1990, 1–27.

7. Cardwell 1844 [2000], 167, cited at Evenden 2000, 30; see also Forbes 1966, 148.

8. Bonner [1555] 1815, 165–166.

9. Stock-Morton 1996, 60–69.

10. Petrelli 1971 XXVI (3), 276–292; Stock-Morton 1996, 60–95; Wiesner 2004, 70–71.

11. Pollard 1910, 211.

12. Bonner [1555] 1815, 165.

13. A steady stream of infanticide cases, mostly involving bastard children, appears in English court records from 1558 to 1624. See Hoffer and Hull 1981, 128.

14. The International Federation of Social Workers and the International Association of Schools of Social Work state bluntly that social work ethics is constructed around a series of conflicts including "the fact that social workers function as both helpers and controllers." See International Federation of Social Workers 2012.

15. Expectations of confidentiality may have been common prior to Bonner's oath. Aveling observes that a midwife, Johane Hammulden, became notorious during the reign of Henry VIII (1491–1547, reigned 1509–1547) for breaching confidentiality by "divulging a remark made by a woman she had delivered, relating to the conjugal proceedings of Henry VIII." See Aveling [1872] 1967, 17.

16. Aveling [1872] 1967, 17. The original source appears to be Garnet [1649] 1995, 212–214.

17. There was a lively Puritan debate over whether the female midwives should be allowed to baptize in an emergency. See Neal 1817, 38–39; Bicks 2003, 131.

18. Garnet [1649] 1995, 212–213, emphasis added. In contrast, neither Bonner's oath nor his Articles of Visitation ascribe the virtue of honesty to midwives.

19. Garnet [1649] 1995, 212–213: Evenden remarks, "one puritan mother thought that she was doomed when a male midwife appeared" (Evenden 2000, 80, note 7).

20. In 1646, for example, a surgeon in Puritan Massachusetts was arrested and fined fifty shillings for acting as a midwife. See Gregory 1850, 26.

21. Garnet [1649] 1995, 212.

22. The distinction was officially declared invalid by the Roman Catholic Church when Vatican Council I (1869–1870), called by Pope Pius IX (1792–1878, reigned 1846–1878), officially rejected it and made intentional termination of pregnancy at any stage an excommunicable offense.

23. Calvin, John [1563] 1852, 41–42.

24. Thompson 1986, 10–11.

25. Aveling reads the requirement that midwives attend to every woman in labor as a measure of religious toleration. He traces this provision to an oath sworn by midwife Jane Scarisbrycke, a "Papist [Catholic] midwife," licensed to practice by an Anglican bishop in 1578. Scarisbrycke's oath required her to attend to "any woman laboring of childe, being married and professing the reformed faith, whether the wife of a minister or otherwise." Aveling further supports his interpretation with a statement from the "later writings of Bishop George Hooper (1640–1727, enthroned 1704–1727)" forbidding "any midwife to refuse to come to any woman labouring of child for religion's sake, or because she is wife unto a minister of the church that hath married and doth marry both by God's law and the king's" (Aveling [1872] 1967, 19). Nonetheless, since this provision was an interrogatory in Bonner's Articles of Visitation, it also served as an instrument of religious repression in the campaign to reestablish Roman Catholicism.

26. Packard 1901, 18–23.

27. The earliest known text of a colonial American midwife's oath is the New York oath prefacing this chapter—a secular oath that hews closely to the text of English Puritan oaths. Later North American oath texts can be found in municipal statutes or from the archives of the more centralized Roman Catholic Church (see Biggs 2004, 40). In the absence of a written text of a Puritan midwife's oath, historians Peter Hoffer and N. E. H. Hull identify the Canterbury oath sworn by Eleanor Pead (1567) as a prototype for New England Puritan oaths. See Hoffer and Hull 1981, 156–157. Their claim is plausible since, as historian Doreen Evenden has observed, these oaths change very little over time. Thus, in 1713, midwife Mary Cooke swore virtually the same oath that Pead swore in 1567. See Evenden 2000, 29. It is also probable that the text of any American Puritan oath would parallel the texts of known English oaths since in Francophone colonies, Roman Catholic midwives' oaths are similar to the oaths sworn in France (obligating the midwife, for example "to serve the pregnant women of each parish, to take no needless medical risks, to reveal no family secrets, and to 'sprinkle' [holy water] only when necessary.") See Johnston 1996, 112. Nonetheless, the text of the Pead oath is problematic as a model for a New England Puritan oath both because the New England Puritans were in fact, Puritans, and so would likely have sworn a Puritan oath, and also because standards of midwife conduct enforced in Massachusetts are those characterized in English Puritan oaths. Thus, one of the charges leveled against midwife Ann Hutchinson (1591–1643) at her excommunication trial in 1638 included the secret burial of a stillborn infant. Such secret burials are in clear violation of the seventeenth-century Puritan oath, but are not a violation of the Canterbury oaths sworn by Pead or Cooke. Finally, the only known text of a colonial American midwife's oath, the eighteenth-century New York oath that prefaces this chapter, is modeled on the text of a Puritan oath, not on the text of Peade's Canterbury oath. It seems likely that any seventeenth-century New England Puritan oath would also be based on the text of an English Puritan oath.

A note on the paucity of oath texts: save for the enthusiasm of a nineteenth-century British obstetrician, James Aveling (1828–1892), we might have no English-language oath texts. A reformer who believed that women were better suited to serve as midwives than as obstetricians, Aveling campaigned for the civic licensing of midwives. Believing it "proper to introduce every subject with its history" (Thorton 1967, xvi), Aveling prefaced his book on licensing midwives with a history that included almost all the known examples of English oath texts. His work laid the foundation for later scholarly studies.

28. Hutchinson settled in Pelham Bay, now in the New York City borough of the Bronx. A river, a parkway, and an elementary school, P.S. 78, are named in her honor. The author, an alumnus of P.S. 78, as a school boy was fascinated by the elaborate murals adorning the walls of the school, celebrating Hutchinson's exile, her flight to New York, and her fight for female equality and religious freedom.

29. The Duke of York's laws of 1665 placed the New Jersey and Massachusetts settlements under British law and were extended to the New York settlements after 1675. These laws would have made Anglicanism the official religion of the New York colony had not a special dispensation permitted the Dutch tradition of religious toleration to continue. See Hoffer and Hull 1981, 156–157.

30. Walsh 1907, 11.

31. Evenden 2000, 53.

32. A reproduction of Mary Cook's oath (1713), with her signature at the bottom, is in Evenden 2000, appendix C. The signature indicates that Cook was literate.

33. Evenden 2000, 30.

34. See note 27.

35. Ulrich 1990; Burns 2008, 414–417.

36. Winthrop [1630–1649] 1908, 317–318.

37. Ibid.

38. Hoffer and Hull 1981, 38.

39. James I, c. 27 (1624), cited in Hoffer and Hull 1981, 20.

40. As one legal historian remarked, this presumption of guilt rather than innocence is "a significant departure from common law for it created a legal presumption whereby a woman who had concealed the death of her bastard child was presumed to have murdered it." See Jackson 1994, 67.

41. Chamblit [1733] 1753.

42. *People v. Clarissa Davie* 1818, 45–46.

43. Common Council of the City of New York 1905, 121–123.

44. Ibid.

45. New York City 1731, 27–29.

46. For a discussion of the role of poverty in infant abandonment and infanticide, see Gilje 1983, 580–590.

47. Evenden 2000, 174.

48. Smellie 1754.

49. Shippen, January 31, 1765, 45.

50. MSCNY, October 3, 1808, 94.

51. City of Albany [1773] 1972, 53. Excised from this version of the oath was the provision prohibiting males to be in attendance at childbirth.

52. Bonner [1555] 1815, 165–166.

53. Ibid.

54. Ibid.

55. Aveling [1872] 1967, 8–10. See also Forbes 1966, 145.

56. Common Council of the City of New York 1905, 121–123.

Chapter 3: The Medical Ethics of Gentlemanly Honor and Oaths

1. MSSNY 1868, 90.

2. *Minutes of the Comita Minora of the Medical Society of the State of New York* Founding meeting September 18, 1806. The *comita minora* of the MSCNY conducted ceremonial oath signings for new members; emphasis added.

3. Ryan 1832, 50–51. The full oath is prefaced with the following. "*Ego A___ B___ Doctoratus in arte medica titulo jam donaudus, sancte coram Deo, cordium scrutatore,*

spondeo, me in omni grati animi officiis erga Academiam Edinburgenam ad extremum caste vitae habitum perseveraturum; tum porro..." The letters "A. B." are placeholders for the graduate's name. Emphasis in English language text added.

4. Gaps in the records and indecipherable handwriting make it difficult to discern many signatures in oath books. Moreover, students like Benjamin Rush signed an "affirmation" rather than an oath. Affirmations are identical to oaths except that the preamble reads as follows: "I, A. B. worthy of the title Doctor of Medicine, seriously and solemnly before the Academic Senate, pledge that I will persevere in every duty of a worthy mind towards the University of Edinburgh until the last breath of my life." For Rush's objections to oaths see, Rush 1789. "An Inquiry..."

5. Bard [1765] 1931, 120.

6. Buchan 2003, 1, 40.

7. American medical apprenticeships were formal arrangements. Upon completion, apprentices received written certificates attesting to the areas of instruction covered. For examples and a description of the labors of an apprentice, see Packard 1901, 158–164.

8. For a discussion of Edinburg's influence on colonial American medicine, see Koblenzer 1982, 143–158.

9. Bard [1763] 1822, 54.

10. Rush 1948, 43.

11. Bard [1762] 1931, 122–123.

12. Morgan [1765] 1965, 28–30.

13. Ruschenberger 1887.

14. For further discussion of Edinburgh's influence, see Sloan 1971, 12–13; Koblenzer 1982, 143–158.

15. For a variety of reasons, including the cost of tutelage in Latin, large numbers of Edinburgh medical students did not complete degrees. Samuel Bard complains that he had to hire private tutors and "spend an hour ever day in writing and speaking Latin" (Bard [1764] 1931, 120). For further discussion, see Rosner 1991.

16. Peters 1845, vol. I, 23.

17. Rush 1789, "An Enquiry" 104–108.

18. The authorship of oaths, codes, and other organizational documents is typically obscured by a utilitarian retrograde amnesia enabling institutions to attribute these documents to collective wisdom. Monro *primus* probably drafted the Edinburgh oath either as sole author or as a member of a committee. *Primus* prided himself on devising regulations for institutions and had a Latin/Greek edition of the Hippocratic Corpus—which included the Hippocratic oath—in his family library. Veatch observes that, "In my rather extensive search of medical and philosophical writing of eighteenth-century Scotland, the Monro library is the only place I encountered any mention of the Hippocratic Oath" (Veatch 2005, 26). The presence of a copy of the Hippocratic oath is a strong reason for favoring *Primus* as author or co-author of the oath. *Primus* also authored an unpublished ethics manuscript in which he espoused a belief in representative democratic government and nondenominational rational Christianity of the sort that would embrace the "*Deus*," of the oath in preference to the more personal "Jehovah" or "Jesus." In the oath, as in *Primus*'s other writings,

the older expression, "the sick," is used rather than the newer term "patient." See Monro, Alexander *Primus* 1739, 342–243; [1739] 2004 vol. II, 84–85; Veatch 2005, 26.

19. Monro, *Primus* [1739] 2004 vol. II, 167.

20. Ibid., 139.

21. Dalzel 1862, 90.

22. Universities of Oxford and Cambridge Act of 1859.

23. Bower 1817, vol. I, 282; Dalzel 1862, vol. II, 194–195.

24. Dalzel 1862, vol. II, 200.

25. Monro, Andrew 1691, preface, 2; Dalzel 1862, vol. II, 209.

26. Lawson 1843, 121.

27. Andrew Monro changed the *sponsio* so that students only had to pledge loyalty to "the Christian Religion" rather than to the "Reformed" Presbyterian version of Christianity. When the Presbyterians regained power, they reworded the *sponsio* to "oblig[e] every Principal and Professor to swear allegiance to William and Mary and sign [a Presbyterian] Confession of Faith" (Grant 1884, vol. II, 255).

28. Monro, Andrew 1691, 28.

29. The charges were trumped up. As one historian wrote, "The Presbyterians ... resorted ... to their old accusations against their opponents of Popery and Atheism. Dr. Pitcairne, already mentioned as one of the most celebrated physicians of Scotland, was branded with the latter epithet, because he wrote a satirical poem on the General Assembly, which annoyed and incensed the members in no ordinary manner. It has even been stated in various recent Presbyterian publications that Dr. Pitcairne entertained infidel principles, while it is well known, for the evidence is undeniable, that this distinguished man, like thousands of others in Scotland, was in religion a decided and determined member of the Episcopal Church, and in politics a Jacobite, or adherent of the exiled sovereign" (Lawson 1843, 164).

30. Recent scholarship indicates that Pitcairne was neither an atheist nor an orthodox Episcopalian; he was a Newtonian—a correspondent and follower of Sir Isaac Newton (1642–1727). Newton and Pitcairne held that it was impossible for a scientist to accept the mathematical nature of the universe without accepting a creator who imposed rationality upon it. Purged with Pitcairne was his friend and fellow Newtonian, the mathematician David Gregory (1659–1708), who left Edinburgh in 1692 to become Savilian Professor of Astronomy at Oxford University. David Gregory was great uncle to the physician-ethicist John Gregory. See Guerrini 1987, 70–83; Bower 1817, vol. I, 316.

31. Monro, Alexander 1691, 39.

32. In the words of the Commission of Inquisition, "Doctor Monro being asked ... did judicially in presence of the said Commission, refuse to sign the said Confession of Faith.... Therefore the said Commission ... deprives the said Doctor Alexander Monro of his place, as Primar of the said College of Edinburgh" (Dalzel 1862, vol. II, 229–230).

33. Sibbald signed the loyalty oath.

34. Stewart 2003, 34–35.

35. Howell 1817, 918–940. See also Hill accessed 2009.

36. Ibid., 936.

37. Buchan 2003, 40.

38. Although the Enlightenment has been considered a single movement, more recent scholarly work characterizes it as a European movement questioning received religious, political, and intellectual traditions that took root at different times in various European national cultures, from the seventeenth through the early nineteenth centuries. Enlightenment values include ideals of religious toleration, political rights, intellectual and scientific freedom, and the interrogation of the received religious, political, and intellectual ideas. In some cultures (e.g., Scottish), toleration was embraced in the name of sentiment, in others (French and German), in the name of reason. What informed them all, to cite the quotation from Samuel Johnson that prefaces Roy Porter's book on the English Enlightenment, was "Distrust" and rejection of their past, which as Johnson remarks is "a necessary qualification of a student of history" (Porter 2001, xiii).

39. Haakonssen 1996, 1.

40. Ibid., 2.

41. Sloan 1971, 14.

42. Emerson 2004, 183–218.

43. Wright-St. Clair 1964.

44. The source of this attribution is *Primus's* autobiography. For a more nuanced account, see Emerson 2004, 183–218.

45. Rosner 1991.

46. Veatch 2005, 34.

47. Scholars set different dates for the Edinburgh physician's oath. Cantor dates it from 1705, i.e., before Monro *Primus*, but he seems to conflate the 1730s oath with the earlier liberalized 1705 version of the *sponsio*. All other scholars date the oath to *Primus*'s tenure. Stirling dates the oath from 1735; Nutton dates it at 1731; Veatch dates the oath from 1762, an outlier date. See Cantor 2005, 361; Nutton 1995, 522; Stirling 1904, 400–406; Veatch 2005, 33–35.

48. Cantor 2005, 361.

49. The absence of these words in the Latin original and English translation of it speaks volumes about the oath. The earliest translation of the oath dates to 1803 or earlier and reads as follows: "Whereas the distinction of a degree in Medicine is now to be conferred upon me, I solemnly promise before God, the Searcher of Hearts, that I will to my latest breath abide steadfastly and loyally to the University of Edinburgh. Further that I will practice the art of Medicine with care, with purity of conduct, and with uprightness, and, so far as in me lies, will faithfully attend to everything conducive to the welfare of the sick. Lastly that, whatever things seen or heard in the course of medical practice which ought not to be spoken of, I will not, save for right reason, divulge. This I promise, as I hope for the gracious blessing of Heaven" (Veatch 2005, 33–35).

50. The *Dictionary of National Biography* lists Ryan as a Roman Catholic born in Burrisoleigh, Tipperary, which is a Catholic county. Nonetheless, because the *Dictionary* has the date of Ryan's death wrong, and because Ryan dedicated his doctoral dissertation to an Anglican clergyman, Brody, Meghani, and Greenwald (2009, 17) argue that he was not Catholic. It appears to this commentator that since Ryan is a Catholic family name—a shortened version of O'Ryan—the *Dictionary* has it right: Ryan was Catholic.

51. Ryan 1832, 50–51.

52. The Quaker refusal is justified by Matthew 5:34–37, which in the King James version of the Bible is rendered as "(34) But I say unto you, Swear not at all; neither by heaven; for it is God's throne: (35) Nor by the earth; for it is his footstool: neither by Jerusalem; for it is the city of the great King. (36) Neither shalt thou swear by thy head, because thou canst not make one hair white or black. (37) But let your communication be, Yea, yea; Nay, nay: for whatsoever is more than these cometh of evil."

53. The Quaker version reads: "I, A. B. worthy of the title Doctor of Medicine, seriously and solemnly before the Academic Senate, pledge that I will persevere in every duty of a worthy mind towards the University of Edinburgh until the last breath of my life. Furthermore indeed that I will exercise the Art of Medicine cautiously, purely, and honourably, and, as far as I can, to take care faithfully that all [my actions] are conducive to [effecting] health in sick bodies. And finally that it behooves [me] to keep silent on all matters seen and heard during the course of healing, unless there is a pressing need to reveal these matters" (Cantor 2005, 361).

54. Sixty-eight Quaker physicians formally signed the pledge between 1772 and 1867, and an unknown number before that date. Edinburgh alumnus Dr. Lawson Whalley cites the oath in proudly proclaiming his alma mater's liberal nondenominationalism. See Whalley 1818, [1823] 1825.

55. Cantor 2005, 362.

56. Ibid., 361.

57. Brody, Meghani, Greenwald 2009, 157–158.

58. Ryan, Michael [1831] 2009, 156.

59. Common Council of the City of New York 1905, 121–123, emphasis added.

60. Nutton 1995, 518–524; Veatch 2005, 32–35.

61. Aberdeen first changed its traditional *sponsio* in 1888. See Aberdeen University Court1888; Veatch 2005, 32–33.

62. Glasgow first changed the traditional *sponsio* for medical students in 1868; Rancich, Pérez, Morales et al. 2005, 211–220.

63. Parker 1715, 129.

64. Fissell 1993, 19. Fissell had in mind the works of acknowledged Scottish Enlightenment figures like John Gregory, not the Edinburgh medical oath.

65. Pellegrino 2008, 163.

66. "Nazi doctors ... told me directly that the oath of loyalty to Hitler they took as SS military officers was much more real to them than was a vague ritual performed at medical school graduation.... An oath for Germans especially can be experienced as an absolute commitment to an immortalizing principle, an association of self with a transcendent morality. (Lifton 1986, 207).

67. "Oath of Soviet Physicians" [1971] 2004, vol. 3, 2719; see also, Lichterman 2009, 611.

68. Even today, some physicians occupy roles that do not prioritize obligations to their patients. Physicians working for insurance companies, for example, prioritize the interests of their corporate employers over the interests of those they examine. For further discussion, see Applbaum 1999, 144–157.

69. Fox, Daniel 1988.

70. Dekker [1603] 1925, 36–37.

71. Baker 2006, 93–134; Fox, Daniel 1988, 5–9.

72. Rolls 1984, 1132–1134.

73. Fissell 1993, 28.

74. Cleland 1743, cited at Fissell 1993, 31.

75. Fissell 1993, 32.

76. Ibid., 28.

77. Governors of the General Hospital in Bath 1744, cited at Fissell 1993, 28. Emphais in the original.

78. Sibbald 1706.

79. Referring to Edinburgh and other universities in his graduation address of 1771, John Morgan said that "the 'oath' which is prescribed by Hippocrates to his Disciples has been generally adopted by Universities and Schools of Physic" however, the medical college of Pennsylvania "laying aside the form of oaths … is of a free spirit, wishes only to bind its Sons and Graduates by ties of Honour and Gratitude." Cited in Packard 1901, 210.

80. Stirling observed that the Edinburgh Oath is "very similar to the Hippocratic Oath." See Stirling 1904, 400–403; Veatch 2005, 34.

81. Von Staden 1996, 407 (line 7.i.i); Edelstein 1943, in Temkin and Temkin 1967, 36–42. John Securis 1566, quoted in Larkey 1936, cited in Burns 1977, 223.

82. Monro *Primus* [1739] 2004, vol. 2, 34.

83. Ibid., 71.

84. Erlam 1955, 92.

85. Ibid.

86. Ibid., 97.

87. Ibid.

88. The eighteenth-century English philosopher Jeremy Bentham (1748–1832) introduced the neologism "deontology" into the philosopher's lexicon, intending the term to apply to any moral theory emphasizing duties, including his own utilitarian theory of ethics. English-language philosophers narrowed their use the term when another British philosopher, C. D. Broad (1887–1971), designated ethical theories as deontological if they emphasize concepts of duty so strongly that they preclude utilitarian considerations. On Broad's use of the term "deontological," even though Bentham invented the term to describe his own utilitarian theory of duty, Bentham is not a deontologist. In another twist of linguistic history, "deontology" acquired a different meaning for historians of medicine. The source of this twist is an 1845 monograph, *Déontologie Médicale ou les Devoirs et les Droits des Médecins dans l'État Actuel de la Civilisation,* in which the French physician Maxmilien Isidore Amand Simon (1807, fl. 1845–1865) appropriated Bentham's concept of deontology to characterize the rights and duties of physicians. Following Simon's usage, "deontology" became the French correlate of what in English became known as "medical ethics." Thus, in many countries, the field characterized as "medical ethics" in English texts is characterized as "medical deontology." In this book, I use the term "deontology" in Bentham's original sense: an ethical system is

deontological to the extent that it focuses on duties. Thus, a variant of the Hippocratic oath will be classified as deontological if its primary emphasis is on duties and prohibitions, not motivations and character. See Broad 1930.

89. Bard [1765] 1931, 120.

90. Defoe [1729] 1890, 21. See also Defoe 1725.

91. Johnson [1755] 1818

92. Jewson 1974, 382–383. See also Jewson 1976, and Porter and Porter 1989.

93. One eighteenth-century physician described the dilemma of patronage as follows: "Princes are too apt to look upon the Liberty of doing what no Body else must do, as one of the Richest Jewels in their Crowns, and to run riot accordingly. If any harm comes of the Extravagance, they find a way to tax their Doctors with it; and if none, they ascribe their Escape to their good Stars; all this by Virtue of their Prerogatives. On the other hand, a Physician's oblig'd to exert his Authority, yet with all the Decency and Deference he can, and to rule his Betters, tho' with an Air of Duty rather than Tuition.... Bashfulness is a very proper quality in Courtiers. You'll find yourself mistaken, if you think to Rivet your Interest by such Compliances as wou'd do very well elsewhere" (Parker 1715, 129).

94. Parker 1715, 130.

95. Ibid.

96. Ibid., 37. Parker's interchangeable use of "patient" and "sick man" indicates that his tract was written during a period of linguistic transformation.

97. Medical *Sponsio Academica*, University of Edinburgh 2004:

"I declare that I will practise my profession to the best of my knowledge and ability, in good conscience and with integrity. In my practice the care of my patients will be my first consideration. I will strive to prevent and treat disease, improve quality of life, provide support in times of suffering. I will respect the autonomy, confidences and dignity of all my patients in their living and in their dying. I will promote the health and welfare of the community. I will treat with respect my colleagues and all who contribute to the well-being of my patients. I will constantly seek to gain in knowledge and understanding, and to pass on the art and science of medicine to others, as my teachers have done before me. I will treat all patients equally and without prejudice. I will not breach these obligations, or abuse the trust placed in me, either under threat or for personal gain. I make this declaration solemnly, freely and upon my honour."

98. Cleland 1743, cited in Fissell 1993, 31.

99. Cleland 1743. See also Harley 1990, 138.

100. William Withering studied in Edinburgh from 1762 to 1766 and would have signed the oath upon matriculation.

101. Robert Darwin studied medicine in Edinburgh for two years and would have signed the oath on matriculation, but he received his medical doctorate from Leyden.

102. Harley 1990.

103. Darwin 1789, 4. See also Posner 1975.

104. Darwin 1789, 5.

105. Ibid., 4.

106. Ibid., 3.

107. Ibid., 5.

108. Parks 1989, 23; see also Nye 1993.

109. Parks 1989, 27.

110. Ibid., 36–37.

111. Ibid., 6.

112. Kiernan 1988, 155–156.

113. A flyte between two nineteenth-century American physicians at the New Orleans Charity Hospital, Dr. Samuel Chopin and Dr. John Foster, erupted because, as in the Darwin-Withering flyte, Chopin changed a prescription without properly consulting his colleague, Foster. Their flyte ended in a pistol duel in which Chopin was killed. Two Philadelphia physicians, Doctors Jeffries and Smith, also dueled to their mutual deaths; but with his dying breath Jeffries "bore honorable testimony to [his opponent's] character as a man of science and a gentleman." See Baldick 1965, 120, 128; Kiernan 1988, 309–310.

114. Originally the "University of the City of New York."

115. Pattison 1987, 95.

116. Ibid., 90–127.

117. Baldick 1965, 120.

118. Hosack 1804.

119. Erlam 1955, 97.

120. Struthers 1867, 21–23.c

121. Chambers 1885, vol. III, 501–502.

122. The event of half-hangit Maggie Dickson resurrection is remembered by the distribution of free pints of beer. Maggie lived to have other children, not stillborn.

123. Moore 2005, 33–34.

124. For an outline of *Primus's* course, see Taylor 1986.

125. Guerrini 2006, 3; Lawrence 1988, 195–196.

126. Richardson 2000, 53.

127. Erlam 1955, 97.

128. Ibid., 84.

129. Cristensen 1997.

130. The possibility of resuscitation was recognized in the eighteenth-century medical literature. Cardiopulmonary criteria were not considered definitive of death; only putrefaction was definitive. Greater emphasis was placed on cardiopulmonary criteria in the nineteenth century, as the stethoscope came into common usage.

131. Houlbrooke 1998, 292–293. Although this passage describes English funerals, the same appears true of eighteenth-century Scottish funerals. See Graham 1899, vol. I, 52–53.

132. Graham 1899, vol. I, 52–53.

Chapter 4: The Lecturers: Samuel Bard and Benjamin Rush

1. Bard [1769] 1996, 20–21.

2. Gregory [1772] 1998, 17.

3. [1801] 1811, "On Vices...," 130.

4. Bard's last year at Edinburgh overlapped John Gregory's first year. For a comparison of their lectures see Truman 1997, 29–32.

5. A few English-language texts that could be characterized as "medical ethics" were published prior to 1769. After a Latin edition of the Hippocratic corpus was published in 1525, several medical practitioners translated the oath into English. These often loose translations are of interest because of what they reveal about the preoccupations and mind-set of the translators; however, they were not cited in the later literature and had little impact on the development of "medical ethics." A seminal 1715 essay on the physician–patient relationship by English physician Samuel Parker published during this period was a source for Rush's 1808 lecture "On the Duties of Patients to their Physicians," which, in turn, provided some of text for the AMA code of ethics. With one notable exception, however, a faculty member or an alumnus of the Edinburgh medical college wrote every other known English-language text on "medical ethics" published to this point. The singular exception is Thomas Gisborne (Gisborne 1794), an Evangelical Anglican minister and a member of the social reform Clapham sect. Gisborne's work influenced and was influenced by Percival. It was reprinted in 1847 as part of W. A. Greenhill's influential series on medical ethics and etiquette. The oath texts cited can be found in Larkey 1977, 218–236. Other works referenced in this note are Parker 1715; Rush [1808] 1811, "On the Duties of Patients...," 318–330.

6. Schleiner 1995.

7. Deists believe that a deity created the universe and does not meddle with the natural laws governing it. Newtonian deists (like Pitcairne) share with Isaac Newton the notion that studying the mathematical laws of nature brings one closer to the "mind" of the deity. Proponents of both forms of deism hold that church-based religions corrupt and distort humanity's relationship to the deity; they also hold that any suspension of natural law, including the miracles mentioned in holy texts, must be explicable in terms of natural law or dismissed as superstition.

8. Bard, John 1941, 26

9. Bard 1765, "*Tentamen...*"

10. Bard was indicted as a British spy but was never tried. McVickar [1822] 1931; Thomas 1931, 127.

11. Thomas 1931, 127.

12. Bard [1769] 1996, 24.

13. Ibid., 27.

14. Ibid., 27–28.

15. Duchamp 1821, 620.

16. Bard [1769] 1996, 14–15.

17. Ibid., 16. This translation of the Sixth Commandment is from The King James Translation of the Holy Bible (1611). Interestingly, Bard's Edinburgh classmate, Thomas Percival, also dwells on physician's duties to learn from their errors; see Percival 1803, chapter 2, section XXVIII.

18. Bard [1769] 1996, 19.

19. Von Staden 1996, 406–408.

20. New Jersey Medical Society [1766] 1966, 309.

21. Gregory [1767–1768] 1998, 70, 77, 82.

22. Ibid., 115–116.

23. Other Edinburgh alumni shared Bard's view that secret nostrums violate the duty of beneficence toward the sick. Bard's classmate Thomas Percival argued against "dispens[ing] a secret *nostrum*.... For if it be of real efficacy, the concealment of it is inconsistent with beneficence and professional liberality" (Percival 1794, section 2, article 19). Nicholas Romayne offered a similar argument; Romayne, 1809, 32–33; see also Walsh 1907, 101.

24. Bard [1769] 1996, 20.

25. Monro *Primus* [1739] 2004, 34.

26. Bard [1769] 1996, 20–21.

27. McVickar [1822] 1931, 158–159.

28. Percival 1794, section 1, article 1.

29. Ibid. Note that Percival, a hospital practitioner, adopts the argot of the wards, referring to patients as "cases."

30. Cantor 2005, 361.

31. The authors envision the good physician as a "Friend [or] Father ... and were it not for the Light of Religion, [the sick person] could scarce refrain from adoring him as a Deity. [The good physician] appears, in short, in the most amiable and endearing Light. 'Tis his Office to relieve the Sick, assuage our Pain, and distribute Health, Felicity, and Joy: He even combats for us the greatest of all Evils, and, for a While, retards the mortal Attacks of the *King of Terrors*. This is his proper Duty; but he may at the same Time ... support our Patience, banish our Fears, or improve them to our best Interests, by raising our Hopes ... and ... if ... Death must come, he can soften us into a Compliance with, and Resignation to, the Will of our Common Creator" (Anonymous 1753, 47).

32. Bard [1769] 1996, 21–22.

33. McVickar [1822] 1931, 153.

34. Rush [1801] 1811, "On Vices" 123–124.

35. Percival 1794, section 2, article 3; comparable section in Percival 1803, chapter 2, section III. Gregory shares this view; see Gregory [1770] 1998, 107–108.

36. Bard [1769] 1996, 24.

37. Ibid.

38. Rush [1789] 1815, 260.

39. Hunter 1784, 72.

40. Percival 1794, section 1, article 3; see also Percival 1803, chapter 1, article III.

41. McVickar 1822 [1931], 150–151.

42. In a series of tracts beginning with *An Address to the Inhabitants of the British Settlements in America upon Slave Keeping* (Rush [1773] 1997, 247–254), Rush became the first prominent American to argue publicly, not merely for the abolition of the slave trade, but also for the emancipation of slaves. He was also the first American scientist to argue against scientific racism, publicly proclaiming black Africans the mental, physical, and moral equals of white Europeans. In 1787, Rush and Benjamin Franklin drafted the constitution of America's first abolitionist society, the Pennsylvania Society for Promoting

the Abolition of Slavery and for the Relief of Free Negroes Unlawfully Held in Bondage. Practicing what he preached, Rush freed his own slave, William Grubber, whom he had purchased in 1775 in preparation for establishing a household with his future wife, Julia Stockton (1759–1848) in the following year. See Franklin 1813; 1818.

43. One notable exception was an early lecture (Rush 1786) credited with laying the groundwork for American psychiatry.

44. Rush [1789] 1815, "Observations on the Duties…," 251–264.

45. Ibid. Compare with Gregory [1770] 1998, 112–114 and Gregory [1767–1768] 1998, 182–183.

46. Rush [1789] 1947, precept XI, 314. Compare Gregory [1770] 1998, 106. See also Percival 1794, section 2, article 2; Percival 1803, chapter 2, article II.

47. Rush [1789] 1947, precept XIII, 315. Compare Gregory [1770] 1998, 108.

48. Rush invokes learned authority on this point. "The poor should be the objects of your peculiar care [because as] Dr. Boerhaave used to say, 'they were his best patients, because God was their paymaster" (Rush [1789] 1947, precept XV, 316).

49. Rush [1789] 1947, precept IX, 313. For an excellent analysis of Rush on the mind and its role in the physician–patient relationship, see Haakonssen 1997.

50. Rush [1789] 1947, precept IX, 313.

51. The "Great Awakening" of the 1730s and 1740s swept through the Calvinist religions of British North America (Congregationalism, Presbyterianism), introducing an emotional connection to God into highly cerebral Calvinist services. Rush's first mentor, his pastor, the Reverend Gilbert Tennent (1703–1764), was a leader of the Great Awakening movement and a key figure in fomenting a schism in American Presbyterianism between "New Siders," who favored emotional "Awakened" services, and the "Old Siders," who were reluctant to embrace them.

52. Rush 1811, "On the Vices…," 121–122, 128–129.

53. Ibid.

54. The Golden Rule is translated as follows in the popular King James Version of the New Testament (1611), "As ye would that men should do to you, do ye also to them likewise" (Luke 6:31); alternatively, "whatsoever ye would that men should do to you, do ye even so to them" (Matthew 7:12). In the Challoner translation of the Catholic Bible (1752), another likely source for Ryan, Luke 6:31 is translated as, "And as you would that men should do to you, do you also to them in like manner."

55. Ryan then quotes "*sic enim medicina orta; subinde aliorum salute, aliorum interritu perniciosa discernans a salutaribus.*" Roughly translated this means: "So the art of medicine fearlessly attempts to discover medicines, sometimes bringing forth health, and other times doing harm."

56. Ryan [1831] 2009, 156–157.

57. Ryan 1831, "Letter from Dr. Ryan," 222–224. Ryan, who lectured on medical jurisprudence, may have had in mind such laws as the Duke of York's law of 1665, which states: "That no person or persons employed about the bodies of men, women, or children, for the preservation of life or health as chirugeons, midwives, physicians, or others, presume to set forth *or exercise any act contrary to the known approved rule of art …*

without the advice and consent of such as are skillful in the same art (if such may be had) ... *and consent of the patient or patients if they be mentis compotes, much less contrary to such consent*, upon such severe punishment as the nature of the fact may deserve; which law, nevertheless, is ... to inhibit and restrain the presumptuous arrogance of such as, through confidence of their own skill, or any other sinister respects, dare boldly attempt to exercise any violence upon or towards the body of young or old, one or other, to the prejudice or hazard of the life or limb of man, woman, or child" (Walsh 1919, 24–25, emphasis added).

58. For an assessment of human subjects experiments at the Edinburgh Royal Infirmary and other eighteenth-century medical centers, see Maehle 1999.

59. Gregory [1771] 1998, C36, 9, 249. Gregory is citing the Golden Rule, see note 54.

60. Gregory [1766] 1998, lecture 1, 13, 248.

61. Gregory [1771] 1998, C36, 10, 249.

62. McVickar [1822] 1931, 73.

63. Ibid., 153. Emphasis on "cautious" added.

64. In his most influential medical publication, *A Compendium of the Theory and Practice of Midwifery*—the first obstetrics text written by an American physician—Bard translates the duty of caution into the rule that "a practitioner of midwifery ... *is never to interfere with the natural course of labour*, unless where some untoward circumstance or obstacle ... put nature out of her course" (Bard [1807] 1819, 176, emphasis in the original).

65. Cullen 1772, noted by Dr. Stuart, 791.

66. Ibid., 788–789. Emphasis on the first use of "cautious" added.

67. Cullen (circa 1772). Notes by Dr. Rhodes, 6th lecture, section 2, 10a-247.

68. See Percival 1803, chapter 1, article XII. Note the Cullenesque requirement for "well authenticated facts."

69. Rush [1789] 1947, precept XIV, 315–316.

70. For further discussion of Rush's reputation, see Haakonssen 1997, 216–226; Holmes 1966, 246–260; Kopperman 2004, 539–574; Powell 1970; Shryock 1971, 507–552, especially, 516–519.

71. Sullivan 1994, 211–234.

72. Rush 1948, 87.

73. Ibid., 3–9. As was customary in the eighteenth and nineteenth centuries, Rush, like *Primus*, wrote an autobiography intended solely for his descendants. Because of Rush's fame, many publishers sought to publish the autobiography but Rush's descendants declined, fearing that publication might undermine Rush's reputation. The American Philosophical Society ultimately acquired rights to the autobiography, which was first published in 1948.

74. Rush 1948, 87.

75. Rush [1796] 1979, 3.

76. Rush 1948, 88.

77. Ibid., 89.

78. Ibid., 88.

79. Cullen 1770. The current International Classification of Diseases (ICD) system descends not from Cullen's work, but from a statistical classification system designed by

Jacques Bertillon (1851–1922) that was adopted by the International Statistical Institute in 1899. The WHO undertook supervision of the ICD in 1946.

80. Rush [1801] 1811, "Upon the Causes…," 150–154.

81. Rush 1948, 89.

82. John Mitchell (1711–1768), a distinguished Virginia physician and Edinburgh alumnus, wrote the manuscript.

83. Rush 1794, *An Account…*, 199.

84. Ibid.

85. Ibid.

86. Kuhn [1793] 1794, 207–208.

87. Ibid.

88. The reference is to a story in the Hebrew Bible about three Israelites thrown into a fiery furnace on the orders of a Babylonian king as punishment for their refusal to worship a pagan god. Miraculously, however, their faith in the true god enabled them to survive unharmed. See Burdick, Stek, and Youngblood 1995, 1291–1295.

89. Rush [1793] 1951, "Letter to Julia Rush," 657–658.

90. Rush 1794. *An Account…*, 211.

91. Rush [1793] 1794, 211–212. Rush had a curious habit of projecting his own faults onto others. It was actually Rush who ignored climatological factors because the disease described as "yellow fever" in the manuscript that inspired his "cure" occurred in the *winter*, and thus could not have been the (mosquito-borne) *summer* disease plaguing Philadelphia. Nonetheless, as one historian put it, with all the zeal of "a religious bigot [Rush] pursue[d] his bleedings and purging" and tried to convert other physicians to his beliefs. See Jones 1962, 43–48 and King 1958, 149–150.

92. Rush [1793] 1951, "To Mrs. Rush," 659.

93. Rush [1793] 1951, "To His Fellow Citizens," 660–661.

94. Ibid.

95. Ibid, 660, note 1.

96. Rush [1793] 1951, "To the College of Physicians," 661–662.

97. Rush 1794, *An Account…*, 203.

98. Rush [1807] 1811, 245.

99. Rush [1793] 1951, "To John R. B. Rodgers," 697.

100. Rush [1801] 1811, "Upon the Causes…," 157–158.

101. Cullen 1827, 476–477.

102. Ruschenberger [1813] 1887, 91.

103. Ibid., 94.

104. Cobbett 1801, *The Rush-Light*, No. I, 49.

105. Among these was Dr. William Currie (1754–1828), a dissenting member of the Episcopal Church (i.e., one who refused to sign the thirty-nine articles of faith) who had rebelled against his Tory father to serve as a military surgeon in the American Army during the revolution. Currie's patriotic credentials enabled him to publicly criticize Rush, who played the patriotism card to silence Tory physicians. See Currie [1793] 1794.

106. Cobbett 1801, "The American Rush-Light No. II," 264–270. Emphasis in the original document.

107. Shryock 1971, 541. Untreated yellow fever may have a mortality rate of between 15 and 95 percent; Vainio and Cutts 1998, appendix I, 62–65.

108. Cobbett 1801, "The American Rush-Light No. II," 310.

109. Ibid. Emphasis in the original passage.

110. Ibid., 311–312

111. Moreover, when Rush himself came down with yellow fever he did not follow the Golden Rule by submitting himself to the same massive bleeding and purging regimen that he used on his patients. See Rush 1794, *An Account…*, 343–345.

112. Rush recommended to his students that they collect any unpaid bills at the end of the year and collect from the estates of the deceased—practices that presume that students would keep a register with patients' names and addresses, like their master. See Rush [1808] 1811, 336–337.

113. Rush 1794, *An Account…*, 345–346.

114. The Royal Society of London for Improving Natural Knowledge (founded in 1661, now known simply as The Royal Society) debated inoculation starting in 1699, and papers on the subject were published in *Philosophical Transactions of the Royal Society* in 1714 and 1716.

115. Gregory [1771] 1998, C36, 10, 249.

116. Montagu, Lady Mary [1718] 1763, 61–63.

117. Maitland 1722.

118. The prisoners were released as compensation for serving as test subjects. Glynn and Glynn 2004, 54.

119. The inoculation of the Royal family came too late to prevent a major controversy over inoculation during a major outbreak of smallpox in Boston in 1721.

120. Rush 1781.

121. Maitland 1722, 21.

122. Northerners tended to treat house slaves as lesser members of their extended family, and so it was natural for Boylston to inoculate the son of his house slave alongside his own son.

123. Marvin 1892, 480.

124. Barquet and Domingo 1997, 635–642.

125. The original texts are available online, courtesy of the Harvard University Library; see Boylston 1730; Douglass, Alexander, and James Franklin 1722; and Mather et al. 1721. See also Colman 1721; and Mather, Dummer, and Tumain 1722.

126. This title is not to be confused with "Treasurer of the United States"; it is instead the title of the director of an office in charge of minting U.S. currency. The office was established in the U.S. capital, which was then in Rush's hometown, Philadelphia, and during this period reported to the Department of State. In 1835, it was transferred to the Department of the Treasury. For an excellent account of this incident, see Butterfield 1951, "Appendix II…," 1209–1212.

127. Rush [1808] 1951, 975. Emphasis in the original.

128. Rush [1807] 1811, 232–236.

129. Rush 1794, *An Account….*

130. Rush [1803] 1811, 212–213.

131. Ibid., 226–227.

132. Rush [1801] 1811, "Upon the Causes...," 141.

133. Butterfield 1951, vol. I, lxi.

134. Rush [1801] 1811, 120–140; Rush [1808] 1811, 318–330.

135. Rush [1801] 1811, 121–122.

136. Ibid., 319.

137. Rush, [1808] 1811, 324.

138. Rush's dictatorial paternalism contrasts with the views of his teacher, see Gregory [1770] 1998, 107.

139. Rush [1808] 1811, 320.

140. Ibid.

141. Ibid.

142. Ibid.

143. Ibid., 330.

144. Ibid., 336.

145. Ibid., 322.

146. Ibid., 322

147. Rush [1801] 1811, 125–126.

148. Ibid.

149. Ibid., 124.

150. Bard [1807] 1819.

151. Ibid., iii.

152. Ibid., vi, emphasis added.

153. At one point, more than half the members of the South Carolina medical society were his students: figures from Goodman 1934, 132–133; cited in Brodsky 2004, 277–278.

154. Brodsky 2004, 278

155. Rush 1809, 31.

156. AMA, *PHD* 1895, 648, 757.

157. New York Times 1902.

158. Wilson 1904, 10.

159. Ibid., 11.

160. Butterfield 1951, Letters. vol. II, 1197–1208.

161. Quoted by former President John Adams in a letter to Benjamin Rush. Cited in Butterfield 1951, Letters. vol. II, 1207.

162. Wilson 1904, 18–19.

163. Hartley 1953.

Chapter 5: Oaths and Codes of Medical Police and Ethics, 1806–1846

1. Percival 1985 [1803], article XXI, XXII, 44–45.

2. MSSNY 1823, 8–9.

3. A medical society's bylaws, proceedings, oaths, and codes of medical police/ethics were recorded in a transaction book, a large volume, often bound in leather, into which a professional scribe officially transcribed entries from rough notes. Separate pages were set

aside for members' pledge signatures. Larger societies sometimes printed their transactions, often combining several years' transactions into a single publication. Some societies had their codes of police/ethics printed as a small pamphlet to which fee scales or bylaws might also be appended. When there was a print run, extra copies of codes like would be printed for distribution to "such other Physicians of the State as [members] may think proper."

4. For example, the Boston Medical Association's bylaws state that VI, *No member* of this Association shall consult with, or voluntarily meet in a professional way, or aid or abet any practitioners in this city, who is not a member of this Association.VII. *If any member* becomes acquainted with the conduct *of another member*, which he considers as a breach of the rules and regulations of the Association, it shall be his duty to make the same known to the Standing Committee, who shall inquire into the case, and decide upon the same as they may think proper.

5. AMA *Transactions* 1874, 29.

6. Ibid., 30.

7. MSCNY December 5, 1832.

8. Only fellow medical practitioners—other physicians and surgeons—had standing to bring charges before the censors or *comita minora* of a medical society. Thus, a complaint by a midwife, Louisa Kastner, had to be presented to the censors by Valentine Seaman, a member of the society who (as noted in Chapter 2) ran a training program for midwives. See MSCNY 1808, vol. 1, 94.

9. A code of medical ethics appears to have been published by the Manchester Medical Society (UK) after its founding in 1834. This is the only known case of a non-American medical society issuing a code of medical ethics prior to the 1880s.

10. Morrice 2002, 15.

11. Styrap 1878, 1886, 1899, 1895; Styrap [1878] 1995, 149–171; Bartrip 1995, 145–148.

12. Nye 2009, 418–426.

13. Maehle and Tröhler 2009, 432–438; Maehle 2009.

14. Haber 1991.

15. Brodie 1843, 30.

16. Smith, R. G. 1995, 206. See also Smith, R. G. 1994.

17. Smith, R. G. 1995, 207.

18. Ibid., 210; emphasis added. For an account of the GMC process by a Scottish physician, see Cronin [1937] 1965, 350–368.

19. In 1902, as part of a general reorganization, the BMA established a Central Ethics Committee (CEC) to address "medico-ethical" and "medico-political" problems. Yet, even though the head of the CEC, Robert Saundby (1849–1918), published codes of ethics, neither the CEC, nor the BMA—nor, to reiterate, the GMC—would officially accept any formal code of professional conduct until the 1980s. See Morrice 2002, 11–36; Saundby 1902; Saundby 1907.

20. James J. Walsh dates the meetings of the society from 1749 on the basis of a note by John Bard (Walsh 1919, 50–59). This date conflicts with the view that the earliest American medical societies were modeled on the gatherings of British military surgeons quartered in the American colonies during the French and Indian War, which first started five years

later in 1754, ending in 1763. Multiple sources, however, refer to a New York medical society associated with the Bard family that had a medical library and that they played a role in founding King's College Medical School. The number and variety of these references support Walsh's claim that such a society was functioning in New York City from the mid-eighteenth century. See Annan 1948, 117–123; Bard [1769] 1996; McDaniel 1958, 134; McVickar [1822] 1931, 135; Walsh 1907, 34, 59.

21. In 1794, however, Charlton became the first president of the Medical Society of the State of New York County, i.e., Manhattan (MSCNY). He advocated raising educational requirements for physicians and developing public health measures to control yellow fever (Minute Book Medical Society of the State of New York [County]).

22. MSCNY 1806, *Minute Book,* November 14, 1794—Samuel Bard was one of the censors.

23. MSCNY 1806, *Minute Book,* February 9, 1796; Walsh 1906, 219–220.

24. MSCNY 1806, *Minute Book,* February 14, 1797.

25. New York State, then and now, has an upstate-downstate divide. *Downstate* refers to the counties in and around New York City; *upstate* refers to the rest of the state. Until 1797, the state legislature met in various locations, primarily Albany, Kingston, and New York City. In 1797, upstate counties persuaded the legislature to make Albany its permanent home and the state capital. Propinquity aided by a newfound sense of clout enabled the upstate medical societies to lobby the legislature effectively—forcing downstate medical societies to play catch-up.

26. MSCNY 1806, *Minute Book*, February 14, 1797; Walsh 1907, 37–46; Walsh 1919, 66.

27. At its June 28, 1806 meeting, the New York City society reconstituted itself as MSCNY, but still found many other aspects of new state law "highly objectionable" (MSCNY 1806, *Minute Book*; Walsh 1919, 78).

28. Rogers 1960, 258–263; Stookey 1967, 579–581.

29. Walsh 1907, 116.

30. MSSNY 1806. *Minutes of the Comita Minora of the Medical Society of the State of New York.*

31. MSSNY 1868, 11; emphasis added.

32. MSSNY 1868, 13.

33. Vonnegut 1976, chapter 48.

34. A Boston "Confederacy of Physicians" was founded on May 14, 1780, at the Green Dragon Tavern in Boston, "[f]or our mutual Advantage and Improvement in the Art of Physick. Also for the Satisfaction of the Sick that shall fall under our Care." The confederates were committed to freely sharing their knowledge and advice with each other and to supporting the dignity of physic, by "[k]eep[ing] Peace and Harmony … with [each] other," so that "[a]ny difficulty or misunderstanding arising between any two members of the Confederacy, and they not being able to Settle the Matter, it shall Finally be Submitted to the Decision of the Other members" (Countway Library of Medicine 1780). This organization may have morphed into the Massachusetts Medical Society incorporated by *An Act to Incorporate certain Physicians, by the Name of The Massachusetts Medical Society* (1781). The act gave the "Fellows of said Society full Power and Authority to make and enact such Rules and Bye-laws, as are not repugnant to the Laws of this Commonwealth; and to annex

reasonable fines and penalties to the Breach of them … in any Court Record within this Commonwealth." The society was also given licensing authority: "whereas it is clearly of Importance, that a just Discrimination should be made between such as are duly educated and properly qualified for the Duties of their profession, and those who may ignorantly and wickedly administer Medicine, whereby the Health and Lives of many valuable Individuals may be endangered, or perhaps lost to the Community. Be it therefore enacted by the Authority aforesaid, That the President and Fellows of said Society … shall have full Power and Authority to examine all Candidates for the Practice of Physic and Surgery." Harvard University graduates became exempt from the requirement of passing an examination by the society's censors in 1806. For details, see Burrage 1923.

35. The Association may instead be a descendant of a Boston society established perhaps as early as May 1780 or as late as 1803, when Boston physicians associated with the Harvard Medical College, John Collins Warren (1778–1856), James Jackson (1777–1867), and John Fleet, founded the Medical Improvement Society (not to be confused with the Boston Medical Improvement Society founded in 1828), whose purpose was to provide a common medical library for the physicians of the city of Boston. This association may have morphed into the Association of Boston Physicians by 1806, which published the first American medical police in 1808. It is unclear whether the John Warren who was on the committee that drafted the medical police was John Warren (1753–1813), founder of Harvard Medical College, or his son, John Collins Warren (1778–1856).

36. Rosen 1974, 154.

37. The modern sense of the noun "police," as "[t]he organized body of civil officers in a city, town, or district, whose particular duties are the preservation of good order, the prevention and detection of crime, and the enforcement of the laws," was first introduced in the 1913 edition of Webster's *American Dictionary of the English Language* ("Police" 1913).

38. Johnson [1755] 1818.

39. "Police" 1913.

40. Members of the standing committee might also have been exposed to the expression "medical police" through the writings of Professor Andrew Duncan (1744–1828) of Edinburgh University, who founded a journal, *Medical and Philosophical Commentaries* (known as the *Edinburgh Medical and Surgical Journal* after 1805). Duncan was inspired by a book written by the German physician-hygienist Johann Peter Frank (1745–1821), *A Comprehensive System of Medical Police* (1779), and he began to explore various meanings of the concept of "medical police" as part of his 1795 lectures on medical jurisprudence, in various writings, and in his journal (Frank 1779–1827). Another influence many have been Fodéré's *Treatise on Forensic Medicine, Public Hygiene, and Medical Police* (Francois Emmanuel Fodéré (1764–1835). For more background on the various meanings of "medical police," see Carroll, Patrick 2002, 461–494; Rosen 1953, 21–42; Rosen 1974, 120–141; see as well Rosen 1974, 142–158.

41. Boston Medical Association 1808, 41–46.

42. Ibid., 41; emphasis added.

43. Ibid., 11.

44. Boston Medical Association 1885.

45. Boston Medical Association 1808, 7; this volume, Appendix I.

46. Percival, Thomas [1803] 1985.

47. Percival prefaces *Medical Ethics* with the following Latin quotation from Cicero's *De Officiis*, "On Duties" (book I, section ii.): "For no phase of life, whether public or private, whether in business or at home, whether one is working on what concerns oneself alone or dealing with another, can be without its moral duty; on the discharge of such duties depends all that is morally right, and on their neglect all that is morally wrong" (Percival [1803] 1985, vi. Translation from Cicero [44 BCE] 1921, 7).

48. Percival [1803] 1985, title page.

49. Percival [1803] 1985, article XXIII, 45–46. See also Boston Medical Association 1808, 8. Note: "Laudable" is defined in Webster's *American Dictionary of the English Language*, 1828, as: "Praiseworthy; commendable; as laudable motives; laudable actions" ("Laudable" 1828).

50. Some philosophical treatments of punishment hold that the verb "punish" is only properly used when a pain or harm is meted out to a malefactor by those *legally* authorized to do so. Webster's Dictionaries of 1828 also characterized "to punish" as "to chastise; as, a father punishes his child for disobedience." The 1913 definition similarly does not presume legal authority as requisite for punishment: viz.: "To impose a penalty upon; to afflict with pain, loss, or suffering for a crime or fault, either with or without a view to the offender's amendment; to cause to suffer in retribution; to chasten; as ... a father *punishes* his child for willful disobedience." There is no presumption of legal authority in the nineteenth-century use of the verb "punish." For recent philosophical discussion of these issues, see Zaibert 2006, 24–29.

51. MSSNY 1823, 8–9.

52. Ibid.

53. Medico-Chirurgical Society of Baltimore 1832, section III, article X, 15.

54. The Connecticut Medical Society was founded as the New Haven medical society in 1784 and was chartered as a state society in 1792.

55. The paragraphs dealing with exemptions and vicarious offices were deleted; see Connecticut Medical Society 1817, 1824, 1832.

56. In the 1830s, the Medical Association of the District of Columbia issued codes that, although substantively identical to traditional codes of medical police, had "System of Ethics" in their title. See Medical Association of Washington 1833, 1837.

57. The original Boston Medical Police had two additional sections: Exemption from Charges (three paragraphs); Vicarious Offices (one paragraph).

58. Fees were usually listed in a table delineating the range of standard fees for a visit or for a specific procedure. For example, the charge for a first visit to a patient at the patient's home would often be set at between $1.00 and $2.00, with subsequent visits at $1.00, except if the visit was out of town. Additional charges were added for specific procedures: thus, extracting a tooth might cost $.50; vaccinations between $2.00 and $5.00; and cases of midwifery between $25 and $50. There was typically a note reminding physicians that the poor should either be treated gratuitously or billed at less than full price. The rich, who would naturally demand and receive more attention, should be billed at higher fees. Moreover, if a code of medical police was printed as a separate document, a fee scale was typically appended.

59. Boston Medical Association 1808, 4.

60. Ibid. Compare with Percival 1803, chapter II, articles VI and VII.

61. Unlike Britain, where sharp class distinctions were drawn between apothecaries, physicians, and surgeons, who were represented by different organizations, in colonial and postcolonial America, physicians and surgeons tended to have equal status and were members of the same medical societies.

62. Boston Medical Association 1808, 6–7.

63. Ibid., 4. Compare with Percival 1803, chapter II, articles VI and VII.

64. Benjamin Rush, who had little use for compromise, offers the following disdainful description of such orchestrated consultations:

"A Mahometan [sic] and a Jew might as well attempt to worship the Supreme Being in the same temple, and through the medium of the same ceremonies, as two physicians of opposite principles and practice, attempt to confer about the life of the same patient. What is done in consequence of such negotiations … is the ineffectual result of neutralized opinions; and whenever they take place, would be considered as the effect of a criminal compact between physicians, to assess the property of their patients [i.e., to extort extra fees from patients], by a shameful prostitution of the dictates of their consciences" (Rush 1794, 359).

65. Hamilton [1804] 1965, 120.

66. Appiah 2010, 16. Emphasis in the original.

67. Lazare 2005, 35.

68. MSCNY 1832.

69. "I am sorry" is often taken as equivalent to "I apologize." It is not. "I apologize" is a performative utterance—to write or speak the words is to perform the act—whereas "I am sorry" is merely a statement about one's emotional state. One might infer contrition from a statement about sorrow, but it is neither an explicit admission of wrongdoing nor an implicit commitment not to repeat the wrongful act. Thus, I am often sorry that I must fail a student who, despite earnest effort, did not earn a passing grade but I will unapologetically flunk her or him. "I am sorry," might pass as an apology in current American usage, but it falls short.

70. Fines were levied for late payments of dues and other violations of the bylaws but seem not to have been regarded as appropriate in resolving issues of gentlemanly honor—including stealing patients. When a breach was framed as an issue of honor, financial compensation appears to have been considered inappropriate.

71. As in the passage from the New York System of Ethics prefacing this chapter: "… with honor to all its members" (MSSNY 1823, 8–9).

72. Committee on Ethics of the New York Academy of Medicine, date unknown.

73. Finnell 1869.

74. Sims 1870.

75. Committee on Ethics of the New York Academy of Medicine 1870.

76. Cushman rejected Sims's "excellent advice" of watchful waiting because "it was impossible for her to sit still under the thought that she might be helped to a quicker means to an entire relief." She went to Sir James Simpson (1811–1870), famous for initiating use of chloroform as a form of anesthesia (1847). Simpson removed the tumor from her

breast but, as Cushman put it, the "the snake was only scotched, not killed," and she would ultimately die of the disease under the care of her lover and biographer Emma Stebbins (1815–1882). See Stebbins 1879, 229–230.

77. Committee on Ethics of the New York Academy of Medicine 1871.

78. Ibid.

79. Ibid.

80. Committee on Ethics, New York Academy of Medicine 1867.

81. Massachusetts Medical Society 1881, vol. 2, 62.

82. Ibid.

83. Committee of the Massachusetts State Legislature 1830, 32–33.

84. Ibid., 19.

85. Unrepentant, Bartlett contended that a degree from the Harvard Medical College served as a license to practice. That issue was not resolved by this case; a Harvard degree was later recognized in Massachusetts as conferring a license to practice. See Committee of the Massachusetts State Legislature 1830, 15; see also Boston Medical Surgical Journal Editors 1836, 277–292.

86. MSSNY 1823, section XIX, 16.

87. Medico-Chirurgical Society of Baltimore 1832, 5, emphasis in the original. This statement is from the *System of Ethics* issued by the Medico-Chirurgical Society of Baltimore in 1832. It echoes a line from the ur-text of the genre, Percival's *Medical Ethics*, which states as the first of the physicians' moral obligations that their duty is to "minister to the sick, with due impressions of the importance of their office; reflecting that the ease, the health and the lives of those committed to their charge depend on their skill, attention and fidelity" (Percival [1803] 1985, chapter II, article I, 30).

88. Percival [1803] 1985, viii.

89. MSSNY 1868, 192.

90. MSSNY 1823, 3–4.

91. Nonetheless remnants of the code's origin as a system of *police* remain in its text. Thus, the fourth division of the code is characterized as "Specifications of Medical *Police* in Practice" in the table of contents but titled "Specifications of Medical *Ethics* in Practice" in the code's text.

92. Kahn and Kahn 1997, 1926–1930.

93. Mitchell and Pascalis were on the editorial board when this letter was published in 1821, but Steele would not join until the next year.

94. Percival [1803] 1985, chapter I, article XII, 15.

95. This is a nearly verbatim quotation from Percival's *Medical Ethics* chapter II, article XXIII, Percival [1803] 1985.

96. Mitchell, Manley, Pascalis, and Drake 1821, 95–100.

97. Percival [1803] 1985, chapter I, article XII, 15; numbers added.

98. College of Physicians of Philadelphia [1787] 1887, 175–176.

99. MSSNY 1868, 90 and appendix: By-laws

100. MSSNY 1823, 6–7.

101. Ibid., 22.

102. Ibid., 23—appended as note to the *System of Medical Ethics*.

103. Gregory [1772] 1998, 174–175.

104. Percival [1803] 1985, chapter II, article III, 31–32.

105. With respect to legal affairs, the MSSNY *System of Medical Ethics* stipulates that "[p]hysicians should not interfere in the final settlement of their patients worldly affairs" (MSSNY 1823, 23).

106. Porter, Roy 1989, 89.

107. Jalland 1996, 108–118.

108. MSSNY 1823, article XII, 12–13.

109. Rush [1808] 1811, 322.

110. MSSNY 1823, articles XVI, XVII, 14–15.

111. Ibid., article XXII, 20.

112. Ibid., article XXIII, 21.

113. Ibid., 10.

114. Ibid., articles XIII, XIV, 13–14.

115. Ibid., article XV, 14

116. Ibid., article XVI, 14.

117. Ibid., article XXI, 19–20.

118. Records of the society between 1838 and 1848 are missing. So, the society may have ceased to function after 1838 and then been revived to participate in the founding meeting of the AMA, which also occurred in 1848.

119. MSCNY 1825, various meetings from July 6–October 11, 1825.

120. MSCNY 1827, various meetings from July 16–August 13, 1827, 49–50.

121. Ibid., August 20, 1827, 50–51; MSCNY 1827, Report of the Committee on Quack Medicines.

122. Beck and Peixotto 1827, 426–442.

123. MSCNY 1827, Report of the Committee on Quack Medicines 4–5.

124. Rush's students and other practitioners of "heroic" medicine prescribed mercury chloride, popularly known as "calomel," as a medical laxative in dangerously large amounts. This practice was less common in the Northeast, and in New York City, where Bard's cautious, expectant approach to medicine was more common.

125. The *Merck Manual,* first published in 1899, is the first "beeper book," so to speak, and the oldest continuously published medical textbook in America; see Merck & Company 1899, 49, 172.

126. This paraphrases a famous line from the *Pogo Papers* (Kelly 1953) by cartoonist Walt Kelly, "We have met the enemy and he is us."

127. MSCNY, August 9, 1824; numbers added.

128. Swaim 1822, 1824. For a classic account of the panacea, see chapter 5 of Young 1961.

129. For example, Swaim published a pamphlet in which eminent Philadelphia physicians like Nathaniel Chapman (1780–1853), who became the first president of the AMA, extolled the virtues of his panacea. See Swaim 1822, 1824.

130. MSSNY 1823, 8–9

131. MSCNY, December 12, 1831.

132. Ambrose 2005, 45–56 cited at 52. Webster's 1828 dictionary offers the following definition: "Wight, n. [g., a living being. L., to live.] A being; a person. It is obsolete, except in irony or burlesque" ("Wight" 1828).

133. Hurd 1912, 57–58.

134. Serving on the committee were (names listed in the order in which they appear occur in the *Report*) E. Geddings (1799–1878), Thomas H. Wright, John Fonerden (1804–1869), H. Willis Baxley (1803–1876), and John Jasper Graves; see Medico-Chirurgical Society of Baltimore 1832, 31.

135. The journal became the *North American Archives of Medical and Surgical Science* in 1834–1835.

136. Medico-Chirurgical Society of Baltimore 1832, 1.

137. King James Translation of the Holy Bible, 1611, Psalm 91:6—often attributed to King David.

138. Medico-Chirurgical Society of Baltimore 1832, 6.

139. MSSNY 1823, article XIX, 16.

140. Medico-Chirurgical Society of Baltimore 1832, section I, article VIII, 10.

141. Medico-Chirurgical Society of Baltimore 1832, 5–6.

142. Percival, Thomas [1803] 1985, chapter II, article XI, 37–38; emphasis added.

143. Medico-Chirurgical Society of Baltimore 1832, section II, article X, 10–11.

144. AMA [1847] 1999, 329.

145. Medico-Chirurgical Society of Baltimore 1832, 6.

146. Ibid.

147. Ibid., 19. The version of Rush's lecture that the authors of the Baltimore *System of Ethics* used was appended to R. Eglesfeld Griffith's 1832 American edition (Ryan 1832), the first American edition of Ryan's, *A Manual of Medical Jurisprudence*.

148. Medico-Chirurgical Society of Baltimore 1832, section V, article I, 19–20.

149. Ibid., section V, article V, 21.

150. Ibid.

151. See chapter I, article II, sections 1, 6, 10 in AMA [1847] 1999, full text in Appendix IV.

152. The claim that the professionalization of American medicine is a function of a loss of licensing authority is widely accepted and draws on the work of sociologists such as William Rothstein whose *American Physicians in the Nineteenth Century: From Sects to Science* was a standard text published by a leading publisher in the history of medicine, Johns Hopkins, in 1972, and that was considered important enough to be reissued two decades later, in 1992; see Rothstein 1972. For a similar account, see Starr 1982.

153. See Appel 2010, 153–186.

154. Haller 2000, 131.

155. This is often labeled the first licensing law in British America. The passage relevant to midwives, physicians, and surgeons is quoted in full below. Note that the parenthetical remark, "if such may be had," opens the door to amateur practitioners and that this law places official licensing authority in the hands of experienced practitioners, not government officials.

Chirugeons, Midwives and Physicians: That no person or persons employed about the bodies of men, women, or children, for the preservation of life or health as chirugeons, midwives, physicians, or others, presume to set forth or exercise any act contrary to the known approved rule of art in each mystery or occupation, or exercise any violence or cruelty upon or towards the body of any, whether young or old, without the advice and consent of such as are skillful in the same art (if such may be had), or at least some of the wisest and gravest then present, and consent of the patient or patients if they be mentis compotes, much less contrary to such consent, upon such severe punishment as the nature of the fact may deserve; which law, nevertheless, is not intended to discourage any from the lawful use of their skill, but rather to encourage and direct them in the right use thereof, and to inhibit and restrain the presumptuous arrogance of such as, through confidence of their own skill, or any other sinister respects, dare boldly attempt to exercise any violence upon or towards the body of young or old, one or other, to the prejudice or hazard of the life or limb of man, woman, or child. (Walsh 1919, 24–25)

156. Walsh 1907, 14–15. The colony of New Jersey passed a similar law in 1772. See Shryock 1967, 17.

157. The article was published in a newspaper, the *Independent Reflector: or, Weekly essays on sundry important subjects. More particularly adapted to the province of New-York*, a weekly newspaper of opinion edited by William Livingston (1723–1790) and fellow lawyers John Morin Scott (1730–1784) and William Smith (1728–1793). The newspaper claimed to be dedicated to "truth and liberty" and opposed tyranny and dishonesty in public office. It was "tyrannically suppressed" by censors in 1754. As was traditional, the article was unsigned; however, it is generally accepted that its three authors were the paper's chief editor, William Livingston, who later became governor of New Jersey, and the paper's co-editors: John Morin Scott, who later served in the Continental army, the Continental Congress, and in the New York State legislature; and William Smith, who became Chief Justice of the Province of New York (1763–1782) and later Chief Justice of the Province of Quebec and lower Canada (1786–1793). Walsh 1907, 14–15; see also, Thomas 1931, 116.

158. Anonymous 1753, 47.

159. Ibid., 49–50.

160. Walsh 1907, 20–22.

161. Ibid., 116. The absence of any official role for physicians appears to have frustrated medical societies, who regarded this law as a bad precedent.

162. Abbott 1988.

163. Medico-Chirurgical Society of Baltimore 1832, 6.

164. Kaufman 1971, 55; citations from American Institute of Homeopathy 1846, 3.

165. Haller 2000, 263.

166. Baker 2009, "The Discourses…," especially 449–451.

167. Nye 2009, 418–426.

168. Maehle 2009; Maehle and Tröhler 2009

169. This characterization does not suit Thomsonians—who were initially anti-intellectual, egalitarian, and trade-oriented. However, they had difficulty with professionalizing for this reason. See Appel 2010, 153–186.

Chapter 6: A National Code of Medical Ethics

1. AMA 1847, 2.
2. MSCNY 1808, 186.
3. The proposal to the state was made after the MSCNY "opened a correspondence with several of the leading medical Characters in the different States and Territories in the Union on the necessity and propriety of forming an American Pharmacopoeia and their corresponding concern … that a National Pharmacopoeia would be a work of the highest importance" (MSCNY 1808, 186).
4. MSSNY 1868, 131–134.
5. Spalding's letters indicate that he was riven with feelings of unfulfilled ambition; see Spalding 1916.
6. The first *Pharmacopoeia of the United States of America*, "by the authority of the Medical Society and Colleges," was published in Boston by Wells and Lily in 1820. For information on its descendant, the U.S. Pharmacopeia, see http://www.usp.org/aboutUSP/ (accessed September 5, 2010).
7. Walsh 1919, 136.
8. Ibid.
9. AMA 1847, 2–3.
10. America's national telegraph system would not be created for another decade and a half, in the 1860s. In the 1840s, news had to travel by means of the U.S. postal service which, at that time, transported mail by means of a system of coaches traveling along post roads, supplemented by a handful of steam-powered vehicles—some riverboats and a few railroad lines—both traveling at speeds of less than twenty miles per hour.
11. AMA 1847, 15.
12. Davis 1903, 142.
13. AMA 1847, 17.
14. Ibid.
15. On anti-Irish attitudes during this period, see Hoeber 2001, 191–232; Prince 1985, 1–19; Wilson and Coval.
16. The Bell Family Papers are in the Tennessee State Library. A finding aid is available online; see Bell Family Papers 1796–1927.
17. For an account of the challenges facing Jewish intellectuals in academia and the professions in the 1840s, see Feuer 1984, 151–201.
18. The reference is to Jonah 3:1–14 from The King James Translation of the Holy Bible 1611.
19. Letter of Gertrude Gouverneur Meredith to William Meredith, September 30, 1805, in Ashton 1997, 72, emphasis in the original.
20. According to Ashton, Gratz dealt gently but directly with the "anti-Semitism she encountered among gentile women, [and] she attacked their prejudices directly, hoping to eliminate them" (Ashton 1997, 79).
21. Ashton 1997, 66.
22. Ibid., 205.

23. Originally, the journal's title was the *Philadelphia Journal of the Medical and Physical Sciences* (1820–1827). Its first editor was Nathanial Chapman, but, in 1825, Chapman began sharing the editorial work with W. P. Dewees and J. D. Godman. Because this arrangement proved unmanageable, Hays was brought in as an editorial assistant. After two years, in 1827, Hays renamed the journal *The American Journal of the Medical Sciences* and took over all editorial tasks—without publicly acknowledging his role as sole editor.

24. Ebert 1952, 243–276; quote from *Lancet* at 255.

25. Billings, John Shaw 1876, 332.

26. Ibid., 333.

27. Stillé 1880, 36. A brief biography of Isaac Hays can be found at Baker 2009, "Hays..." 704–705. The quotation is from Alexander Pope's *Essay On Man,* Epistle iii, line 303. Hays' papers are primarily in the library of the American Philosophical Society, but some are in the library of the College of Physicians of Philadelphia.

28. Kappa Lambda Society 1822–1835, January 8, 1823, 36. All extant papers of the Kappa Lambda society of Philadelphia are in the archives of the library of the College of Physicians of Philadelphia.

29. For an excellent review of the literature on Kappa Lambda, see Shultz 2008, 415–418. For further information on the fraternal nature of Kappa Lambda and of the connections between Kappa Lambda and the AMA, see Ambrose 2005, 45–56; see also Baker 1997.

30. An earlier Greek letter society, Phi Beta Kappa was founded at the College of William and Mary in 1776.

31. In addition to Jackson, the founding members of the Philadelphia branch of Kappa Lambda were Franklin Bache (1792–1864), J. H. Gordon, Thomas Harris (1784–1861), Thomas Hesson, Hugh H. Hodge (1796–1873), Charles Meigs (1792–1869), and René La Roche (1795–1872).

32. Kappa Lambda Society 1822–1835.

33. Ibid., January 8, 1823, 7.

34. Kappa Lambda Society of Hippocrates 1821.

35. Kappa Lambda Society 1822–1835, December 11 and 25, 31–33.

36. Kappa Lambda Society 1823.

37. The third member was Dr. Benjamin Ellis (1798– 1831), a University of Pennsylvania graduate and author of the first two editions of *The Medical Formulary*; Ellis 1829, 1834; Kappa Lambda Society 1822–1835, January 29 and February 26, 1823, 40–41.

38. Kappa Lambda Society 1823, article 18; which replicates Percival 1803, chapter II, article 18.

39. The minutes read as follows:

> The committee on additions to Percival's Medical Ethics, to whom was refereed the last section of their report, reported the same with amendment, this sections was further amended and adopted....
> 3rd What ought to be the rule as regards charges to the clergy? Your committee think that the clergy should be placed upon the same footing as any other class of people;

> that is, when able to pay the charges for medical attendance, they should be presented with their respective bills for payment, but if poor, to be treated as any others who may be poor. (Kappa Lambda Society 1822–1835, January 8, 1823, 160–161)

40. During this period, Hays participated in a parallel codification and Americanization project: drafting an English-language version of the charter and bylaws of a Sephardic congregation Kaal Kadosh Micve Israel [The Holy Congregation and Hope of Israel] of the City of Philadelphia, Kaal 1824.

41. Kappa Lambda Society 1822–1835, September 13, 1826, 159.

42. Emerson was admitted in 1823. Kappa Lambda Society 1822–1835, December 10, 1823, 77.

43. Ruschenberger 1891, 60–78; quotation on 73.

44. The report is signed in this order: "John Bell, Isaac Hays, G. Emerson, W. W. Morris, T. C. Dunn, A. Clark, R. D. Arnold." Only two first names are given—those of Bell and Hays. If the order reflects participation, and if Bell's role was primarily that of spokesperson for the committee, then, as Emerson's note indicates, in all likelihood he worked closely with Hays—as he had in providing healthcare to charities and during the 1832 cholera epidemic—and the two together probably edited the document working from the amended 1826 Kappa Lambda text of Percival and adding material from other sources. See this volume, Appendix VI.

45. As a secret society, Kappa Lambda was unable to publicize censures and so physicians forced out of the society felt free and motivated to reveal the fact of its existence and malign it. A letter of censure for public flyting had this format.

> By the publication which has appeared with your signature and which the Board have carefully read, they are of [the] opinion that you have taken your cause beyond the cognizance of the guardians, and carried it before a tribunal from which there is no appeal.
>
> In that publication they perceive with regret, that you have preferred very heavy charges against a fellow member. In the case of your having any cause of complaint against such an individual it was incumbent upon you to have sought the mediation of some mutual friend, or to have brought the subject before the board of Guardians. By pursuing a different course, you have not complied with one of the expressed provisions of the Constitution [Signed 3 guardians] (Kappa Lambda Society 1822–1835, November 17, 1826, 171)

46. At the urging of Hays and others, the Philadelphia branch of Kappa Lambda launched an investigation into members who were "encouraging, either by verbal or written recommendations the sale and use of secret nostrums," such as Swaim's Panacea. The resulting expulsions created a reservoir of ill will from expelled physicians and pharmacists; see Kappa Lambda Society 1822–1835, August 11, 1824, 102.

47. Kappa Lambda Society 1822–1835, August 8, 1826, 158.

48. Ibid., July 11, 1827, 194.

49. Morgan, William 1827.

50. Medical Examiner 1839.

51. Philosophical Hall, February 5th 1835:

> 3 1/2 PM: A special meeting of the Kappa Lambda was convened this afternoon by order of the President, Dr. Otto, at the request of Drs. Branch, Bond and Wood for the purpose of settling and closing the concerns of the institution.
> Present: Doctors Otto (President), Bache, Bell, La Roche, Hodge, Remington, Wood, Walton, Meigs and Bond.... Resolved that from and after the termination of this meeting the Kappa Lambda Society of Philadelphia be held to be *dissolved* ... unanimously approved. On Motion adjourned *sine die*. Henry Bond, Secy. (Manuscript: Philadelphia: Library of the College of Physicians of Philadelphia)

52. Kappa Lambda Society 1822–1835, December 11, 1822, 4–5.

53. AMA 1847, 17.

54. Ibid.

55. Hamilton 1889, 22

56. Michigan physician and former Union Army military surgeon William Brodie (1823–1890) acknowledges Hays' role in the formation of the AMA in his presidential address of 1886 (Brodie, William 1886, 506); however, in his essay honoring Davis on his retirement as founding editor of *JAMA*, John Hamilton accepts Davis's self-anointed title as "father" of the AMA (Hamilton, John 1889, 22), and this claim, repeated in The President's Address of 1891, became commonplace at the AMA's jubilee celebration of 1897 (Briggs 1891, 650). For further analysis of the construction of the myth of Nathan Smith Davis as the AMA's founding father, see Baker 1999, 23–25.

57. In addition to Bell, Emerson, and Hays, Richard. D. Arnold of Georgia (1808–1876), Theophilus C. Dunn, M.D. of Rhodes Island (1800–1871), and William W. Morris of Delaware were University of Pennsylvania alumni. Clark received his doctorate from the College of Physicians and Surgeons (Columbia).

58. Hays 1847, "Note to Convention," 92; this book, Appendix IV.

59. Ibid.; this book, Appendix IV.

60. In turning to the Webster dictionaries, I follow the advice of historian Samuel Haber, who observes that "the American professions ... are ... social artifacts fashioned by public events and usage; and ... [t]he historian forfeits too much if he or she loses touch with popular use and wont. Historians must start with the self-understanding of the people they are studying" (Haber 1991, x).

61. Specifically, Webster 1828, Webster 1913, Webster 1948 [1978].

62. Bell [1847] 2013, 83; this book Appendix V.

63. Ibid.

64. Bell 1847, 85; this book Appendix V.

65. Ibid.

66. "That [the midwife] shall be diligent and ready to help any woman in labor, whether she be poor or rich; that in time of necessity she will not forsake the poor woman and go to the rich." Common Council of the City of New York 1905, 121–123.

67. "Always most readily and cheerfully, when applied to, assist gratis, by all means in our power, the distressed poor and indigent in our respective neighborhood" (New Jersey Medical Society [1766] 1966, 310).

68. "In urgent cases of sickness, or of injuries occasioned by accidents, a call for medical or surgical help should be obeyed immediately, unless such compliance be to the detriment of some other sufferer." The New York code disparages the character of a physician reluctant to respond to the calls of the indigent stating that "not affording some attention to the poor, stands as a proof of [a physician's] selfishness or want of humanity." See MSSNY 1823, articles XVIII, XIX, 19.

69. "[T]he office of a physician is not exclusively one of emolument, but also of benevolence and humanity. As, therefore, [a physician] may be often summoned, in haste, to afford assistance in urgent cases of sickness, or of recent accidents and injuries, it always behooves him to obey such calls with promptitude" (Medico-Chirurgical Society of Baltimore 1832, 6; preface and section I article VIII, 10).

70. Civilian ambulance services were introduced around 1900. Arnold Griswold (1898–1972) opened the first American emergency department (ED or ER) at the University of Louisville hospital in 1911. The American ED had evolved into something approximating its present form by the 1940s.

71. Cabell [1856] [1981] 2002, 283; note 2.

72. One could argue that the 1986 Emergency Medical Treatment and Active Labor Act (EMTALA), which obligates hospital emergency departments to treat all patients irrespective of their ability to pay, perpetuates America's frontier tradition of answering the "call" for anyone in need—except that care is now provided in the emergency department, rather than in people's homes.

73. Bell, Hays, Emerson, Morris, Dunn, Clark, and Arnold 1847, chapter III, article I, §1, §4, 105–106; this volume, Appendix VI.

74. The quotation from Gregory states that physicians "have no established authority to which we can refer doubtful cases. Every physician must rest on his own judgment which appeals for its rectitude to nature and experience alone." Gregory [1770] 1998, 100–101. Cited as a note to third division, article 8, MSSNY 1823, this volume, Appendix II.

75. The 1910 Flexner report and Dr. Ernest Codman's (1869–1940) End Result Hospital Reports, which he started issuing in 1911, are generally considered the first major quality assurance initiatives in American medicine—although the AMA had been seeking what we would today consider QA standards since its founding, as had various state and municipal societies. See Luce, Birdman, and Lee 1994, 263–268; Flexner [1910] 1972; Neuhauser 2002, 104–105.

76. De Ville 1990, 3.

77. Bell, Hays, Emerson, Morris, Dunn, Clark, and Arnold 1847, 84, 93; this volume, Appendix VI.

78. See discussion, Kappa Lambda Society 1822–1835, December 11 and 25, 31–33.

79. See the discussion in the New York System of Ethics, MSSNY 1823, 10; and in Webster's 1828 Dictionary entry for "physician."

80. Bell, Hays, Emerson, Morris, Dunn, Clark, and Arnold 1847, chapter I, article II, section 1; note the use of the word "duties" rather than "obligations."

81. Rush [1808] 1811, 318–330.

82. Bell, Hays, Emerson, Morris, Dunn, Clark, and Arnold 1847, chapter I, article II, section 4; this volume, Appendix VI.

83. Bell, Hays, Emerson, Morris, Dunn, Clark, and Arnold 1847, chapter I, article II, section 6; this volume, Appendix VI.

84. The 1828 edition of Webster's dictionary defined pecuniary as "relating to money; as pecuniary affairs or losses."

85. Bell, Hays, Emerson, Morris, Dunn, Clark, and Arnold 1847, chapter I, article II, section 10; this volume, Appendix VI.

86. Emerson's experience on the Philadelphia Board of Health is likely to have influenced chapter III, article I, section 1. On his recommendation, the Board led a publicity campaign encouraging vaccination and instituted new quarantine regulations that successfully reduced deaths from smallpox. From 1827 through 1847, Emerson published a series of papers on vital statistics in various Hays' journals, culminating in "Medical and Vital Statistics," published in the July 1848 issue of Hays' *American Journal of the Medical Sciences*. Emerson also served on the AMA's Committee on Medical Sciences and helped to compile the organization's first report on vital statistics. In 1857 and 1858, he was a delegate to the national quarantine and sanitary convention. Hays worked side by side with Emerson in providing care for the victims of the cholera epidemic of 1832, but these issues were a primary focus of Emerson's life. See Ruschenberger 1891.

87. Webster's 1828 Dictionary defines "eleemosynary" as "1. Given in charity; given or appropriated to support the poor; as eleemosynary rents or taxes. 2. Relating to charitable donations; intended for the distribution of alms, or for the use and management of donations, whether for the subsistence of the poor or for the support and promotion of learning; as an eleemosynary corporation. A hospital founded by charity is an eleemosynary institution for the support of the poor, sick and impotent."

88. Emphasis added.

89. Wakely 1824, 135–138; cited in Shultz 1992, 20.

90. Emphasis added to underline parallel with AMA code. Wakely 1824, 135–138; cited in Shultz 1992, 20.

91. Smith, Thomas Southwood 1827. Originally published as a review of William Mackenzie's *An Appeal to the Public and the Legislature, on the Necessity of affording Dead Bodies to the Schools of Anatomy, by Legislative Enactment*. It was republished in America by the Albany medical textbook publisher Websters and Skinners in an, ultimately unsuccessful, effort to persuade the New York State legislature to pass a Smith-style anatomy act.

92. Wakely 1824, 135–138; cited in Shultz 1992, 20.

93. William Mackenzie actually proposed the act. In my view, Smith anticipated contemporary bioethics: i.e., he diagnosed which aspects of the innovation made it morally disruptive and provided a public justification for initiating a remedy that permitted the innovation to be implemented in a nondisruptive manner. It is noteworthy that although

Mackenzie proposed the legal act, when the anatomy act became law, it was identified with the ethicists rather than the lawmaker because the real challenge was its moral disruption.

94. Smith, Thomas Southwood 1827, 30.

95. Ibid., 32.

96. Ibid.; emphasis in the original.

97. Ibid.

98. Ibid., 32–33. Smith implies that anatomists typically purchase cadavers from professional resurrectionists. In both Britain and America, however, anatomists' assistants were responsible for procuring cadavers from resurrectionists, and these assistants sometimes robbed graves themselves—as did anatomists themselves, their sons, and their medical students. See Moore 2005, 31–33; 234–235; Warren 1860, 404–410. More generally, see Shultz 1992.

99. Smith, Thomas Southwood 1827, 36–37. Emphasis in the original.

100. Smith also responds to the objection that his proposal would "make the bodies of the poor public property." His response is that, one way or another, the poor serve as experimental subjects for physicians and surgeons. A better argument might have been that grave robbers preferred to rob the graves of the poor and lower classes (and, in America, the graves of African Americans) because these depredations were less likely to raise the ire of the authorities. On race and grave robbing, see Savitt 2007, 82–83.

101. In the context of lobbying for an anatomy act Smith, a Benthamite, publicly dissected the corpse of the philosopher Jeremy Bentham: for an excellent study of the passage of the anatomy act in Britain, see Richardson 2000, 159–160.

102. Anatomy acts were least disruptive in jurisdictions that also repealed laws that stigmatized dissection by meting it out as punishment. Removing the stigma of dissection as punishment and creating mechanisms for the voluntary donation of bodies by individuals and families made dissection a less forbidding prospect for those whose bodies were most at risk to be dissected postmortem.

103. Sappol 2002, 121–122.

104. Medico-Chirurgical Society of Baltimore 1832, 6, preface, section III, article X; this volume, Appendix III.

105. *Boston Medical Surgical Journal*. 1843, 181; cited at Coulter [1973] 1982, 181.

106. Berlant 1975.

107. Kaplan 1971, 54.

108. Wolpe 1999, 222–223.

109. Warner 1999, 54–55; see also Warner 1991, 454–478.

110. The data on the growth of homeopathy are drawn from Haller 2005, 65–66.

111. The North American Academy of Homeopathic Healing in Allentown, Pennsylvania, closed its doors in 1841/42. Haller 2005, 369.

112. Warner 1999, 55.

113. Wolpe 1999, 222–223.

114. Whewell 1840.

115. Whewell 1847, vol. II, 54. Whewell developed what would later be called a hypothetical-deductive model of scientific confirmation emphasizing the creative nature of science

in developing conjectures and the importance of winnowing out hypotheses by means of experimentation.

116. Whewell 1847, vol. II, 57.

117. Ibid., 205.

118. Ibid., 62–63.

119. In Whewell's view, Newtonian-Copernican heliocentric theory properly supplanted Ptolemaic theory because its laws explain both mechanics and physics on Earth as well as interplanetary motion, i.e., these laws explained phenomena in seemingly unrelated areas. As Whewell puts it, hypotheses that predict or explain "classes of facts altogether different" from those that "the hypothesis was originally intended to explain" are "the best established theor[ies] that the history of science contains.... No example can be pointed out, in the whole history of science ... in which Consilience ... has given testimony in favor of an hypothesis that was afterwards discovered to be false" (Whewell 1847, vol. II, 67–68).

It is noteworthy that Whewell's protégé, Charles Darwin, emphasizes consilience throughout *Origin of Species*, demonstrating time and again how a few simple laws of natural selection, although designed to explain the origin of species, also explain seemingly unrelated phenomena, such as differences between birds. Darwin's deft use of consilience is one reason why many readers find *Origin of Species* extraordinarily persuasive on first reading. The philosopher of science, Sir Karl Popper (1902–1994) and sociobiologist Edmund Wilson later appropriated aspects of Whewell's theory of consilience. In this book, the term "consilience" is used in its original nineteenth-century sense.

120. Darwin, Charles 1859.

121. Laennec [1821] 1827.

122. Louis [1835] 1836, 59–60; 75–76.

123. Louis [1835] 1836, 75–76. C. G. Putnam, trans., 59–60.

124. For an excellent summary of these experiments, see Haller 2005, 104–108.

125. Holmes [1842] 2007, 21–94.

126. Quotation from Holmes [1843] [1855] [1891] 2007, 118.

127. Holmes [1843] [1891] 2007, 141.

128. Holmes 1842.

129. Coulter [1973] 1982, 180.

130. "Allopath" is defined in Richard Hoblyn's *A Dictionary of Terms Used in Medicine and the Collateral Sciences* (Hoblyn 1844) as "[t]he art of curing founded on differences, by which one morbid state is removed by inducing a different one." It was Hahnemann's term for regular medicine, which he contrasted with "homeopathy," the cure of disease by substances inducing the same morbid states (Hahnemann 1810). Even though the term "allopathic" was a misnomer—since curing by opposites was not the nature of regular therapeutics, even in the nineteenth century—the term has been widely adopted as a characterization of "regular" medicine.

131. Forbes, J. 1846, 47.

132. Holmes [1860] [1891] 2007, 166.

133. Forbes reveals his motives by citing "the clinical researches of Louis and others [which shows] that patients recover as well ... without" medical interventions. See Forbes, J. 1846, 49.

134. The leading obstetricians of the day, the Rush acolyte and Kappa Lambda founder, Charles Meigs, professor of obstetrics at Jefferson Medical College in Philadelphia, joined with fellow Kappa Lambda founder Hugh L. Hodge, of the University of Pennsylvania, in denouncing Holmes's claims about the iatrogenic spread of puerperal fever. "Contagionists," Meigs protested, "will say that [doctors] carried the poison from house to house.... But a gentleman's hands are clean" (Meigs 1854, 104). Undeterred by being dismissed as a "jejune and fizenless ... sophomore writer," Holmes published a rebuttal, condemning the Pennsylvania professors for teaching "doctrines which lead to professional homicide.... [T] he pestilence-carrier of the lying-in chamber must look to God for pardon, for man will never forgive him" (Holmes [1843] [1855] [1891] 2007, 113).

135. Forbes' suggestion that regular medical therapeutics was ineffective and unscientific provoked a defense of regular medicine in a rival journal, *Lancet*, that culminated in a fall in subscriptions that forced Forbes to close his journal. As Forbes remarked in a Postscript to the final issue of his journal, his articles on homeopathy prompted a "cry ... by some of the weekly Journals [*Lancet*]—pretty loud for a month or two.... [Yet] in no instance since the publication of the Review have I had more cause to be satisfied with the effect produced by any articles, than by these.... I believe, indeed, that they have been the means of exciting a spirit of philosophical inquiry into the present state of therapeutics, which cannot fail to end in consequences most beneficial to medical science" (Forbes, J. 1847, 594–595).

Within half a decade, Forbes received an honorary degree from Oxford (1852) and was knighted by Queen Victoria (1853). He reiterated his critique of regular medicine in *Of Nature and Art in the Cure of Disease* (Forbes, J. 1857). An obituary in the *Proceedings of the Royal Society* paid him this accolade: "Although Sir John Forbes can not be ranked among those who have advanced the science of medicine by the discovery of new facts ... he must be regarded as having done most essential service to the cause of progress ... by the determined onslaught which he made upon prevalent errors, and the vigorous earnestness with which he pleaded for generally-neglected truths" (Agnew 2008).

136. "Cinchona" is defined in *A Dictionary of Terms used in Medicine and the Collateral Sciences* (Hoblyn 1844) as "[a] genus of plants several species of which yield Peruvian Bark [the natural source of quinine]. The terms *Cinchona Bark* and *Countess's Powder* are derived from the circumstance that the Countess of Chinchon, wife of the Viceroy of Peru brought some back from South America in 1639."

137. Holmes [1842] 2007, 64–65.

138. Another aspect of Hahnemann's theory that lacked consilience with other nineteenth-century theories, specifically physiology and pathology, was his account of pathology in which all disease symptoms were reduced to the status of an itch.

139. Holmes [1842] 2007, 61–62. The National Center for Complimentary and Alternative Medicine summarized this criticism as follows: "Critics think it is implausible that a remedy containing a miniscule amount of an active ingredient (sometimes not a single molecule of the original compound) can have any biological effect—beneficial or otherwise. For these reasons, critics argue that continuing the scientific study of homeopathy is not worthwhile."

140. Holmes [1842] 2007, 61–62.

141. Forbes, J. 1846, 39.

142. Ibid.

143. Anonymous 1846, 105–107.

144. Hays 1843, "Prospectus," 1.

145. Hays 1843, "Homeopathic Fictions," 13; Hays 1843, "Victim to Homeopathy," 46. Although Hays treated homeopathy in the Quackery section of *Medical News,* he distinguished delusional medical movements, whose followers sincerely believed in what they propounded, from the usual run of quacks and charlatans whose aim was to deceive the public for a profit.

146. Bell [1847], 2013, "Introduction to the Code of Ethics." This volume, Appendix V.

147. The primary focus of these remarks is the need to exclude from medicine the morally unfit and those untrained in science and its methods. However, the remark follows Bell's comments on other "pretenders to science" and would also exclude CAM practitioners. See Bell [1847], 2013, "Introduction to the Code of Ethics"; see also this volume, Appendix V.

148. Hays 1847, "Medical Reform," 49–54. See also, Hays 1847, "Infinitesimal Morality," 62.

149. Kappa Lambda Society of Hippocrates 1823.

150. Friendly Thomsonian Botanic Society of the United States [1837] 2000, 263.

151. International Hahnemann Association, June 26,1880, cited at Haller 2005, 239–270. This was aimed at the American Institute of Homeopathy, which counseled against public critiques of the regulars and whose members often presented themselves as practicing a branch or specialty practice within regular medicine.

152. Whewell 1847, vol. II, 57.

153. Harkness 2002, 732–733.

154. "Considering it desirable that the Codes of Ethics adopted by the various associations of physicians in our country should be uniform in scope and arrangement, and as nearly identical in language as possible, the committee have used the arrangement, and to a great extent, the language of the Code adopted by the American Medical Association, and published in volume xvi of their "Transactions" (for 1865), modifying it where changes seemed to be demanded by a proper regard for liberality and justice, both to patient and to physicians, or by a due concern for the freedom of medical education, opinion, and action" (American Institute of Homeopathy 1884, 681; see text in the appendix to this volume, Appendix VIII).

155. American Osteopathic Organization 1905, 35–39; see text in the appendix to this volume, Appendix X.

156. AMA 1995–2012, "The Founding of AMA" and "Our History."

157. Both the Academy of Natural Sciences and the College of Physicians of Philadelphia have portraits of Isaac Hays.

158. Stillé 1880, 36. Other obituaries are Brinton 1879, 259–260; Gross 1879, 281–292.

159. Bell 1850, 6.

160. "Medicine is [now] demonstrative, not didactic; it has entered into the circle of the positive sciences. Had Dr. Bell devoted himself to science and not to idle dialectics …

and had he confined himself to the substantial, and not vainly wasted his efforts to seize the shadow, he might have reaped the same success that others, inferior to himself, have secured" (Jackson 1850, 21–22).

161. Jackson 1850, 21–22.

162. Shrady 1872, 432.

163. Ruschenberger 1891, 19–20.

164. Ibid., 20.

165. Ibid.

Chapter 7: Professional Medical Ethics 1848–1873: Abortion, Inquisition, and Exclusion

1. Miller, Henry 1860, 57.

2. Stillé 1871, 91–94.

3. A standard Southern characterization of "slavery" at the time. One of Webster's 1828 definitions of the term "peculiar" derives from "pecus," Latin for "cattle": Exclusive property; that which belongs to a person in exclusion of others. ("Peculiar" 1828.)

4. See Mohr 1978, chapter 3, 46–85.

5. Bard [1769] 1996, 14.

6. Puritans and other strict Calvinist did not accept the consensus view that fetal life began at quickening. Thus, the Puritan-influenced New York Midwives' oath of 1716 forbade midwives to "administer any medicine to produce a miscarriage," but it was unique in prohibiting what later would be considered a first-trimester abortion. See Common Council of the City of New York 1905, 121–123.

7. A key text in this development was by the Estonian-German polymath Karl Ernst von Baer (1792–1876). See von Baer 1828–1837.

8. Percival 1803, chapter IV, article 10, 78–79; see also Percival 1794, section IV, article 8.

9. For Percival and for other nineteenth-century physician scholars, the Hippocratic oath unambiguously prohibited abortion. An 1849 translation of the oath by Francis Adams (1796–1861), an Edinburgh-educated Scottish physician and classicist, that came to be accepted as standard in Anglo-American culture renders the oath as explicitly forbidding a physician to "give a woman a pessary to cause an abortion" (Adams [1849] 1942, 14). By contrast, Heinrich Von Staden's postfeminist translation of the oath renders the relevant passage as, "I will not give a drug that is deadly to anyone if asked [for it].... And likewise I will not give a woman a destructive pessary"—the word "abortion" is notably absent. Since Hippocratic physicians performed abortions and practiced medicine in a pagan society that permitted infanticide by exposure, it seems more likely that the intent of this passage was to protect women against the iatrogenic harm of delivering dangerous or deadly medicines by means of a vaginal pessary, rather than to protect an unborn fetus. The full translation of the oath with commentary is found at Von Staden 1996, 406–408.

10. Hodge [1839] 1854, 7.

11. Ibid., 8. The quotation is from Book 5 of Milton's *Paradise Lost*.

12. Hodge 1864, 263. He expounds on this point, noting that a "craniotomy may be resorted to in any case of tedious labor, at the discretion of the practitioner, where there is full and satisfactory evidence of the death of the child. If the child, however, be living, the resort to this operation cannot be justified, while there be any hope remaining for preserving the life of the child as well as that of the mother" (Hodge 1864, 276).

13. Hodge [1839] 1854, 12–13. Emphasis in the original.

14. Ibid., 19.

15. Foucault [1963] 1973; Reiser 1978.

16. Storer, D. H. [1855] 1872, footnote, 174.

17. Luker 1984, 22.

18. Storer, D. H. [1855] 1872, 6–7. Parts of the lecture are also available in Dyer, Frederick 1999, 80–84.

19. Storer, D. H. [1855] 1872, 6–7; Dyer, Frederick 1999, 82–83.

20. For a provocative and insightful analysis of the socio- and psychodynamics of Storer Sr.'s speech and others like it, see Carroll Smith-Rosenberg's "The Abortion Movement and the AMA, 1850–1880," Smith-Rosenberg 1985, 217–244.

21. Storer, D. H. [1855] 1872, footnote, 174.

22. It has been suggested that the Harvard faculty was "Fearful … lest its pecuniary interests might suffer, whether at the hands of the public, one of whose prevailing sins had been so boldly and directly assailed, or of the profession, whose lethargy in this matter and subservience to expediency had been rebuked." It seems unlikely that this male chauvinist rant would have had any economic impact. Perhaps Storer Sr.'s colleagues were offended because he also directed his moralistic polemic against their own conduct in assisting women seeking abortions. Given Bigelow's characterization of the passages as "injudicious," the offense may also have been public moralizing in a manner more appropriate to the pulpit than the lectern. A lifelong protestor against all forms of exploitation, Bigelow may also have objected to Storer Sr.'s misogynist rhetoric. Quotation is from Editors [1857] 1999, *New Hampshire Journal of Medicine*, 85.

23. Storer, Horatio R. [1911] 1999, 483.

24. Dyer 1999, 127.

25. Storer, D. H. [1855] 1872.

26. Editors 1857, "Reports of Medical Societies: Criminal Abortion," 282–284. Emphasis in the original.

27. Dyer 1999, 110–111.

28. Ibid., 121.

29. AMA 1857, 30

30. Storer, Horatio, Blatchford, Hodge, et al. 1859, 75–76.

31. Ibid., 76.

32. Ibid., 77–78.

33. AMA *Transactions* 1859, 28.

34. Miller, Henry 1860, 57.

35. AMA *Transactions* 1864, 50.

36. Storer, Horatio R. 1865, 722–733.
37. Ibid., 713.
38. Ibid., 724–735.
39. Ibid., 736.
40. Ibid., 736.
41. Ibid., 744–745.
42. Storer, Horatio R. 1866, 65, 84–85.
43. Storer, Horatio R. 1867, "Is it I...," 72.
44. Storer, Horatio R. and Heard 1868.
45. Webster's 1828 edition defines *Profession*, n. [L. professio.] as: "(1) Open declaration; public avowal or acknowledgment of one's sentiments or belief; as professions of friendship or sincerity; a profession of faith or religion....(2) The business which one professes to understand and to follow for subsistence; calling; vocation; employment; as the learned professions. We speak of the profession of a clergyman, of a lawyer, and of a physician or surgeon; the profession of lecturer on chemistry or mineralogy. But the word is not applied to an occupation merely mechanical. The collective body of persons engaged in a calling. We speak of practices honorable or disgraceful to a profession." ("Professional" 1828).
46. "Professional" 1913, 1144; emphasis added.
47. Bell [1847] this volume, Appendix V.
48. Phelps 1854, 462. In what may have been a concerted effort to introduce Christianity into the interpretation of the AMA's code of ethics, another physician, Robert S. Bailey of South Carolina, also read a paper on religion and medical ethics at the same AMA meeting.
49. Atlee, March, and Sayre 1855, 50.
50. Ibid., 51.
51. Smith, J. V. C. 1847, 63.
52. Ibid., 63–64.
53. AMA *Transactions* 1855, 56–57.
54. AMA *Transactions* 1858, 39
55. AMA *Transactions* 1865, 71.
56. Ibid., 71–72.
57. MSCNY 1864.
58. AMA *Transactions* 1865, 45–46.
59. *The American Journal of Insanity* (currently published as the *American Journal of Psychiatry*) predates Homberger's journal by two decades. It was founded in 1844 to publish the reports of the Association of the Medical Superintendents of American Institutions for the Insane (also founded in 1844), but it also published original articles on psychiatry.
60. Snyder 1962, 876.
61. Homberger's roots were in Germany, and, at this time, German physicians, like their British and French counterparts, were developing an "honor court" system, comparable to the medical tribunals conducted by *comita minora*, for enforcing the *unwritten* morality of gentlemanly honor. See Maehle 2009.
62. Homberger [1865] 1868, 7. No copies of the original report are known to survive. Homberger reproduced it in a flyting pamphlet, defending his honor,

Batpaxomyomaxia. The transliteration from the Greek is nonstandard—the title is usually rendered as "Batrachomyomachia or the Battle of the Frogs and Mice." Performances of Batrachomyomachia were popular in Berlin, where the title is usually translated "Froschmäusekrieg"—which is still German for a stupid dispute, a major brouhaha over some minor matter. The pamphlet, a foundational document for the field of ophthalmology, is a rare book. A copy is held by the Francis A. Countway Library of the Harvard Medical School, whose librarians kindly made it available.

63. Homberger [1865] 1868, 7.

64. Ibid., 8.

65. Homberger points out that because general practitioners draw their patients from the neighborhood in which they live, they need only hang out a shingle with their name on it to have a successful practice. The specialist, in contrast, "must spread his name in wider circles … for a … community which would yield a splendid return for the services of a general practitioner would suffice neither properly to support a specialist, nor to secure a practice sufficiently large to stimulate his scientific energy" (Homberger, [1865] 1868, 8).

66. Homberger [1865] 1868, 9.

67. Ibid.

68. Ibid., 10–11.

69. Ibid., 14.

70. Ibid., 14.

71. AMA 1865, 36.

72. Committee reports and prize essays were normally published in *Transactions*. The 1865 edition of *Transactions*, for example, included sixteen reports from committees and various papers, including Storer Jr.'s prize essay *On Criminal Abortion*, as well as the minutes of the meeting. See Storer 1865 "Prize Essay," AMA 1865, 722–733.

73. Storer, David Humphreys 1866, 64–65.

74. Bowditch 1866, 512.

75. Snyder 1962, 876–877.

76. Davis 1868, "Proceedings of the Societies: Annual Meeting of the American Medical Association," 361.

77. Homberger protested his expulsion in a flyting pamphlet, *Batpaxomyomaxia; a fight on "Ethics,"* in which he argued that the AMA violated its own procedures by never "cit[ing] me before a court medical" and by "destroy[ing] my evidence," i.e. refusing to distribute his report to the delegates or publish it in *Transactions*. So Homberger published his report himself and continued to challenge the AMA on the propriety of medical advertising. His efforts might have had an impact had he not come to a sad end in 1872, when he appears to have committed suicide after a brief internment in a psychiatric hospital.

78. AMA 1869. *Transactions*, 112–113.

79. Ibid., 28.

80. Ibid., 28–29.

81. AMA 1870, *Transactions*, 40.

82. *Goldfarb v. Virginia State Bar* 1975.

83. *American Medical Association v. Federal Trade Commission* 1980.

84. Bowditch 1868, 89–20.

85. AMA 1868, *Transactions,* 25.

86. Davis 1868, "Proceedings...," 358.

87. Ibid.

88. Ibid., 358–359.

89. Ibid., 359.

90. Ibid., 359–360.

91. Davis 1886, "The Higher Education of Women," 267.

92. Article One of the Fourteenth Amendment reads, "All persons born or naturalized in the United States, and subject to the jurisdiction thereof, are citizens of the United States and of the State wherein they reside. No State shall make or enforce any law which shall abridge the privileges or immunities of citizens of the United States; nor shall any State deprive any person of life, liberty, or property, without due process of law; nor deny to any person within its jurisdiction the equal protection of the laws" (U.S. Constitution, Fourteenth Amendment).

93. Davis 1868, "Proceedings...," 359.

94. AMA *Transactions* 1870, 61–62.

95. AMA *Transactions* 1871, 23, 30, 32, 33–34.

96. Ibid., 41–42.

97. Stillé 1871, 91.

98. Ibid., 94.

99. Ibid., 95.

100. Ibid., 95.

101. Ibid., 95–96.

102. Reyburn, Stephenson, Augusta, et al. [1870] 1967, 215–216; Nickens 1985, 2549–2552.

103. Miller and Lovejoy 1870, 173–174.

104. AMA *Transactions* 1870, 29.

105. Ibid.

106. Ibid., 30.

107. Ibid., 54.

108. Ibid., 55.

109. Ibid., 55–56.

110. Ibid., 59.

111. Ibid., 66.

112. Anonymous 1870. "The Doctors...," 3.

113. AMA *Transactions* 1870, 65.

114. Ibid., 66–67.

115. Anonymous 1870. "The Doctors...," 3.

116. Anonymous 1870. "Medical ...," 344.

117. Stillé 1871, 95–96.

118. M. D. 1871, 174.

119. Ibid., 174–175.

120. Ibid., 178.

121. AMA *Transactions* 1872, 56.

122. AMA *Transactions* 1873, 34; AMA 1874, 34.

123. The Medico-Chirurgical Society of the District of Columbia was founded in 1884; the Lone Star State Medical, Dental, and Pharmaceutical Association of Texas in 1886; the Old North State Medical Society (ONSMS) of North Carolina in 1887.

124. Roman 1909.

125. Davis, Ronald 2008 "Letter..."

126. Ibid., "Achieving...," 323–325.

127. The Writing Group members are Robert B. Baker, Ph.D., the Union Graduate College-Mount Sinai School of Medicine Bioethics Program and Department of Philosophy, Union College; Janice Blanchard, M.D., Department of Emergency Medicine, George Washington University School of Medicine; Clarence Braddock, M.D., M.P.H., Stanford Center for Biomedical Ethics; Giselle Corbie-Smith, M.D., M.Sc., Department of Social Medicine, University of North Carolina at Chapel Hill; LaVera Crawley, M.D., M.P.H., Stanford University Center for Biomedical Ethics; Eddie Hoover, M.D., editor, *Journal of the National Medical Association*; Elizabeth Jacobs, M.D., M.P.P., Stroger Hospital of Cook County & Rush University Medical Center; Thomas A. LaVeist, Ph.D., Department of Health Policy and Management, Johns Hopkins Bloomberg School of Public Health; Randall Maxey, M.D., Ph.D., National Medical Association; Kathryn L. Moseley, M.D., University of Michigan Medical School; Todd L. Savitt, Ph.D., Department of Medical Humanities, Brody School of Medicine, East Carolina University; Harriet A. Washington, B.A., visiting scholar, DePaul University College of Law; David R. Williams, Ph.D., Department of Society, Human Development, and Health, Harvard School of Public Health, as well as AMA project staff; Matthew K. Wynia, M.D., M.P.H., study director; and Ololade Olakanmi, B.A., project research assistant.

128. The sections on the AMA and African-American physicians in this chapter were profoundly informed by my collaboration with the Writing Group. The views expressed in this chapter are mine and should not be attributed to other members of the Writing Group, except insofar as they mirror positions taken in the collaborative articles referenced in the next three footnotes.

129. Baker, Washington, Olakanmi, et al. 2008 "African...," 306–313.

130. Davis, R. 2008, "Achieving Racial Harmony...," 323–325; Davis R. 2008, "Letter of Apology."

131. The research and various articles by the Writing Group are available on the website of the AMA's Institute for Ethics, http://www.ama-assn.org/ama/pub/physician-resources/medical-ethics/about-ethics-group/institute-ethics/research-projects/the-history-african-americans-organized-medicine.page? Other relevant articles available on the website are Baker, Washington, Olakanmi, et al. 2008 "Creating...," 501–512; and Washington, Baker, Olakanmi 2008 "Segregation...," 513–527.

Chapter 8: The Anti-Code Revolt: Laissez Medical Faire Ethics, 1876–1979

1. "Woe unto you, scribes and Pharisees, hypocrites! for ye devour widows' houses, and for a pretence make long prayer: therefore ye shall receive the greater damnation" (The King James Translation of the Holy Bible 1611, Matthew 21:14).

2. AMA *Transactions* 1873, 32.

3. Ibid., 35.

4. AMA *Transactions* 1874, 28–29.

5. Ibid., 29.

6. Ibid., 29.

7. Ibid., 30.

8. Ibid.

9. Ibid.

10. Morghenstern 2004.

11. Homberger's "scandalous" advertisement that he had trained in eye surgery in Paris would have been routine in France and uncontroversial in Berlin. See Homberger, Julius 1869, cover.

12. AMA *Transactions* 1874, 31.

13. Fissell 2009, 536.

14. AMA *Transactions* 1869, 41.

15. AMA *Transactions* 1877, 46.

16. AMA *Transactions* 1874, 32.

17. Ibid., 33.

18. Ibid.

19. New York Times 1894, "Sims Statue Unveiled." Sims became a controversial figure in the late twentieth century; see Chapter 9.

20. Sims 1876, 93. There was a motion to deny Stevenson admission, but that was squelched by a vote (numbers not recorded). See AMA 1876, 46.

21. Sims 1876, 93.

22. Ibid., 96.

23. Ibid., 96–97.

24. Ibid., 97.

25. Ibid., 98. The reference is to John 8:7, King James' translation, *The Holy Bible.*

26. Simms 1876, 98.

27. Ibid.

28. AMA *Transactions* 1876, 46.

29. Delafield 1886, 16.

30. The applicant, Henry Goldman M.D., was a graduate of the Homeopathic Medical College of New York.

31. Carrie L. Black, M.D. was a graduate of New York Medical College and the Hospital for Women.

32. In 1880, the New York Legislature passed "An Act to regulate the licensing of physicians and surgeons." Section 5 stated that, "[t]he degree of doctor of medicine lawfully

conferred by any incorporated medical college or university in this State shall be a license to practice physic and surgery within the State." Since both the female and the homeopathic applicants had M.D. degrees from state-recognized medical colleges, they were properly licensed to practice in New York.

33. MSSNY *Transactions* 1881, 53–59.
34. Ibid., 54.
35. Ibid.
36. Bailey 1881, 110.
37. Ibid.
38. Ibid.
39. Ibid., 112.
40. MSSNY *Transactions* 1882, 26.
41. Ibid., 29.
42. Ibid., 30–31. See also Vanderpole 1883, 26–41.
43. Dalton 1881, 26, 29–30.
44. Jacobi 1882, 10–11.
45. Ibid., 11. See also Jacobi 1883, 156–175.
46. AMA 1882. "Minutes of Judicial Council," 60.
47. Lane 1885, 8.
48. The debate was richer than the Flint-Post exchange. See, e.g., Hamilton, Frank 1884.
49. Flint 1882, 2–3.
50. Ibid., 4.
51. Ibid., 11.
52. Ibid., 12.
53. Ibid., 14.
54. Ibid., 16.
55. Post, Ely, Vanderpole, et al. 1883.
56. Roosa and St. John 1883, 106, emphasis in the original; see also Vanderpole 1883, 26.
57. Flint 1882, 18.
58. Ibid., 20.
59. See Vanderpole 1883, 26; Pilcher 1883, 42–43, for a reiteration of these themes.
60. Post, Alfred 1883, 1.
61. Ibid., 4.
62. Pilcher 1883, 52–53.
63. Ibid., 53.
64. Ibid., 44.
65. Ibid., 55.
66. Davis 1868. "Give...," 115.
67. Chastened by Davis's editorial, the syphologists publicly apologized, evinced contrition, "suspend[ing] further publication" of offending material, and contended that the publication of names had been "contrary to [their intention or desire" (Brown and Higgins 1868, 187).
68. Storer, Horatio R. 1868, 189–190.

69. Solis-Cohen 1892, 682–683.
70. Solis-Cohen 1894, 95–96.
71. A Conservative Member 1892–1893 .
72. Inquirer 1892.
73. Medicus 1894, 438–439.
74. Kaumheimer 1894, 480.
75. Journal of the American Medical Association Editors 1895, "Anonymous…," 141.
76. Davis stepped down as editor of *JAMA* in 1893.
77. Journal of the American Medical Association Editors 1895, "Report…," 760.
78. Holton 1894, "Report…," 950.
79. Ibid.
80. Ibid.
81. Holton 1894, "Code…," chapter II, articles I, II, 508.
82. Holton 1894, "Report…," 950.
83. Ibid.
84. Ibid., 950–951
85. Ibid.
86. Didama 1894, 951.
87. Ibid. Emphasis in the original.
88. AMA 1894, "Proceedings," 952.
89. AMA 1895, "Official Report of the Proceedings," 762.
90. Ibid., 766
91. Harris 1901, 1545.
92. Harris 1902, 1649–1652.
93. Harris 1903, 1381.
94. Holton 1894 (Code Proposal 1894, part I, chapter I, article II, section 1), "Report…," 950–951.
95. AMA 1903, "Galley proof of draft…," chapter I, article I, section 1: similar but not identical to AMA 1847 *Code of Medical Ethics*, chapter I, article I, section 1. See this volume, Appendices VI and IX.
96. Harris 1903, 1379.
97. Harris 1902, 1649; Harris 1903, 1379.
98. AMA 1903, "Galley proof of draft…," 82.
99. AMA 1903, "Galley proof of draft…," Preface. See also Harris 1902, 1649.
100. Ibid. This is essentially the same devolutionist policy that Davis adopted to prevent debates over the admission of African-American and female physicians from disrupting the harmony of AMA meetings in the 1870s.
101. Harris 1903, 1379.
102. Shattuck 1910, 30.
103. Pilcher 1883, 52–53.
104. Ibid., 53.
105. Ibid., 55.
106. *AMA Minutes of the House of Delegates…* 1911, 3

107. Ibid.

108. AMA *PHD* Judicial Council 1912, 3.

109. AMA *PHD* 1900, June 1900; see also, Journal of the American Medical Association 1900, "Report," 34 (1900), 1553, 1557, 1559.

110. AMA 1902, "PHD Resolution from the Section on Surgery and Anatomy," June; AMA 1902 "Report," *JAMA* 38, 1661.

111. Harris 1903, 1381; AMA *Principles* 1903, chapter II, article VI, section 4; Appendix IX, this volume.

112. Levy, Anderson, Chapin, and Hill 1912, 275.

113. AMA *PHD* 1911 "Proposed…," 43.

114. AMA *Principles* 1903, chapter I, section 3; Appendix IX, this volume.

115. Soper 1907, 2019–2022.

116. Leavitt 1996, 66–68; New York Times, November 12, 1938; Mary Mallon (Typhoid Mary) 1939.

117. AMA *PHD* 1912, "Principles of Medical Ethics: A Proposed Revision," 12–16; Billings, Frank, et al., *PHD* 1912, 11.

118. AMA *PHD* 1912, "New Principles Adopted," 46–47.

119. AMA *Principles*, 1912, chapter I, section 1, *PHD* 1912, 12.

120. AMA *PHD* 1912, 12.

121. Ibid., 15.

122. Although Percival's 1803 code attempts to replace the concept of gentlemanly honor with a notion of professional ethics, his American followers failed to appreciate his approach and, as argued in Chapter 7, the 1847 code was interpreted through the prism of ideals of gentlemanly honor. The 1912 *Principles* is thus the AMA's first formal step away from this conception, portraying professional ethics as a guide to implementing medicine's primary goal—service to humanity. It is also, as noted in the text, the first official ethics document to use "unprofessional" as a term of moral condemnation equivalent to any other disservice to humanity.

123. Flint 1882, 14.

124. For a well-documented study of this generational shift in conceptions of medicine, see Warner 1991, 454–478.

125. AMA *PHD* 1912, 59.

126. Ibid., 57.

127. AMA *Principles* 1912, 15, chapter III, section 2,

128. Ibid., 12, chapter I, section 2, emphasis added.

129. Ibid., 12, chapter II, section 4.

130. Ibid., 12, chapter II, section 4.

131. Ibid., 15, chapter II, article VI, section 2.

132. Ibid., 13, chapter II, article I, section 5

133. Ibid., 12,chapter I, section 4.

134. Ibid., 15, chapter II, article VI, section 6

135. Lambert, Cooke, Moore et al. 1913 *PHD*, "Report," 12.

136. Ibid., 14.

137. Ibid., 12.

138. Ibid., 13.

139. Ibid., 15.

140. Ibid., 13.

141. Ibid., 14.

142. Ibid., 15.

143. Ibid.

144. Flexner [1910] 1972.

145. Doukas, McCullough, and Wear 2010, 318–322.

146. Lambert, Cooke, Moore et al. 1913 *PHD*, "Report," 15.

147. AMA *PHD* 1924, 21–22, 40.

148. AMA *PHD* 1926, 28; AMA *PHD* 1929, 24–25, 34–35; AMA *PHD* 1934, 11, 50.

149. *AMA PHD* 1935, 1936, 1954, 1955: Resolution from the Section on Laryngology, Otology, and Rhinology, June 1935, 63; May 1936, 45, 56, 63–64, 67; Section on Ophthalmology, Nov.–Dec. 1954, 54–55, 99, 100; June 1955, 40, 50, 52, 53, 64.

150. *AMA PHD*, Resolution from the Section on Laryngology, Otology, and Rhinology, June 1935, 63; May 1936, 45, 56, 63–64, 67; Section on Ophthalmology, Nov.–Dec. 1954, 54–55, 99, 100; June 1955, 40, 50, 52, 53, 64; Dec. 1953, 58, 99, 100; Dec. 1959, 135–136; Nov–Dec. 1960, 112–113; Nov. 1961, 132–134; June 1963, 75. More recently, see a 1992 CEJA "Report," *JAMA* 267 (1992), 2366–2369.

151. AMA *PHD* (CEJA Resolution 21), Nov.–Dec.1969, 243, 313. CEJA 1992 "Report," *AMA* 267, 2366–2369.

152. See, for example, AMA *PHD* Nov.–Dec., 1970, 125, 126, 171.

153. Through the remainder of the twentieth century, the AMA continually had bully pulpit campaigns against fee splitting, steering, and commissions. For a sample, see *PHD*, June 1942, 65,70; June 1947, 58, 94, 96; June 1951, 15–16, 39. In response to a Congressional report issued by the Truman Committee on Medical Practices, a Committee on Medical Practices was formed to investigate complaints of fee splitting; see AMA *PHD* Dec. 1953, 80–81, 99, 100; June 1954, 12; Nov.–Dec. 1954, 51, 90, 91; June 1955, 12–13, 53, 54. On "gifts" from manufacturers and distributors, for example, see AMA *PHD* June 1971, 295, 345; Nov.–Dec. 1971, 208; 235–236.

154. Cunniffe 1946, 15. Internal constituencies, like ophthalmologists, lobbied the committee, "submit[ing] practically every conceivable plan to circumvent the section of the Principles of Medical Ethics concerning rebates" (Cunniffe 1947, 39).

155. Cunniffe 1947, 40.

156. Watson 1850, 25.

157. Cunniffe 1949, 38; AMA *PHD "Report of the Judicial Council," Principles* 1949, 38.

158. AMA *PHD "Report of the Judicial Council," Principles* 1949, chapter I, section 1, 38–39.

159. AMA 1958, Judicial Council, introduction.

160. Ibid., 5; section 1

161. Woodhouse, Ward, Hutcheson, Buie, and Pearson 1957

162. AMA 1958, Judicial Council, 50.

163. Ibid.,

164. Ibid., 51.

165. AMA 1958, 1, Judicial Council.

166. Fox 1979, 81–97; Veatch 2005.

167. Journal of the American Medical Association Editors 1887, "Physicians…,"; Journal of the American Medical Association Editors 1887 "Indirect…"; Journal of the American Medical Association Editors 1888 "Unethical…"; Journal of the American Medical Association Editors 1888 "Doctors…" ; Journal of the American Medical Association Editors 1888 "To Be Tried…" ; Solis-Cohen 1892.

168. Journal of the American Medical Association Editors 1883, "Address" *1*(2), July 21, 37; (8), Sept. 1, 247; (13), Oct. 6, 398–400.

169. Graham 1886, 477–480; Davis 1886 "Dr. Graham's Address," 491–492; Davis 1886, "The Higher Education of Women" 267–269.

170. Davis 1885, "The Moral Side of Euthanasia," 382.

171. Davis 1888, "Medical Colleges and Medical Ethics."

172. Journal of the American Medical Association Editors 1887, "Clergymen…"

173. Journal of the American Medical Association Editors 1887, "Sects…"

174. Journal of the American Medical Association Editors 1883, *1*(2), July 21, 38; (17) Nov. 3, 511–512; 1888, *11*(21), 741–742.

175. Journal of the American Medical Association Editors 1883, 1(14), 430; Journal of the American Medical Association Editors 1885, "Domestic…"; Davis 1886, "The Division…" .

176. Journal of the American Medical Association Editors 1885, "Domestic Correspondence."

177. Journal of the American Medical Association Editors 1883, *1*(2), July 21, 37; (8) Sept. 1, 246; (17), Nov. 3, 511–512; Journal of the American Medical Association Editors 1885, 5(20), 551–552; Journal of the American Medical Association Editors 1886, "What Constitutes a Consultation" ; 1887 *7*(22), 616; Journal of the American Medical Association Editors 1888, *10*(3), 94; Journal of the American Medical Association Editors *15*(19), 698–699; Journal of the American Medical Association Editors 1888, "To Be Tried…"; Briggs 1891; 1892, "The Code of Ethics," *18*(13), 396; "Revision of the Code of Ethics," 19(10), 293.

178. Davis 1888, "Humanity…," 114–115.

179. Parvin 1890, 369–373.

180. Journal of the American Medical Association Editors 1891.

181. Journal of the American Medical Association Editors 1886, "Letter From London."

182. Journal of the American Medical Association Editors 1892, "Honesty…"

183. Journal of the American Medical Association Editors 1888, 11(25), 850.

184. Early 1891, 758.

185. Journal of the American Medical Association Editors 1886, "Book Reviews."

186. Journal of the American Medical Association Editors 1890, "Antivivisection Bitterness"; Journal of the American Medical Association Editors 1891, "The Ethics of Experimentation Upon Living Animals."

187. Journal of the American Medical Association Editors 1886, "Gynecological Society"; Journal of the American Medical Association Editors 1887, "Criminal Abortions"; Steele

1887; Journal of the American Medical Association Editors 1888, "The Ethics of Marriage" ; Journal of the American Medical Association Editors "Criminal Abortion and State Laws" ; (14), 502; (16), 573; Journal of the American Medical Association Editors 1888, "Professional Abortionists."

188. Davis 1888, "The Ethics...," 309–311; Parvin 1890, 370–371.

189. Markham 1888, 805–806; Parvin 1890, 371–373.

190. Davis 1885, 382–383.

191. Davis 1886, "Is Life...," 323–324.

192. *Buck v. Bell, Superintendent of the Colony for Epileptics and the Feeble Minded*, May 2, 1927, 247 US 200, in Lombardo 2008, 285–287.

193. AMA 1928, *PHD*, 62.

194. AMA 1933, *PHD*, 41.

195. AMA 1936, Report Committee to Study Contraceptive Practices, *PHD*, 54.

196. Myerson, Ayer, Putnam, et al. 1936. The ANA, however, did not condemn compulsory sterilization for purported "imbeciles" like Carrie Buck. The classic case on compulsory sterilization for criminality is *Skinner v. State of Oklahoma, ex. rel. Williamson*, 316 U.S. 535 (1942), in which the U.S. Supreme Court struck down Oklahoma's compulsory sterilization law. See Nourse 2008.

197. Emanuel 1994, 796.

198. Pernick 1996, 5–6.

199. Ibid., 7.

200. Davis 1885, 382–383; Davis 1886, "Is Life...," 323–324.

201. AMA *PHD (Clinical Conventions)* December, 1973. "Report of the Judicial Council." *PHD*, 139–140.

202. Ibid., 140.

203. In February 1973, the MSSNY adopted the following: "The use of euthanasia is not in the province of the physician. The right to die with dignity, or the cessation of the employment of extraordinary means to prolong the life of the body when there is irrefutable evidence that biological death is inevitable, is the decision of the patient and/or the immediate family with the approval of the family physician" (AMA *PHD (Clinical Convention)* December, 1973, 137–139).

204. Pius XII 1957.

205. See Wildes 1996, 500–512.

Chapter 9: American Research Ethics, 1800–1946

1. Osler, Sir William 1907, 7, 8.

2. Hornsby, Schmidt 1913, 281–282

3. Ibid., 465.

4. Katz, Jay [1984] 2002, 2.

5. Fletcher wrote this in a commentary on the infamous Tuskegee Syphilis Study; see Fletcher 2000, 280.

6. Walsh 1919, vol. 1, 24–25.

7. Other bioethicists and historians of medical ethics have made similar observations about the long history of informed consent practices; see Beauchamp, Faden 1986; Lederer [1995] 1997; Pernick 1982; Powderly 2000.

8. Walsh 1919, vol. 1, 24–25.

9. The classic British case is *Slater v. Baker and Stapleton* (1767); influential twentieth-century U.S. cases prior to *Schloendorff* include *Mohr v. Williams* (Minnesota Supreme Court 1905), *Pratt v. Davis* (Illinois Supreme Court 1906), *Rolater v. Strain* (Oklahoma Supreme Court 1913).

10. Malpractice lawsuits were not a significant factor in the practice of American medicine in the eighteenth or early nineteenth century. By the end of the nineteenth century, however, they began to assert a significant influence on the minds of practitioners. See De Ville 1990; Mohr 2000, 1731–1737.

11. Osler, Sir William, second edition, [1897] 1898, 183.

12. Osler, Sir William, third edition, [1897] [1898] 1901, 183–184.

13. Osler, Sir William [1897] [1898] 1901, 183–184. These experiments were commemorated in Dean Cornwell's (1892–1960) *Pioneers of American Medicine* painting series (1939–1942)—copies of which were circulated in a pamphlet by John Wyeth Pharmaceuticals during this same period. The passage accompanying the painting of Walter Reed and colleagues emphasizes his use of "volunteers."

14. Hornsby, Schmidt 1913, 281–282.

15. Goffman 1958, 43–84.

16. Anonymous 1866; Grier 2006, 45.

17. Beaumont's granddaughter, Lucretia Beaumont Irwin, presented these journals, his letters, and other papers to the Becker Medical Library at the Washington University School of Medicine in St. Louis in 1915. Many are available at http://beckerarchives.wustl.edu/index.php?p=collections/findingaid&id=8636 . Yale University holds a collection of Beaumont's early papers.

18. Meyer 1912, 23. Beaumont copied out passages that he found personally significant from various texts as part of a continuing self-improvement project. This is likely to have been such a passage, but the source is not known.

19. In the context of flytes and duels, to "post" someone is, quite literally, to post a written statement, often printed, in which one maligned an opponent as lacking the virtues of a true gentleman. Thus, Beaumont's post charges Richards with being a liar, a villain, and poltroon, and thus lacking the gentlemanly virtues of honesty, honor, and courage. Had Richards refused to apologize and accepted the challenge, the two officers would have dueled off the post with pistols; other officers would have officiated as seconds.

20. Meyer 1912, 58; Horsman 1996, 71, 78.

21. Meyer 1912, 57–60.

22. The newspaper article probably summarized the moral perfection section of Benjamin Franklin's (1706–1790) biography from one of several American editions published around that period.

23. Meyer 1912, 78.

24. Beaumont 1826–1830. *Case Book and* Aphorisms. The emphasis is in the original; however, the numbers in parentheses were added for ease of analysis. They are not in the original.

25. Numbers 1979, 134.

26. Beaumont [1823] 1825.

27. Meyer 1912, 57–59.

28. Beaumont November 18, 1822–January 12, 1825, 22–23. The emphasis is in the original; no specific date in June 1824 indicated.

29. Historian Numbers suggests that "science may have motivated Beaumont more than charity, that his successful administration of medicine through the fistula [i.e., the abnormal opening into the stomach] triggered the notion that other, more interesting, experiments could be performed. In short, he recognized St Martin's potential for science" (Numbers 1979, 114).

30. Beaumont January 1834, Memorial to 23rd Congress. Emphasis in the original.

31. Beaumont, Deborah, and William, December 18, 1823.

32. Dr. Beaumont's entries about St. Martin's age were off by a decade. He was probably 30 years old at the time Mrs. Beaumont's letter was written; however, since neither Dr. Beaumont nor his wife spoke French, and since St. Martin spoke little or no English, miscommunication was always a problem in their relations. Nonetheless, by this time, Mrs. Beaumont is likely to have appreciated that she was dealing with a mature man; her reference to St. Martin as a "boy" is likely to have been an indicator of his social status as a servile dependent.

33. Beaumont, William 1824, Beaumont, Surgeon, U.S.A. [Ft. Niagara, NY] to Joseph Lovell, Surgeon General [Washington, DC] September 1824. "A singular case …

34. Matthews, W. August 13, 1827, "Letter…Regarding encounter with St. Martin…." Emphasis in the original.

35. Matthews, W. August 13, 1827, "Letter…Regarding reimbursement…."

36. Green 2010.

37. Beaumont, William 1832, "W. Beaumont and St. Martin, Four Articles of Agreement."

38. Calculation from Measuring Worth website.

39. Meyer 1912, 148.

40. Numbers 1979, 132.

41. Ibid., 118–120.

42. Bliss 1999, 113.

43. Committee of Commemoration of Alexis Bidagan dit St. Martin of the Canadian Medical Society 1963, 63–65.

44. Sims 1854, 1.

45. World Health Organization 2010.

46. Sims [1858] 1990, 55.

47. In 1884, the year after Sims's death in 1883, his autobiography, *The Story of My Life*, was edited and published by the New York house of Appleton and Company by Sims' son, Harry Marion-Sims, over the objections of Sims' widow and daughters. Sims had dictated

the incomplete typescript draft from memory over a two-month period, apparently inspired by reminiscences he recounted to amuse and distract a dying patient. See Harris, Seale 1950, 361–364.

48. Sims [1884, 1885] 1898, 227.

49. Ibid., 229–230.

50. Ibid.

51. Ibid., 231.

52. Ibid., 234–235.

53. AMA 1849, *Transactions* 33, 211–218; 34, 241–251.

54. As late as 1857, Sims did not recommend using anesthetics for operations correcting obstetric fistulas because "they are not painful enough to justify the trouble and risk" (Sims [1858] 1990, 31). See also Pernick 1985.

55. Sims [1858] 1990, 245.

56. Sims 1852.

57. Sims [1884, 1885] 1898, 259.

58. Ibid., 266. The implication of this surprising remark is that, until this time, Sims believed that his slaves willingly accepted their enslaved status.

59. Sims [1884, 1885] 1898, 266.

60. Sims 1854, 1. A shortened version of this statement is given in the Silver Sutures lecture, Sims [1858] 1990, 52, and in *The Story of My Life,* Sims [1884, 1885] 1898, 236.

61. Sims 1854, 1.

62. Sims [1884, 1885] 1898, 241–242.

63. Sims [1858] 1990, 55.

64. Sims [1884, 1885] 1898, 227.

65. Ibid., 229–230.

66. Sims 1854, 1; Sims [1858] 1990, 52; Sims [1884, 1885] 1898, 236.

67. Sims [1884, 1885] 1898, 241–242.

68. Sims 1854, 1; Sims [1884, 1885] 1898, 241–242.

69. Sims [1884, 1885] 1898, 241–242.

70. Ibid., 229–230.

71. Goldner 2001.

72. Digital History.

73. Sims 1854, 1; Sims [1858] 1990, 52; Sims [1884, 1885] 1898, 236.

74. Sims [1884, 1885] 1898, 234–235, emphasis added.

75. Mays 2011; New York Times, October 21, 1894.

76. J. Marion Sims Statue, Montgomery Alabama (http://www.panoramio.com/photo/66424080); Sims statue in New York's Central Park, opposite the New York Academy of Medicine (http://www.centralparknyc.org/visit/things-to-see/north-end/dr-j-marion-sims.html [accessed August 10, 2011]); Sims statue in South Carolina: Marion Sims–Columbia, SC–Statues of Historic Figures on Waymarking.com (http://www.waymarking.com/waymarks/WM9JW3_J_Marion_Sims_Columbia_SC). All sites accessed November 12, 2012.

77. Ojanuga 1993, 30.

78. Axelson 1985; quoted at Ojanuga 1993, 30.

79. McGregor 1998, 51, 54.

80. Washington 2007, 67.

81. Wall 2006, "Did J. Marion Sims...Addict," 336–356.

82. Beauchamp and Faden 1986, 76–82; Pernick 1982, 1–35; Powderly 2000, 12–27.

83. Sims [1866] 1990, 330.

84. Ibid., 331–332.

85. Ibid., 332.

86. Ibid., 333. Note that, as a prelude to divorce, the young lady in question was no longer living with her husband but rather with her mother, who had assumed the role of her guardian and thus had the prerogative of consenting or refusing to consent to an experiment.

87. Sims uses the term "experiment" more broadly than does Beaumont. Beaumont's does not describe surgical innovations designed to save his patient's life as "experiments." He reserved the term "experiment" for efforts designed to create generalizable new knowledge. Sims, in contrast, characterizes any form of surgical innovation as an "experiment," irrespective of whether the effort is simply a nonstandard therapy designed to benefit a particular patient or an effort to create generalizable new knowledge.

88. Sims [1866] 1990, 331–332.

89. Ibid.

90. Sims 1854, 1; Sims [1858] 1990, 52; Sims [1884, 1885] 1898, 236.

91. Sims [1858] 1990, 55

92. Ibid., 333.

93. Sims [1866] 1990, 333.

94. Gruenewaldt 1854; cited at Numbers 1979, 130–131.

95. Kollock 1857; cited at Wall "Medical Ethics..." 2006, 347.

96. World Health Organization 2010.

97. Sims [1884] [1885] 1898, 88.

98. Cartwright 1851, 703; see also Faust 1981.

99. Sims [1884] [1885] 1898, 266.

100. Sims 1876, 93.

101. National Commission for the Protection of Human Subjects of Biomedical and Behavioral Research 1979, section B.3.

102. Wall 2006, "Medical Ethics," 349.

103. Cirillo 2004.

104. New York Times Editors 1898, cited in Malkin 1993, 677.

105. Rowton 2009, 2.

106. Sternberg, May 14, 1900, Letter to Agramonte.

107. Lederer [1995] 1997, 21–22.

108. Ibid.

109. Gallinger [1900] 1995; in Lederer [1995] 1997, 143–146, at 143.

110. Gallinger [1900] 1995, section 5; in Lederer [1995] 1997, 145.

111. Gallinger [1900] 1995, section 6; in Lederer [1995] 1997, 145.

112. Carroll, James, November 22, 1900, Letter from Major James Carroll to Jenifer Carroll.

113. Reed, Walter. November 22, 1900. Letter from Walter Reed to Emilie Lawrence Reed.

114. Sternberg 1901, 233. Cited by Lederer 2008, 13.

115. Reed, Carroll, Agramonte Feb. 4–7, 1901. Cited in McCaw 1904, 110. Later published as Reed, Carroll, Agramonte 1901.

116. Carroll, August 18, 1906, *Report to the Surgeon General*; see also Leon, Letter to Hench October 10, 1940; and Hench October 26, 1940.

117. Carroll, August 18, 1906, *Report to the Surgeon General.*

118. Ibid.

119. Reed, Walter. September 25, 1900. Letter... to Kean, September 25, 1900. For another perspective, see Altman [1987] 1998, 129–158.

120. Some experiments on volunteers had been conducted before this; however, they were less formal than the experiments devised at this later point under Reed's supervision.

121. Moran 19??, 7–9.

122. Measuring Worth.com.

123. Moran 19??, 8.

124. Measuring Worth.com.

125. Benigno, Antonio. November 26, 1900. Spanish language version available at Archives of the Philip D. Hench Walter Reed Collection, University of Virginia http://yellowfever.lib.virginia.edu/reed/collection.html

126. Carroll, August 18, 1906, *Report to the Surgeon General.*

127. McCaw 1904, 110.

128. Ibid., 21–22. Emphasis in the original.

129. Carroll, August 18, 1906, *Report to the Surgeon General.*

130. Lederer 2008, 12–13. More generally, see Lederer [1995] 1997.

131. See Turner 1980 and, for a different perspective, Rudacille 2000.

132. The classic study of the impact of antivivisectionism on research ethics is Lederer 1995.

133. Bigelow 1871, 42.

134. Ibid.

135. Ibid., 44.

136. Ibid.

137. Ibid., 44–44.

138. Ibid., 43.

139. Cannon 1922, 190.

140. Taber 1906, 3.

141. Ibid.

142. Ibid.

143. Barthlow 1874, 310–311.

144. Taber 1906, 17–19.

145. Ibid., 20.

146. Taber 1907, 1–2.
147. James [1875] 1987, vol. 15, 11.
148. James [1909] 1987, vol. 15, 191.
149. AMA 1900, "Association News."
150. AMA 1908, "PHD, Annual Session."
151. AMA 1909, "PHD 1909." 2073.
152. AMA 1910, *PHD*, 24.
153. Ibid.
154. See Bliss 1982 [2007]; Cooper and Ainsberg 2010.
155. Bigelow 1871, 44.
156. Cannon 1916, 1373.
157. Ibid.
158. Flexner [1910] 1972.
159. Doukas, McCullough, Wear 2010.

Chapter 10: Explaining the Birth of Bioethics, 1947–1999

1. Kipling 1902.
2. Stowe [1852] 1853, 266.
3. Rothman 1991; Jonsen 1998; Stevens 2000; Fox and Swazey 2008; Evans 2012.
4. See, e.g., Stevens 2000, ix.
5. Stevens 2000, 47.
6. The tale is associated with Buddhist, Jain, and Hindu philosophy. It probably made its way into American culture through a poem by American poet John Godfrey Saxe (1816–1887), "The Blind Men and the Elephant." See Saxe, John Godfrey.
7. Thalidomide Trust.
8. Gaw 2012, 150–155.
9. Campbell 2000, 195–198.
10. Ibid., 195.
11. For a detailed chronology, see Baker and McCullough 2009, "A Chronology...," 77–97.
12. History of Soft Drinks.
13. New York Times, May 27, 2007.
14. AMA [1957] 1999, 355–356; emphasis added.
15. Thomasma, Kushner, Kimsma, et al. 1998.
16. Aaron and Schwartz 1984.
17. Headlines from the *New York Times* and the *Saturday Review* in 1962, cited in Carpenter 2010, 247. For accounts of Kelsey and the thalidomide story, see Carpenter 2010, 238–256; Jonsen 1998, 140–142; Rothman 1991, 63–64.
18. Subcommittee of the [New York State] Committee on Grievances [1965] 1972, 54. The physicians were Chester Southam (1919–2002), professor of medicine at Cornell University and division chief at the Sloan Kettering Institute for Cancer Research, and Emanuel Mandel, director of medicine at Jewish Chronic Disease Hospital.

19. Beecher 1966, 1354–1360.

20. Harkness, Lederer, and Wikler 2001, 365–2366.

21. According to the U.S. Department of Agriculture webpage, two articles in the popular press inspired the act. The first, by "Coles Phinizy [which appeared] in the November 29, 1965, issue of *Sports Illustrated*, details the story of Pepper the Dalmatian. [After realizing that Pepper had been dognapped] U. S. Representative Joseph Resnick (D-New York) was contacted.... Unfortunately, Pepper had been euthanized in an experimental procedure at a New York hospital and thus never returned to her owners. On July 9, 1965, Rep. Resnick introduced H.R. 9743, a bill that would require dog and cat dealers, and the laboratories that purchased the animals, be licensed and inspected by the USDA." A second article, published in 1966 by *Life Magazine* was titled "Concentration Camp for Dogs" and featured pictures of skeletal dogs; see Adams and Larson 2012.

22. Carpenter 2010, 549.

23. Washington, Baker, Olakanmi, Savitt, Jacobs, Hoover, and Wynia 2009, "Segregation...," 513–527.

24. Senator Edward Long. May 10, 1966. F 0273–04 (FDA Correspondence 1959–1972); cited in Carpenter 2010, 370.

25. Percival 1794, section 1, article XII.

26. Percival 1803, chapter I, article XII, 14–15; emphasis in the original.

27. Beecher 1970, 218.

28. Kappa Lambda Society of Hippocrates 1823. "Extracts...."

29. Statements about the "first" are hazardous since few things are without precedent. However, insofar as the distinctive feature of the research ethics committees proposed by Percival and exemplified by contemporary IACUCs and IRBs is review and approval *prior* to initiation of an experiment, the NEHW committee is the earliest hospital research ethics committee known to the author.

30. Storer, Horatio R. 1867, "Female...," 191.

31. Zakrzewska 1924, 340. The NEHW committee differs from that proposed by Percival in some important respects. Percival's committee assessed only proposed "*new remedies [or] new methods of chirurgical treatment*"; the scope of the NEHW committee is said to be "unusual or difficult cases ... where a capital operation in surgery is proposed," so it would appear to apply not only to innovative surgery, but to all "difficult cases." What proved most controversial was that, whereas Percival's committees have surgeons as the sole judges of surgical cases, the NEHW committee allows physicians to assess the benefits of a surgical procedure.

32. Storer, Horatio R. 1867, "Female...," 191.

33. Ibid.

34. Ibid., 192.

35. Ibid., 191.

36. Storer, Horatio R. 1867, *Is it I*, 89–90.

37. Senator Edward Long, May 10, 1966. F 0273–04 (FDA Correspondence 1959–1972); cited in Carpenter 2010, 370.

38. Jonsen 1998, 142–143.

39. Rothman 1991, 56.

39. U.S. Senate Subcommittee on Government Research 1968. See Jonsen 1998, 90–94; Rothman 1991, 168–184.

40. Barnard [1968] 1991, 173.

41. Wangensteen [1968] 1991, 173.

42. Ibid., 173–174.

43. The "Belmont Report" is named for the Maryland conference center at which it was drafted. The conference center was formerly part of the Smithsonian Institution.

44. U.S. Department of Health and Human Services 1978. For further background, see Childress, Meslin, and Shaprio, eds. 2005.

45. Osler 1907, 8.

46. Rothman 1991, 56.

47. Taylor, Telford [1946] 1992, 67. The formal indictment states that the accused "were principals in, accessories to … medical experiments, without the subjects' consent, upon German civilians and nationals of other countries, in the course of which experiments the defendants committed murders, brutalities, cruelties, tortures, atrocities, and other inhuman acts." See Nuremberg Trials: The Doctors' Trial.

48. U.S. Department of Health and Human Services 1978.

49. Barnett 1974, 28.

50. U.S. Public Health Service 1973, 166, 172–173; emphasis added.

51. Ibid., 166, 172.

52. Kampmeier 1972, 1247–1251.

53. Buxton 1968, 105.

54. Buxton 1973, 154.

55. To qualify this point, it should be noted that in his influential proto-bioethical book, *The Patient As Person*, Methodist theologian Paul Ramsey (1913–1988) attempted to translate Christian ethics into a secular medical ethics based on fidelity (Ramsey 1970, xii), in which consent was "a canon of loyalty" (Ramsey 1970, 5). At one point, however, Ramsey remarks that "a rule governing medical experimentation on human beings is needed to insure that no person shall be degraded and treated as a thing or as an animal in order that good may come of it" (Ramsey 1970, 9). This captures Buxton's repulsion against "being used." Nonetheless, despite have this important insight into the issue, Ramsey actually justified the practice of consenting to experimentation not in terms of this concept of degrading persons into things, but in terms of the concept of fidelity.

56. National Commission for the Protection of Human Subjects of Biomedical and Behavioral Research 1978.

57. Wittgenstein [1980] 1984, 42e.

58. Engelhardt Jr. 1978, In National Commission for the Protection of Human Subjects of Biomedical and Behavioral Research 1978, Appendix I, Essay 8.

59. Beauchamp 1978, In National Commission for the Protection of Human Subjects of Biomedical and Behavioral Research 1978, Appendix I, Essay 6.

60. Jonsen 2005, 4.

61. Engelhardt Jr. 1978, In National Commission for the Protection of Human Subjects of Biomedical and Behavioral Research 1978, Appendix I, Essay 8, 8.

62. Engelhardt Jr. 1978, In National Commission for the Protection of Human Subjects of Biomedical and Behavioral Research 1978, Appendix I, Essay 8, 4.

63. Engelhardt Jr. 1978, In National Commission for the Protection of Human Subjects of Biomedical and Behavioral Research 1978, Appendix I, Essay 8, 4.

64. National Commission for the Protection of Human Subjects of Biomedical and Behavioral Research 1978, Part B.

65. Wenger [1933] 2000, 85.

66. Beauchamp 1978, In National Commission for the Protection of Human Subjects of Biomedical and Behavioral Research 1978, Appendix I, Essay 6, 17.

67. National Commission for the Protection of Human Subjects of Biomedical and Behavioral Research 1978, Part B.

68. Stillé 1871, 91–94.

69. Governors of the General Hospital of Bath 1744 cited in Fissell 1993 28. Emphasis in the original.

70. Fox and Swazey 2008, 154.

71. National Commission for the Protection of Human Subjects of Biomedical and Behavioral Research 1978, Part B.

72. National Commission for the Protection of Human Subjects of Biomedical and Behavioral Research 1978, Part C.

73. Wittgenstein 1961, statement 7.

74. Jonsen 1998, 83–84.

75. Engelhardt Jr. [1986] 1996, 5.

76. Kuhn, T. 1970, 137.

77. Beauchamp also served on the staff of the National Commission and was involved in the semifinal revision of the text of the Belmont Report; see Beauchamp 2003, 17–46.

78. Beauchamp and Childress 1979, vi.

79. Ibid., ix.

80. Kant [1798] 1998, 2004.

81. Beauchamp and Childress 1979, 56–57.

82. Wittgenstein 1961, statement 5.6; see also 5.61.

83. Jonsen, Rothman, and Stevens discuss some morally disruptive technologies in detail; Evans, Fox, and Swazey focus on other factors in their construction of the history of bioethics; see Jonsen 1998, 107–118, 166–324; Rothman 1991, 144–167, 222–246; Stevens 2000, 75–149.

84. Ad Hoc Committee of the Harvard Medical School to Examine Brain Death 1968, 337.

85. Ibid.

86. Ibid., 339.

87. Pius XII 1957.

88. Ad Hoc Committee of the Harvard Medical School to Examine Brain Death 1968, 340; quotations from Pope Pius XII 1957.

89. Jonsen 1998, 239–240.

90. Ibid.

91. AMA 1977, Judicial Council, 23.

92. This illustration is drawn from a lecture by lawyer-bioethicist George Annas.

93. President's Commission for the Study of Ethical Problems in Medicine and Biomedical and Behavioral Research 1981, 2.

94. Hilberman 1975, 159–165.

95. AMA 1966, Judicial Council; published as Williamson 1966, 793–795.

96. AMA 1968, Judicial Council.

97. Ayd 1968, 9–11.

98. AMA 1977, Judicial Council, 23.

99. Ibid.

100. Ad Hoc Committee of the Harvard Medical School to Examine Brain Death 1968, 337.

101. *In Re Quinlan*, In The Matter Of Karen Quinlan, An Alleged Incompetent. Supreme Court of New Jersey, 70 N.J. 10. 1976. 355 A.2d 647.

102. Teel 1975, 6–9.

103. Stevens 2000, 142.

104. Clinical Care Committee of the Massachusetts General Hospital 1976, 362–364.

105. Younger, Jackson, Coulton, et al. 1983, 443–457.

106. Prosnitz 1983, 439–442.

107. Jonsen 1998, 363.

108. Joint Commission on the Accreditation of Healthcare Organizations 1989.

109. Jonsen 1998, 363–364.

110. Ibid., 338–339.

111. American Association of Medical Colleges 1998, 4–5.

112. Presad, Elder, Sedig, et al. 2008, 4, 89–94.

113. President's Commission for the Study of Ethical Problems in Medicine and Biomedical and Behavioral Research 1983, 3–9.

114. Wittgenstein 1955.

115. President's Commission for the Study of Ethical Problems in Medicine and Biomedical and Behavioral Research 1983, 4.

116. Ibid., 89–90.

117. *Cruzan v. Director* 1990.

118. Queens County (NY) Grand Jury [1984] 1995, 12.

119. President's Commission for the Study of Ethical Problems in Medicine and Biomedical and Behavioral Research 1983, 89–90.

120. Ibid., 250–251.

121. Wallis 2011, 623–624.

122. AMA [1847] 1999, chapter III, article I, section 1.

123. Keen 1900, 1593–1594.

124. AMA 1912, "Principles…," chapter III, section 2.

125. Flexner, Simon, and James Flexner 1941, 377.

126. Taubenberger and Morens 2006, 15–22.

127. AMA CEJA 1958, 55. Some scholars claim that this duty was deleted in 1957. Actually, the provision was demoted from a principle to an annotation, but it remained in the AMA's 1957–1976 *Principles of Medical Ethics*.

128. AMA CEJA 1986.

129. Ibid. This was modified the next year as follows: "Where there is no statute that mandates or prohibits the reporting of seropositive individuals to public health authorities and a physician knows that a seropositive individual is endangering a third party, the physician should: (1) attempt to persuade the infected party to cease endangering the third party; (2) if persuasion fails, notify authorities; and (3) if the authorities take no action, notify the endangered third party" (AMA, CEJA 1987, 4).

130. AMA CEJA 1986.

131. Ibid.

132. International Association of Fire Fighters 2012. The IAFF (founded in 1918) proudly honors firefighters who "*Answered the Call*: On the morning of September 11, 2001, [when] hijacked planes were flown into the World Trade Center towers in New York City, the Pentagon outside Washington DC, and a Pennsylvania field" especially "the 343 IAFF members [who] died." The website memorializes these fallen firefighters as heroes. "*Never Forget.* On October 12, 2001 the IAFF and FDNY held a memorial service for fire fighters who lost their lives on 9/11 … a procession of 356 honor guard members from around the country, each of whom carried a flag for a fallen fire fighter." Although the United Nations and other organizations celebrate physicians who risk their lives treating HIV, SARS, and other epidemic diseases, organized American medicine no longer celebrates them as heroes.

133. AMA 1912, "Principles…," chapter I, section I; AMA 1912 *PHD*, 12.

134. Ibid., chapter III, section 2; AMA 1912 *PHD*, 15.

135. Ibid., chapter II, article VI, section 2; AMA 1912 *PHD*, 15.

136. Ibid., chapter I, section 3; AMA 1912 *PHD*, 12.

137. AMA, CEJA 1958, *Principles of Medical Ethics, JAMA,* 23.

138. Ibid., 55.

139. Ibid., 53.

140. AMA, CEJA 1977, *Principles of Medical Ethics, JAMA*, 1.

141. Centers for Disease Control and Prevention (CDC) estimates of mortality reported on Flu.gov.

142. Some commentators suggest that because, in 1972, the U.S. Surgeon General declared that it was time to "close the book" on infectious diseases, and because, in 1977, the medical profession was preparing to celebrate the global eradication of smallpox, discussions of doctors duties during epidemics may have appeared anachronistic; see Huber and Wynia 2004, W7.

143. Cover 1983, 40–44.

144. Sade and Morin 2001, 72–75.

145. AMA CEJA 1986.

146. AMA, CEJA 1986–1987,,1–8.

147. AMA, CEJA 1987. See also AMA, CEJA 1988, 1360–1361.

148. AMA, CEJA 1987, 1.

149. Ibid., 2; emphasis added.

150. Ibid., 1.

151. Ibid., 2.

152. Wallis 2011, 642.

153. Ibid., 627. See also the entire issue of the *Mount Sinai Journal of Medicine* 1989, vol. 56.

154. Wallis 2011, 627.

155. Annas 1988, 847; cited at Wallis 2011, 642.

156. Freedman 1988, S24.

157. American College of Physicians Ad Hoc Committee on Medical Ethics 1984.

158. Ibid., 34–50. Among the bioethicists cited were Henry Beecher, Howard Brody, Tom Beauchamp, Daniel Callahan, Eric Cassell, James Childress, Charles Curran, Norman Daniels, Joseph Fletch, Samuel Gorovitz, Hans Jonas, Albert Jonsen, Leon Kass, Robert Levine, Ruth Macklin, William May, Stephen Miles, Edmund Pellegrino, Paul Ramsey, Mark Siegler, Stephen Toulmin, and LeRoy Walters, as well as the reports of both the National Commission and the President's Commission.

159. American College of Physicians and Infectious Diseases Society of America 1988, 460–469.

160. American College of Physicians 1989, 10–11.

161. Wallis 2011, 646–647.

BIBLIOGRAPHY

Abbreviations

AMA: American Medical Association. The AMA's archives offer digitized versions of the following materials at http://www.ama-assn.org/ama/pub/about-ama/our-history/ama-historical-archives/the-digital-collection-historical-ama-documents.page?

- *Transactions*: A record of AMA meetings from 1848 to 1882
- *Proceedings of the House of Delegates (PHD)* 1883–1909 (some gaps)
- *Digest of Actions,* which offers a guide to policy development.

CEJA: Reports of the AMA's Council on Ethical and Judicial Affairs: *Journal of the American Medical Association.* These are most easily located by means of the AMA's *Digest of Actions.*

MSCNY: Medical Society of the State of New York (County)/County of New York.

Records of the Manhattan-based MSCNY from the eighteenth and nineteenth centuries are housed at the library of the New York Academy of Medicine (NYAM), including records of the *comita minora.*

MSSNY: Medical Society of the State of New York: Copies of the nineteenth-century *Transactions* of the society and some records of its *comita minora* can be found at the library of the NYAM.

Bibliography

A Conservative Member. 1892. "The Proposition to Revise the Code of Ethics." *Journal of the American Medical Association* 19(24): 706; 1893. *Journal of the American Medical Association* 20(2): 51–52, 20(6): 156–158, 20(7): 183–186, 20(9): 258–260, 20(18): 509–510.

Aaron, Henry, and William Schwartz. 1984. *The Painful Prescription: Rationing Health Care.* Washington DC: The Brookings Institution.

Abbott, Andrew. 1988. *The System of Professions: An Essay on the Division of Expert Labor.* Chicago: University of Chicago Press.

Aberdeen University Court. 1888. Minutes of a meeting held on May 21, 1888 Aberdeen: University of Aberdeen.

Ad Hoc Committee of the Harvard Medical School to Examine Brain Death. 1968. "A Definition of Irreversible Coma." *Journal of the American Medical Association*, 6(205): 337.

Adams, Benjamin, and Jean Larson. 2012. "Legislative History of the Animal Welfare Act." U.S. Department of Agriculture: National Agricultural Library. http://www.nal.usda.gov/awic/pubs/AWA2007/intro.shtml (accessed August 3, 2012).

Adams, Francis. [1849] 1942. "The Oath." In *The Genuine Works of Hippocrates Translated from the Greek with a Preliminary Discourse and Annotation.* London: The Sydenham Society. Selection in *Source Book of Medical History*, edited by Clendening and Logan, 14. New York: Dover Publications.

Agnew, R. 2008. "John Forbes FRS (1787–1861)." *JLL Bulletin: Commentaries on the History of Treatment Evaluation.* From *Proceedings of the Royal Society* (1862–63). http://www.jameslindlibrary.org/illustrating/articles/john-forbes-frs-1787–1861 (accessed January 19, 2011).

Altman, Lawrence. [1987] 1998. *Who Goes First? The Story of Self-Experimentation in Medicine*, Berkeley: University of California Press.

AMA. 1847. "Minutes of the Proceedings of the National Medical Convention, Held in the City of New York, in May, 1846." In *Minutes of the Proceedings of the National Medical Conventions, Held in New York, May, 1846, and in, Philadelphia, May, 1847.* Philadelphia: T. K. & P. G. Collins.

AMA. [1847] 1999. "Code of Ethics." In *The American Medical Ethics Revolution: How the AMA's Code of Ethics Has Transformed Physician's Relationships to Patients, Professionals, and Society*, edited by R. Baker, A. Caplan, L. Emanuel, and S. Latham, 324–334. Baltimore: Johns Hopkins University Press.

AMA. 1857. "Minutes of the Eleventh Annual Meeting of the American Medical Association held in the City of Nashville, Tenn., May 1857." *Transactions*, XI, 30.

AMA. 1859. "Minutes of the Thirteenth Annual Meeting of the American Medical Association held in the City of Louisville, May 3, 1859." *Transactions*, XIII, 28.

AMA. 1864. "Minutes of the Fourteenth Annual Meeting of the American Medical Association held in the City of Chicago, June 1863," *Transactions, XIV*.

AMA. 1882. "Minutes of the Judicial Council," *Transactions*, 33, 60.

AMA. 1894. "Proceedings of the Forty-fifth Annual Meeting," San Francisco, June 8, 1894. *Journal of the American Medical Association* 22(25), 952.

AMA. 1895. "Official Report of the Proceedings in General Session, 1895 of the Forty-sixth Annual Meeting, May 7, 8, 9, and 10, 1895." *Journal of the American Medical Association* 24, 72–76.

AMA. 1900; "Association News." *Journal of the American Medical Association*, 34(24): 1551.

AMA. 1902. "PHD Resolution from the Section on Surgery and Anatomy, PHD, June, 1902; Report." *Journal of the American Medical Association* 38(1902): 1661.

AMA. 1903. Galley proof of draft of 1903 Principle of Medical Ethics with typescript and hand written corrections and addenda, Archives, JC 2209.

AMA. 1908. "PHD, Annual Session 1908." *Journal of the American Medical Association*, 50(23): 2001.

AMA. 1909. "PHD 1909." *Journal of the American Medical Association*, 52(25): 2031–2085.

AMA. 1910. "Report of Committee on Elaboration of the Principles of Ethics," American Medical Association. 1910. *Minutes of the House of Delegates Proceedings of the Sixty-First Annual Session in St. Louis, 30.*

AMA. 1911. *Minutes of the House of Delegates Proceedings of the Sixty-Second Annual Sesssion, Los Angles, California, June 26–30.*

AMA. 1912. *Minutes of the House of Delegates Proceedings of the Sixty-Third Annual Session Atlantic City, N.J., June 3–6, 1912.*

AMA. 1912. "Principles of Medical Ethics: A Proposed Revision," *Minutes of the House of Delegates Proceedings of the Sixty-Third Annual Session Atlantic City, N.J., June 3–6, 1912*, 12–15.

AMA. 1913. *Minutes of the House of Delegates Proceedings of the Sixty-Fourth Annual Session, Minneapolis, Minn. June 16–20, 1913.*

AMA. 1936. Report of the Committee to Study Contraceptive Practices. *Minutes of the House of Delegates, The Eighty-Seventh Annual Session, held at Kansas City, MO. May 11–13, 1936*, 53–55.

AMA. 1949. *Proceedings of the House of Delegates, The Ninety-Eighth Annual Session, held at Atlantic City, N.J., June 6–10, 1949.*

AMA. 1949. *Principles of Medical Ethics.* Chicago: American Medical Association.

AMA. [1957] 1999. *Code of Medical Ethics: Current Opinions with Annotations, 1998–1999.* Chicago: American Medical Association.

AMA. 1958. Judicial Council. "Principles of Medical Ethics: Opinions and Reports of the Judicial Council, Abstracted and Annotated." *Journal of the American Medical Association* (Special Issue) June 7, 1958.

AMA. 1966. Judicial Council. "Program flyer: First National Congress on Medical Ethics and Professionalism," held October 2–3, 1965 and March 5, 1966." Chicago: AMA Archives JC 37.68/1968, JC39.73/1966.

AMA. 1968. Judicial Council. "Program flyer: Second National Congress on Medical Ethics," held October 5–6, 1968. Chicago: AMA Archives.

AMA. 1969. "CEJA Resolution." *PHD*, Nov.–Dec. 1969: 243, 313.

AMA. 1973. *House of Delegates Proceedings, Clinical Convention 1973, New York City,* "Report of the Judicial Council." *PHD (Clinical Convention)*: 139–140.

AMA. 1977. CEJA, *Judicial Council Opinions and Reports Including the Principles of Medical Ethics and Rules of the Judicial Council.* Chicago: American Medical Association.

AMA. 1977. Judicial Council. "5.15 Definition of Death." In *Opinions and Reports of the Judicial Council.* Chicago: American Medical Association.

AMA. 1986. *Council on Ethical and Judicial Affairs.* CEJA-Report B-I-86: Statement on AIDS. Chicago: American Medical Association.

AMA. 1986–1987. CEJA. "Anonymized Quotations from CEJA Correspondence File." Chicago: AMA Archives.

AMA. 1987. *CEJA. Report A–I-87 "Ethical Issues Involved in the Growing AIDS Crisis."* Chicago: American Medical Association.

AMA. 1988. CEJA: "Ethical Issues Involved in the Growing AIDS Crisis." *Journal of the American Medical Association*, 259: 1360–1361.

AMA. 1995–2012. "Our history." http://www.ama-assn.org/ama/pub/about-ama/our-history.shtml (accessed February 2, 2011).

AMA. 1995–2012. "The Founding of AMA." http://www.ama-assn.org/ama/pub/about-ama/our-history/the-founding-of-ama/our-founder-nathan-smith-davis.shtml (accessed February 2, 2011).

AMA. 1999. *Code of Medical Ethics: Current Opinions with Annotations 1998–1999*. Chicago: American Medical Association.

Ambrose, Charles. 2005. "The Secret Kappa Lambda Society of Hippocrates (and the Origin of the American Medical Association's Principles of Medical Ethics)." *Yale Journal of Biology and Medicine*, 78: 45–56.

American Association of Medical Colleges. 1998. *Report I: Learning Objectives for Medical Student Education: Guidelines for Medical Schools*. Washington, DC: American Association of Medical Colleges.

American College of Physicians Ad Hoc Committee on Medical Ethics. 1984. *American College of Physicians Ethics Manual*. Philadelphia: American College of Physicians.

American College of Physicians and Infectious Diseases Society of America. 1988. "The Acquired Immunodeficiency Syndrome (AIDS) and Infection with the Human Immunodeficiency Virus (HIV)." *Annals of Internal Medicine*, 108: 460–469.

American College of Physicians. 1989. "Medical Risk to the Physician." *Ethics Manual*. Philadelphia: American College of Physicians.

American Institute of Homeopathy. 1846. *Transactions of the American Institute of Homeopathy*. Philadelphia: American Institute of Homeopathy.

American Institute of Homeopathy. 1884. "Report on a Complete Code of Medical Ethics." In *Transactions of the Thirty-seventh Session*. Pittsburgh: Stevenson and Foster.

American Medical Association v. Federal Trade Commission. 638 F.2d 443 (2d Cir. 1980), aff'd by an equally divided Court, 455 U.S. 676. 1982.

American Osteopathic Organization. 1905. "The Code of Ethics of the American Osteopathic Organization." In *The Osteopathic Directory*. Minneapolis: William R. Dobbyn & Sons.

Annan, Gertrude. 1948. "The Academy of Medicine of New York.1825–1830, and Its Contemporary, the New York Academy of Medicine." *Bulletin of the Medical Library Association*, 36(2): 117–123.

Annas, George. 1988. "Not Saints, but Healers: The Legal Duties of Health Care Professionals in the AIDS Epidemic." *American Journal of Public Health*, 78: 844–849.

Anonymous. 1753. "The Use and Importance of the Practice of Physic; Together with the Difficulty of the Science, and the Dismal Havoc Made by Quacks and Pretenders." *The Independent Reflector*, February 15, 1753: 49–50.

Anonymous. [1842] 1974. "British and Foreign Medical Review." In *The Fate of the Concept of Medical Police, 1780–1890. From Medical Police to Social Medicine: Essays in the History of Health Care*, edited by G. Rosen, 14, 446. New York: Science History Publications.

Anonymous. 1846. "Young Physic." *Lancet*. IV(48): 105–107. Reprinted in *The Medical News and Library*. Philadelphia: Lea and Blanchard.

Anonymous. 1866. *Book of Household Pets, 45*. New York: Dick & Fitzgerald. See also Grier, Katherine. 2006. Chapel Hill: North Carolina University Press & Orlando (FL) Harcourt Books.

Anonymous. 1870. "Medical Miscellany: The American Medical Association." *Boston Medical and Surgical Journal,* May 5, 1870, 82: 344.

Anonymous. 1870. "The Doctors: The Question of Color." *New York Times.* May 7, 1870: 3.

Appel, T. A. 2010. "The Thomsonian Movement, the Regular Profession, and the State in Antebellum Connecticut: A Case Study of the Repeal of Early Medical Licensing Laws." *Journal of the History of Medicine,* 65(2): 153–186.

Appiah, K. A. 2010. *The Honor Code: How Moral Revolutions Happen.* New York: W. W. Norton & Company.

Applbaum, Arthur Isak. 1999. "Doctor, Schmoctor: Practice Positivism and its Complications." In *The American Medical Ethics Revolution,* edited by Robert B. Baker, Arthur L. Caplan, Linda L. Emanuel, and Stephen R. Latham, 144–157. Baltimore: Johns Hopkins University Press.

Ashton, Dianne. 1997. *Rebecca Gratz: Women and Judaism in Antebellum America.* Detroit: Wayne State University Press.

Atlee, John, Alden March, and Lewis Sayre. 1855. "Report of the Committee on James L. Phelps, 'Religion, as an Element in Medicine; or the Duties and Obligations of the Profession.'" *Transactions,* 1855, 50–51.

Aveling, James Hobson. [1872] 1967. *English Midwives: Their History and Prospects,* edited by John L. Thorton. London: Hugh L. Elliot Ltd. Also reproduced in Forbes, Thomas. 1966. *The Midwife and the Witch.* New Haven: Yale University Press.

Axelson, D. E. 1985. "Women as Victims of Medical Experimentation: J. Marion Sims' Surgery on Slave Women." *Sage,* 2(2): 10–30. Note: quoted at Ojanuga, 30.

Ayd, Frank. 1968. "What Is Death." Typescript of lecture at Second National Congress on Medical Ethics, October 5, 1968. Chicago: AMA Archives JC 39.73/1969.

Bailey, William H. 1881. "Anniversary Address." *Transactions MSSNY.*

Baker, Robert. 1997. "The Kappa Lambda Society of Hippocrates: The Secret Origins of the American Medical Association." *Fugitive Leaves,* Third Series, 11(2). Philadelphia: College of Physicians of Philadelphia.

Baker, Robert. 1999. "The American Medical Ethics Revolution." In *The American Medical Ethics Revolution,* edited by Robert B. Baker, Arthur L. Caplan, Linda L. Emanuel, and Stephen R. Latham, 17–51. Baltimore: Johns Hopkins University Press.

Baker, Robert. 2006. "Medical Ethics and Epidemics: A Historical Perspective." In *Ethics and Epidemics, vol. 9 (Advances in Bioethics),* edited by J. Balint, S. Philpott, R. Baker, and M. Strosberg, 93–133. Oxford: Elsevier Ltd.

Baker, Robert. 2009. "Hays, Isaac." In *The Cambridge World History of Medical Ethics,* edited by R. Baker and L. McCullough, 704–705. New York: Cambridge University Press.

Baker, Robert. 2009. "The Discourses of Practitioners in Nineteenth- and Twentieth-century Britain and the United States." In *The Cambridge World History of Medical Ethics,* edited by R. Baker and L. McCullough, 446–464. New York: Cambridge University Press.

Baker, Robert, Arthur Caplan, Linda Emanuel, and Stephen Latham, eds. 1999. *The American Medical Ethics Revolution.* Baltimore: Johns Hopkins University Press.

Baker, Robert, and Laurence McCullough, eds. 2009. *The Cambridge World History of Medical Ethics.* New York: Cambridge University Press.

Baker, Robert, and Laurence McCullough. 2009. "What Is the History of Medical Ethics?" In *The Cambridge World History of Medical Ethics*, edited by R. Baker and L. McCullough, 3–15. New York: Cambridge University Press.

Baker, Robert, and Laurence McCullough. 2009. "A Chronology of Medical Ethics." In *The Cambridge World History of Medical Ethics*, edited by R. Baker and L. McCullough, 77–97. New York: Cambridge University Press.

Baker, Robert, Harriet A. Washington, Ololade Olakanmi, Todd L. Savitt, Elizabeth A. Jacobs, Eddie Hoover, and Matthew K. Wynia, 2008. "African American Physicians and Organized Medicine, 1846–1968: Origins of a Racial Divide." *Journal of the American Medical Association,* 300(3): 306–313.

Baker, Robert, Harriet A. Washington, Ololade Olakanmi, Todd L. Savitt, Elizabeth A. Jacobs, Eddie Hoover, and Matthew K. Wynia for the Writing Group on the History of African Americans and the Medical Profession. 2009. "Creating a Segregated Medical Profession: African American Physicians and Organized Medicine, 1846–1910." *Journal of the National Medical Association,* 101(6): 501–512.

Baldick, Robert. 1965. *The Duel: A History of Dueling.* New York: Clarkson N. Potter Inc.

Balint, John, Sean Philpott, Robert Baker, and Martin Strosberg, eds. 1988. *Ethics and Epidemics.* Amsterdam: Elsevier.

Bard, John. 1941. Letter, cited in Felix Hirsch. "The Bard Family." *Columbia University Quarterly,* October 1941: 26.

Bard, Samuel. [1762] 1931. Letter to John Bard, December 29, 1762. In "*Doctor Samuel Bard,*" edited by Milton Halsey Thomas. *Columbia University Quarterly*, June 1931: 120, 122–123.

Bard, Samuel. [1763] 1822. Letter to John Bard, November 24, 1763. In *Domestic Narrative of the Life of Samuel Bard, M.D., LL.D*, by John McVickar, 54. New York: Applewood Books.

Bard, Samuel. [1764] 1931. Letter to John Bard, June 2, 1764. In "*Doctor Samuel Bard,*" edited by Milton Halsey Thomas. *Columbia University Quarterly,* June 1931: 120.

Bard, Samuel. [1765] 1931. Letter to John Bard, May 16, 1765. In "*Doctor Samuel Bard,*" edited by Milton Halsey Thomas. *Columbia University Quarterly*, June 1931, 120.

Bard, Samuel. 1765. *Tentamen medicum inaugurale, De viribus opii: quod…pro gradu doctoratus…/ eruditorum examini subjicit, Samuel Bard, Americanus.* Edinburgh: University of Edinburgh, Apud A. Donaldson et J. Reid.

Bard, Samuel. [1769] 1996. *A Discourse upon the Duties of a Physician, with Some Sentiments on the Usefulness and Necessity of a Public Hospital Delivered Before the President and the Governors of King's College, at the Commencement, Held on the 16th of May, 1769. As Advice to Those Gentlemen Who Then Received the First Medical Degrees Conferred by That University*, 14, 20–21. Bedford: Applewood Books.

Bard, Samuel. [1807] 1819. *A Compendium of the Theory and Practice of Midwifery, Containing Practical Instructions for the Management of Women in Labour and in Child-Bed. Illustrated in Many Cases and Particularly Adapted to the Use of Students*, 5th edition. New York: Collins and Co.

Barnard, Christiaan. [1968] 1991. "Testimony at U.S. Senate Subcommittee on Government Research, Committee on Government Operations." Cited in *Strangers at the Bedside: A History of How Law and Bioethics Transformed Medical Decision Making,* by David Rothman, 173. New York: Basic Books

Barnett, Charles. April, 19, 1974. Quoted in "Debate revives on PHS study," *Medical World News*, 37; cited in Brandt, Allan, "Racism and Research: The Case of the Tuskegee Syphilis Experiment," *Tuskegee's Truths: Rethinking the Tuskegee Syphilis Study,* edited by Susan Reverby, 28. Chapel Hill and London: University of North Carolina Press.

Barquet, Nicola, and Pere Domingo. 1997. "Smallpox: The Triumph Over the Most Terrible Ministers of Death." *Annals of Internal Medicine*, 127(8) part I: 635–642.

Barthlow, Roberts. 1874. "Experimental Investigations into the Functions of the Human Brain." *American Journal of the Medical Sciences*, 67: 305–313, quote from 310–311.

Bartrip, Peter. 1995. "An Introduction to Jukes Styrap's *A Code of Medical Ethics* (1878)." In *The Codification of Medical Morality: Historical and Philosophical Studies of the Formalization of Western Medical Morality in the Eighteenth and Nineteenth Centuries: Volume Two: Anglo-American Medical Ethics and Medical Jurisprudence in the Nineteenth Century*, edited by R. Baker, 145–148. Dordrecht: Kluwer Academic Publishers.

Beauchamp, Tom. 1978. "Distributive Justice and Morally Relevant Differences." In "National Commission for the Protection of Human Subjects of Biomedical and Behavioral Research." *The Belmont Report: Ethical Principle and Guidelines for the Protection of Human Subjects of Research*. Part B. Washington, DC: DHEW Publication No. (OS) 78–0013.

Beauchamp, Tom. 2003. "Origins, Goals, and Core Commitments of *The Belmont Report* and *Principles of Biomedical Ethics*." In *The Story of Bioethics: From Seminal Works to Contemporary Explorations*, edited by Eran Klein and Jennifer Walter, 17–46. Washington, DC: Georgetown University Press.

Beauchamp, Tom, and James Childress. [1979] 2009. *Principles of Biomedical Ethics*. New York: Oxford University Press.

Beauchamp, Tom, and Ruth Faden. 1986. *The History and Theory of Informed Consent*. New York: Oxford University Press.

Beaumont, Deborah, and William Beaumont. 1823. *"Letter from W. Beaumont and Deborah Beaumont [Mackinac, MI] to her parents [Plattsburgh, NY] regarding family news. December 18, 1823."* St. Louis: Bernard Becker Medical Library, Washington University School of Medicine.

Beaumont, William. [1823] 1825. *"Journal of Cases in W. Beaumont's Medical Practice, Including Earliest Descriptions of the Wounding of St. Martin, Recorded at Fort Mackinac, MI. November 18, 1822–January 12, 1825."* St. Louis: Bernard Becker Medical Library, Washington University School of Medicine.

Beaumont, William. 1824. *"Beaumont, Surgeon, U.S.A. [Ft. Niagara, NY] to Joseph Lovell, Surgeon General [Washington, DC] September 1824. A singular case and extraordinary recovery from a wound and perforation of the stomach. Manuscript report, June*

6, 1822–September 1824, and first series of experiments, September 1823–August 1826." St. Louis: Bernard Becker Medical Library, Washington University School of Medicine.

Beaumont, William. 1827. "*W. W. (William) Matthews, American Fur Company [Mackinac, MI] to W. Beaumont [Green Bay, WI] Regarding: Reimbursement of Matthews Expenses and Negotiations for Employment of St. Martin and Wife. August 18, 1827.*" St. Louis: Bernard Becker Medical Library, Washington University School of Medicine.

Beaumont, William. 1832. "*W. Beaumont and St. Martin, Four Articles of Agreement [Plattsburgh, NY]. St. Martin to Submit to the Experiments of Beaumont Under Conditions Fully Set Forth. October 16, 1832–November 7, 1833.*" St. Louis: Bernard Becker Medical Library, Washington University School of Medicine.

Beaumont, William. 1834. "*Memorial (with Narrative of Experiments and Expenses Incurred) of Doctor William Beaumont, a Surgeon in the U.S. Army to 23rd Congress Regarding: Request for Government Assistance to Continue Experiments, Remuneration for Expenses Already Incurred. January 1834.*" St. Louis: Bernard Becker Medical Library, Washington University School of Medicine.

Beaumont, William. [1826–1830] 2010. "*Case Book and Aphorisms of W. Beaumont, Second Infantry Regarding: Patients Keefe, Ferguson, and Hinkley. December 2, 1826–1830.*" St. Louis: Bernard Becker Medical Library, Washington University School of Medicine.

Beck, J., and D. Peixotto. 1827. "Review of the Report of the Medical Society of the City of New York, on Nostrums, or Secret Medicines." *The New York Medical and Physical Journal*, 6: 426–442.

Beecher, Henry. 1966. "Ethics and Clinical Research." *New England Journal of Medicine*, 274: 1354–1360.

Beecher, Henry. 1970. *Research and the Individual: Human Studies*. Boston: Little, Brown and Company.

Bell Family Papers, 1796–1927. 1964. Dickson: Tennessee State Library. http://tennessee.gov/tsla/history/manuscripts/findingaids/1200.pdf (accessed November 7, 2010).

Bell, John. 1847. "Introduction to the Code of Medical Ethics." In *Proceedings of the National Medical Conventions Held in New York, May, 1846, and in Philadelphia, May, 1847, 83–90.* Philadelphia: Printed for the American Medical Association, T. K. & P. G. Collins.

Bell, John. 1850. *Memorial to the Trustees of the University of Pennsylvania*. Philadelphia: Edmond Barrington and George D. Haswell.

Bell, John. [1847] 2013. "Introduction to the Code of Ethics." This volume, Appendix nn p. mm.

Bell, John, Isaac Hays, G. Emerson, W. Morris, T. C. Dunn, A. Clark, and R. D. Arnold. 1847. "Code of Medical Ethics." *Proceedings of the National Medical Conventions Held in New York, May, 1846, and in Philadelphia, May, 1847.* Philadelphia: Printed for the American Medical Association, T. K. & P. G. Collins.

Benigno, Antonio. November 26, 1900. "Informed Consent Agreement for Antonio Benigno," English translation © 1998–2004, Rector and Visitors of the University of Virginia, http://etext.lib.virginia.edu/etcbin/fever-browse?id=07004001 (accessed November 19, 2012).

Bergdolt, Klaus. 2008. "Zerbi, Gabrielle." In *The Cambridge World History of Medical Ethics*, edited by Robert B. Baker and Laurence B. McCullough, 719–720. New York: Cambridge University Press.

Berlant, J. 1975. *Profession and Monopoly: A Study of Medicine in the United States and Great Britain.* Berkeley: University of California Press.

Bicks, Caroline. 2003. *Midwiving Subjects in Shakespeare's England*, 131. Aldershot, Hampshire: Ashgate.

Bigelow, Henry J. 1871. *Medical Education in America: Being the Annual Address read before the Massachusetts Medical Society*, 44. Cambridge: Welch, Bigelow, and Company, University Press.

Biggs, Leslie. 2004. "Rethinking the History of Midwifery in Canada." In *Reconceiving Midwifery*, edited by Ivy Lynn Bourgeault, Cecilia Benoit, and Robbie Davis-Floyd, 40. Montreal: McGill-Queen's Press.

Billings, Frank, et al. 1912. "Report of the Judicial Council," "Principles of Medical Ethics: A Proposed Revision," *Minutes of the House of Delegates Proceedings of the Sixty-Third Annual Session Atlantic City, N.J., June 3–6, 1912*, 12–15.

Billings, John Shaw. 1876. "Literature and Institutions." In *A Century of American Medicine, 1776–1876*, edited by E. H. Clarke, et al., 292–366. Philadelphia: H. C. Lea.

Bliss, Michael. [1982] 2007. *The Discovery of Insulin.* Chicago: University of Chicago Press.

Bliss, Michael. 1999. *William Osler: A Life in Medicine*, 113. Toronto: University of Toronto Press.

Bonner, Bishop Edmund. [1555] 1815. "Midwife's Oath." In *Curious Miscellaneous Fragments Of Various Subjects More Particularly Relative to English History From The Year 1050, To The Year 1701, Compiled From British Writers During That Period*, edited by William Helm, 165–166. London: Baldwin, Cradock and Joy.

Bosk, Charles. 1981. *Forgive and Remember: Managing Medical Failure.* Chicago: University of Chicago Press.

Boston Medical Association. 1808. *Boston Medical Police.* Boston: Smelling and Simons. Reprinted in *The Codification of Medical Morality, II*, edited by R. Baker. Dordrecht: Kluwer Academic Publishers.

Boston Medical Association. 1838. *Boston Medical Police/ Rules and Regulations of the Boston Medical Association*, Boston: Dutton and Wentworth.

Boston Medical Association. 1885. *The Medical Police and Rules and Regulations of the Boston Medical Association with a Catalogue of the Officers and Members.* Boston: Franklin Press.

Boston Medical Surgical Journal Editors. 1836. "Medical Impeachment: Doings of the Massachusetts Medical Society in the Case of John S. Bartlett, M.D,. of Boston, One of Its Fellows." *Boston Medical Surgical Journal*, 14: 277–292.

Boswell, James. 1775. *Life of Johnson.* Entry for Friday, April 7, 1775, 615. New Haven: Yale University Press.

Bowditch, Henry I. 1866. "Minority Report." *Transactions of the Eighteenth Annual Meeting of the American Medical Association*, 512.

Bowditch, Henry I. 1868. "Report of the Committee on Medical Ethics." *Transactions of the Nineteenth Annual Meeting of the American Medical Association*, 89–200.

Bowditch, Henry Pickering, and Walter Cannon. 1922. "Bibliographic Memoir Henry Pickering Bowditch: 1840–1911." *Eight Bibliographic Memoirs: Proceedings of the Annual Meeting*, 8, 190. Washington, DC: National Academy of Sciences, Government Printing Office.

Bower, Alexander. 1817. *The History of the University of Edinburgh: Chiefly Compiled from Original Papers and Records, Never Before Published*, vol. 1. Edinburgh: Oliphant, Waugh, and Innes.

Boylston, Zabdiel. 1730. *An Historical Account of the Small-pox Inoculated in New England, Upon All Sorts of Persons, Whites, Blacks, and of All Ages and Constitutions: With Some Account of the Nature of the Infection in the Natural and Inoculated Way, and Their Different Effects on Human Bodies: with Some Short Directions to the Unexperienced in this Method of Practice/Humbly Dedicated to Her Royal Highness the Princess of Wales*. London: Printed for S. Chandler, at the Cross-Keys in the Poultry. http://pds.lib.harvard.edu/pds/view/8290362?n=1.

Briggs, W. 1891. "The President's Address." *Journal of the American Medical Association*, 16(19): 650.

Brinton, Daniel G. 1879. "Obituary Notice of Isaac Hays." *Proceedings of the American Philosophical Society*, 18: 259–260.

Broad, Charles D. 1930. *Five Types of Ethical Theory*. New York: Harcourt Brace.

Brodie, B. C. 1843. *Introductory Discourse on the Duty and Conduct of Medical Students and Practitioners: Addressed to the Students of the Medical School of St. Georges Hospital, October 2, 1843*. London: Longman, Brown, Green, and Longmans.

Brodie, William. 1886. "The President's Address." *Journal of the American Medical Association*, 6(19): 506.

Brodsky, Alyn. 2004. *Benjamin Rush: Patriot and Physician*, 277–278. New York: St. Martin's Press.

Brody, Howard, Zahara Meghani, and Kimberly Greenwald, eds. 2009. *Michael Ryan's Writings on Medical Ethics*, 156–157. Dordrecht: Springer.

Brown and Higgins. 1868. "Medical Advertising." (Letter) *Chicago Medical Examiner*, 9: 187.

Buchan, James. 2003. *Crowded with Genius: The Scottish Enlightenment: Edinburgh's Moment of the Mind*, 1, 40. New York: HarperCollins.

Buck v. Bell, Superintendent of the Colony for Epileptics and the Feeble Minded. May 2, 1927, 247 U.S. 200. Quotation from Appendix A, "The Supreme Court Decision in *Buck v. Bell*, by Justice Oliver Wendell Holmes Jr." In Lombardo, Paul. 2008. *Three Generations No Imbeciles: Eugenics, the Supreme Court and Buck v. Bell*, 285, 287. Baltimore: Johns Hopkins University Press.

Burdick, Donald, John H. Stek, Walter Wessel, and Ronald F. Youngblood, eds. 1995. *The NIV Study Bible 10th Anniversary Edition*, 1291–1295. *The Book of Daniel* 3:27. Grand Rapids, MI: Zondervan Publishing House.

Burns, Chester, ed. 1977. *Legacies in Ethics and Medicine*, 218–236. New York: Science History Publications.

Burns, Chester. 2008. "The Discourses of Practitioners in Eighteenth-Century North America." In *The Cambridge World History of Medical Ethics*, edited by Robert B. Baker and Laurence B. McCullough, 414–417. New York: Cambridge University Press.

Burrage, W. L. 1923. *A History of the Massachusetts Medical Society with Brief Biographies of the Founders and Chief Officers, 1781–1922*. Norwood: Plimpton Press.

Butterfield, L. H., ed. 1951. "Appendix II: John Adams' Appointment of Rush as Treasurer of the Mint," In *Letters of Benjamin Rush*, vol. I, II. Philadelphia: Princeton University Press for the American Philosophical Society.

Butterfield, L. H., ed. 1951. *Letters of Benjamin Rush*, vol. I, II. Philadelphia: Princeton University Press for the American Philosophical Society.

Buxton, Peter. 1968. "Letter to William J. Brown, Chief, Venereal Disease Branch, Communicable Disease Center, November 24, 1968." In *Tuskegee's Truths: Rethinking the Tuskegee Syphilis Study*, edited by Susan Reverby, 154. Chapel Hill and London: University of North Carolina Press.

Buxton, Peter. 1973. "Testimony by Peter Buxton from the United States Senate Hearings on Human Experimentation, 1973." In *Tuskegee's Truths: Rethinking the Tuskegee Syphilis Study*, edited by Susan Reverby, 154. Chapel Hill and London: University of North Carolina Press.

Cabell, N., ed. [1856] [1981] 2002. Letter from Thomas Jefferson to James C. Cabell, May 16, 1824. In *Early History of the University of Virginia as Contained in the Letters of Thomas Jefferson and James C. Cabell*. In *Medicine and Slavery*, by T. Savitt. Urbana: University of Illinois Press.

Calvin, John. [1563] 1852. *Commentaries on the Last Four Books of Moses, Arranged in the Form of a Harmony*, translated by Charles W. Bingham. Michigan: Baker.

Campbell, Alistair. 2000. "My Country Tis of Thee—The Myopia of American Bioethics." *Medicine, Health Care and Philosophy*, 3(2): 195–198.

Cannon, Walter Bradford. 1916. "The Right and Wrong of Making Experiments of Human Beings." *Journal of the American Medical Association*, 67: 1372–1373.

Cannon, Walter. 1922. "Bibliographic Memoir Henry Pickering Bowditch: 1840–1911." In *Eight Bibliographic Memoirs: Proceedings of the Annual Meeting, 8: 190*. Washington, DC. National Academy of Sciences, Government Printing Office.

Cantor, Geoffrey. 2005. *Quakers, Jews and Science: Religious Responses to Modernity and the Sciences in Britain, 1650–1900*. New York: Oxford University Press.

Cardwell, Edward. [1844] 2000. "Documentary Annals of the Reformed Church of England." In *The Midwives of Seventeenth-century London*, edited by Doreen Evenden, 30. Cambridge: Cambridge University Press.

Carpenter, Daniel. 2010. *Reputation and Power: Organizational Image and Pharmaceutical Regulation at the FDA*. Princeton and Oxford: Princeton University Press.

Carroll, James. 1900. *Letter from Major James Carroll to Jenifer Carroll, Camp Columbia, Cuba*. Philip D. Hench Walter Reed Yellow Fever Collection. Charlottesville: University of Virginia.

Carroll, James. 1906. *Report to the Surgeon General.* Philip D. Hench Walter Reed Yellow Fever Collection. Charlottesville: University of Virginia. http://yellowfever.lib.virginia.edu/reed/collection.html

Carroll, Patrick. 2002. "Medical Police and the History of Public Health." *Medical History,* 46: 461–494.

Cartwright, Samuel. 1851. "Report on the Diseases and Physical Peculiarities of the Negro Race." *The New Orleans Medical and Surgical Journal* 7: 691–715.

Chambers, Robert. 1885. *Domestic Annals of Scotland from the Reformation to the Rebellion of 1745*, 3 ed., vol. III, 501–502. Edinburgh: W. & R. Chambers.

Chamblit, Rebekah. [1733] 1753. *The declaration, dying warning and advice of Rebekah Chamblit. A young woman aged near twenty-seven years, executed at Boston September 27th. 1733 according to the sentence pass'd upon her at the Superiour Court holden there for the county of Suffolk, in August last, being then found guilty of felony, in concealing the birth of her spurious male infant, of which she was delivered when alone the eighth day of May last, and was afterwards found dead, as will more fully appear by the following declaration, which was carefully taken from her own mouth.* Boston: Kneeland and Green.

Chapman, Carlton, B. 1984. *Physicians, Law, and Ethics.* New York: New York University Press.

Childress, James, Eric Meslin, and Harold Shaprio, eds. 2005. *Belmont Revisited: Ethical Principles for Research with Human Subjects.* Washington, DC: Georgetown University Press.

Cicero, Marcus Tullius. [44 BCE] 1921. *De Officiis*, translated by Walter Miller. Cambridge, New York: Loeb Classical Library.

Cirillo, Vincent. 2004. *Bullets and Bacilli: The Spanish-American War and Military Medicine,* New Brunswick: Rutgers University Press.

City of Albany. [1773] 1972. *Laws and Ordinances* (Robertson, 61). Cited in *Midwifery in America, 1760–1860: A Study in Medicine and Morality*, by Jane Bauer Donegan. Unpublished doctoral dissertation, 53 (Ph.D., History). Syracuse University, NY.

Cleland, Archibald. 1743. *An appeal to the publick, or, A plain narrative of facts: relating to the proceedings of a party of the governors of the new General-Hospital at Bath, against Mr. Archibald Cleland (one of the surgeons of the said hospital) at an extraordinary meeting of the governors. A. Dodd, . . . London, and by W. Frederick, . . . Bath, 1743.*

Clinical Care Committee of the Massachusetts General Hospital. 1976. "Optimum Care for Hopelessly Ill Patients. A Report of the Clinical Care Committee of the Massachusetts General Hospital." *New England Journal of Medicine,* 295 (7): 362–364.

Cobbett, William. 1801. "The American Rush-Light." In William Cobbett, editor, *Porcupine's Works; containing various WRITINGS AND SELECTIONS, of the UNITED STATES OF AMERICA; of their governments, laws, politics and resources; of the character of their PRESIDENTS, GOVERNORS, LEGISLATORS, MAGISTRATES AND MILITARY MEN; and of the customs, morals, religious, virtues and vices, OF THE PEOPLE; comprising also a complete series of historical documents and remarks from the end of the war, in 1783, to the ELECTION OF THE PRESIDENT, IN MARCH 1801.* London: Cobbett and Morgan

Cohen, I. Bernard. 1985. *Revolution in Science.* Cambridge (MA): The Belknap Press of Harvard University Press.

College of Physicians of Philadelphia. [1787] 1887. "Form of the Constitution of the College of Physicians of Philadelphia, January 2, 1787." In *Transactions of the College of Physicians of Philadelphia, Centennial Volume.* Philadelphia: College of Physicians, 175–176.

Committee on Ethics of the New York Academy of Medicine. Date unknown. Manuscript: "Rules for Courts Medical and Judicial Hearings," New York Academy of Medicine Committee on Ethics, Scrapbook 1867–1884. New York: Library of the New York Academy of Medicine.

Committee of the Massachusetts State Legislature. 1830. *Report of the Evidence in the Case of John Stephen Bartlett, M.D. versus the Mass. Medical Society as given before a Committee of the Legislature, at the Session of 1839*, House Report No. 76. Boston: Dutton and Wentworth State Printers.

Committee of Commemoration of Alexis Bidagan dit St. Martin of the Canadian Medical Society. 1963. "Alexis St. Martin Commemorated." *Physiologist* 6(1): 63–65.

Common Council of the City of New York. 1905. *Minutes of the Common Council of the City of New York. 1675–1766*: 121–123.

Connecticut. Medical Society. 1817, 1824, 1832. *System of Medical Police.* New Haven: Connecticut Medical Society in Convention.

Cooper, Thea and Arthur Ainsberg. 2010. *Breakthrough: Elizabeth Hughes, the Discovery of Insulin, and the Making of A Medical Miracle.* New York: St. Martin's Press.

Coulter, Harris. [1973] 1982. *Divided Legacy: The Conflict Between Homeopathy and the American Medical Association.* Richmond (CA): North Atlantic Books.

Countway Library of Medicine: *Confederacy of Physicians,* NS. D.S.; Mass. 15 Nov. 1780, B MS misc.

Cover, Robert. 1983. "The Supreme Court, 1982 Term—Foreward: Nomos and Narrative." Faculty Scholarship Series Paper 2705 http://digitalcommons.law.yale.edu (Accessed November 30, 2012.)

Cristensen, Clayton. 1997. *The Innovator's Dilemma: When New Technologies Cause Great Firms to Fall.* Boston (MA): Harvard Business School Press.

Cronin, Archibald Joseph. [1937] 1965. *The Citadel.* Boston: Little Brown.

Cruzan v. Director. 1990. Missouri Department of Health 497 U.S. 261 (1990).

Cullen, William. 1772. *Clinical Lectures of Dr. Cullen 1772.* Notes by Dr, Stuart 1772–1775." Manuscript collection of the College of Physicians of Philadelphia, 10a/166.

Cullen, William. (circa 1772). *Clinical Lectures by William Cullen.* Notes by Dr. Rhodes. Manuscript collection of the College of Physicians of Philadelphia, 10a-247, 6th lecture, section 2.

Cullen, William. 1827. *Works of William Cullen, M. D.*, edited by John Thomson, vol. I, 476–477. Edinburgh: John Johnstone.

Cullen, William. 1770. *Synopsis nosologiae methodicae Exhibens Clariss.* Edinburgh: William Creech.

Cunniffe, Edward R. 1946. "Report of the Judicial Council." *Proceedings of the House of Delegates, The Ninety-Fifth Annual Session held at San Francisco June 1–5, 1946*: 33, 62.

Cunniffe, Edward R. 1947. "Report of the Judicial Council." *Proceedings of the House of Delegates, The Ninety-Sixth Annual Session held at Atlantic City N. J., June 9–13, 1947*: 30–40.

Cunniffe, Edward R. 1949. "Report of the Judicial Council." *Principles of Medical Ethics." Proceedings of the House of Delegates, The Ninety-Eighth Annual Session, held at Atlantic City, N. J. June 6–10, 1949*: 38.

Currie, William. [1793] 1794. "Letter to Mr. Brown. September 20, 1793." *Federal Gazette. In An Account of the Bilious Remitting Yellow Fever as it Appeared in the CITY OF PHILADELPHIA in the Year 1793*, edited by Benjamin Rush, 230. Philadelphia: Thomas Dobson.

Dalton, John. 1881. "Report of the Committee on Experimental Medicine." *Transactions MSSNY*, 26: 29–30.

Dalzel, Andrew. 1862. *History of the University of Edinburgh from Its Foundation History*, vol. II, 90. Edinburgh: Edmonston and Douglas.

Darwin, Charles R. 1859. *On the Origin of Species by Means of Natural Selection, or the Preservation of Favoured Races in the Struggle for Life*. London: John Murray. http://darwinonline.org.uk/content/frameset?itemID=F373&viewtype=text&pageseq=1 (accessed January 6, 2011).

Darwin, Robert. 1789. *Appeal to the Faculty Concerning the Case of Mrs. Houlston*, Shrewsbury: P. Sanford, National Library of Medicine, 2168095R.

Davis, Nathan Smith. 1868. "Give an Inch and an Ell is Taken." *Chicago Medical Examiner*, 9: 115.

Davis, Nathan Smith. 1868. "Proceedings of the Societies: Annual Meeting of the American Medical Association." *Chicago Medical Examiner*, 9: 358–360, 361.

Davis, Nathan Smith. 1885. "The Moral Side of Euthanasia." *Journal of the American Medical Association*, 5(14): 382–383.

Davis, Nathan Smith. 1886. "Dr. Graham's address." *Journal of the American Medical Association*, 6(19): 491–492.

Davis, Nathan Smith. 1886. "Is Life Worth Saving." *Journal of the American Medical Association*, 7(12): 323–324.

Davis, Nathan Smith. 1886. "The Division in the Profession of the New York State on Codes of Ethics—Its Bearing on the International Congress Difficulty." *Journal of the American Medical Association*, 6(6): 155–157.

Davis, Nathan Smith. 1886. "The Higher Education of Women." *Journal of the American Medical Association*, September 4, 1886, 7(10): 267–269.

Davis, Nathan Smith. 1888. "Humanity in the Death Sentence." *Journal of the American Medical Association*, 10(4): 114–115.

Davis, Nathan Smith. 1888. "Medical Colleges and Medical Ethics." *Journal of the American Medical Association*, 11(1): 19.

Davis, Nathan Smith. 1888. "The Ethics of Marriage." *Journal of the American Medical Association*, 11(9): 309–311.

Davis, Nathan Smith. 1903. *History of Medicine, with the Code of Medical Ethics*. Chicago: Cleveland Press.

Davis, Ronald. 2008. "Letter of Apology." http://www.ama-assn.org/resources/doc/ethics/ama-apology-african-americans.pdf (accessed March 26, 2011).

Davis, Ronald. 2008. "Achieving Racial Harmony for the Benefit of Patients and Communities." *Journal of the American Medical Association*, 300(3): 323–325.

De Ville, K. 1990. *Medical Malpractice in Nineteenth Century America.* New York: New York University Press.

Defoe, Daniel 1725. *The complete English tradesman in familiar letters; directing him in all the several parts and progressions of trade... Of the Dignity and Honour of Trade in England, more than in other Countries; and how the Trading Families in England are mingled with the Nobility and Gentry, so as not to be separated or distinguished. Calculated for the Instruction of our Inland Tradesmen; and especially of Young Beginners.* London: Charles Rivington.

Defoe, Daniel. [1729] 1890. *The Complete English Gentleman*, edited by Karl Bülbring. London: David Nutt

Dekker, T. [1603] 1925. "The Wonderfull Yeare." In *The Plague Pamphlets of Thomas Dekker*, edited by F. P. Wilson, 36–37. Oxford: Clarendon Press.

Delafield, Francis. 1886. "President's Address: Proceedings of the Association of American Physicians." *Journal of the American Medical Association*, 7(1): 16.

Didama, Henry, D. 1894. "Report of the Minority Committee on Revision of the Code." *Journal of the American Medical Association*, 22(25): 951.

Douglass, William, Alexander Stuart, and James Franklin. 1722. *The Abuses and Scandals of Some Late Pamphlets in Favour of Inoculation of the Small Pox, Modestly Obviated, and Inoculation Further Consider'd in a Letter to A– S– M.D. & F.R.S. in London...; Abuses and Scandals of Some Late Pamphlets in Favour of Inoculation.* Boston: J. Franklin. http://pds.lib.harvard.edu/pds/view/7910092.

Doukas, David, Laurence McCullough, and Stephen Wear. 2010. "Reforming Medical Education in Ethics and Humanities by Finding Common Ground with Abraham Flexner." *Academic Medicine*, 85(2): 318–322.

Duchamp, Henry. 1821. A Biographical Memoir of Samuel Bard, M.D., LL.D., Late President of the College of Physicians and Surgeons of the University of New York; with a Critique Upon His Writings. *The American Medical Recorder*, 4(4): 609–633. Read Before the New York Historical Society, August 14, 1891.

Dyer, Frederick. 1999. *Champion of Women and the Unborn: Horatio Robinson Storer, M.D., 110–111, 121, 127.* Canton: Science History Publications.

"Eleemosynary." 1828. *American Dictionary of the English language.* http://www.1828-dictionary.com/d/search/word, Eleemosynary (accessed October 3, 2010).

Early, C. R. 1891. "Medical Progress." *Journal of the American Medical Association*, 16(22): 758.

Ebert, M. 1952. "The Rise and Development of the American Medical Periodical 1797–1850." *Bulletin of the Medical Library Association*, 40(3): 243–276.

Edelstein L. 1943. "The Hippocratic Oath: Text, Translation and Interpretation." A supplement to the *Bulletin of the History of Medicine*, 1. Baltimore: Johns Hopkins University Press.

Edelstein, Ludwig. 1967. *Ancient Medicine: Selected Papers of Ludwig Edelstein*, edited by O. Temkin and C. L. Temkin, 342. Baltimore: Johns Hopkins University Press.

Edinburgh University. 2004. Medical *Sponsio Academica*. http://www.ed.ac.uk/schools-departments/registry/graduations/medical-sponsio (accessed April 13, 2012).

Editors. [1857] 1999. *New Hampshire Journal of Medicine*, Cited in *Champion of Women and the Unborn: Horatio Robinson Storer, M.D.*, by Frederick Dyer, 85. Canton: Science History Publications.

Editors. 1857. "Reports of Medical Societies: Criminal Abortion." *Boston Medical and Surgical Journal*, 56: 282–284.

Ellis, Benjamin. 1829, 1834. *The Medical Formulary*. Philadelphia: Carey, Lea & Carey.

Emanuel, Ezekiel. 1994. "The History of Euthanasia Debates in the United States and Britain." *Annals of Internal Medicine*, 121(10): 793–802.

Emerson, Roger L. 2004. "The Founding of the Edinburgh Medical School." *Journal of the History of Medicine and Allied Sciences*, 59(2): 183–218.

Engelhardt Jr., H. Tristram. [1986] 1996. *The Foundations of Bioethics*. New York: Oxford University Press.

Engelhardt Jr., H. Tristram. 1978. "Basic Ethical Principles in the Conduct of Biomedical and Behavioral Research Involving Human Subjects." In "National Commission for the Protection of Human Subjects of Biomedical and Behavioral Research." *The Belmont Report: Ethical Principles and Guidelines for the Protection of Human Subjects of Research*. Part B. Washington, DC. DHEW Publication No. (OS) 78–0013.

Erlam, H. D. 1955. "Alexander Monro, Primus [An Autobiography]." *University of Edinburgh Journal*, Summer, 17: 97.

Evans, John. 2001. *Playing God?* Chicago: University of Chicago Press.

Evans, John. 2012. *The History and Future of Bioethics: A Sociological View*. New York: Oxford University Press.

Evenden, Doreen. 2000. *The Midwives of Seventeenth-Century London*. Cambridge: Cambridge University Press.

Faust, Drew. 1981. *The Ideology of Slavery: Proslavery Thought in the Antebellum South*. Baton Rouge: Louisiana State University Press.

Feuer, L. S. 1984. "America's First Jewish Professor: James Joseph Sylvester at the University of Virginia." *American Jewish Archives*, 36: 151–201.

Finnell, T. C. 1869. "Charges Presented to the Committee on Ethics." In *Archives of the NY Academy of Medicine Committee on Ethics, Scrapbook 1867–1884*. Manuscript Collection of the Library of the New York Academy of Medicine.

Fissell, Mary. 1993. "Innocent and Honorable Bribes: Medical Manners in Eighteenth-Century Britain." In *The Codification of Medical Morality*, vol. 1, edited by R. Baker, D. Porter, and R. Porter, 19–46. Dordrecht: Kluwer Academic Publishers.

Fissell, Mary. 2009. "The Medical Market Place, the Patient, and the Absence of Medical Ethics in Early Modern Europe and North America." In *The Cambridge World History of Medical Ethics*, edited by Robert B. Baker and Laurence B. McCullough, 533–539. New York: Cambridge University Press.

Fletcher, John C. 2000. "A Case Study in Historical Relativism: The Tuskegee (Public Health Service) Syphilis Study." In *Tuskegee's Truths: Rethinking the Tuskegee Syphilis Study*, edited by Susan Reverby, 280. Chapel Hill: University of North Carolina Press.

Flexner, Abraham. [1910] 1972. *Medical Education in the United States and Canada: A Report to the Carnegie Foundation for the Advancement of Teaching (Bulletin Number 4)*. New York: Carnegie Foundation for the Advancement of Teaching.

Flexner, Simon, and James Flexner. 1941. *William Henry Welch and the Heroic Age of American Medicine*, New York: Viking Press.

Flint, Austin. 1882. *Medical Ethics and Etiquette: The Code of Ethics Adopted by the American Medical Association with Commentaries by Austin Flint, M.D.* New York: Appleton and Company.

Flu.gov. "Pandemic Flu History." http://www.flu.gov/pandemic/history/index.html (accessed August 29, 2012).

Forbes, Sir John. 1846. *Homeopathy, Allopathy, and "Young Physic."* New York: William Radde.

Forbes, Sir John. 1847. "Postscript to No. XLVIII of the British and Foreign Medical Review by the Editor and Proprietor." *The British and Foreign Medical Review or Quarterly Journal of Practical Medicine and Surgery*, 24: 594–595.

Forbes, Sir John. 1857. *Of Nature and Art in the Cure of Disease*. London: John Churchill.

Forbes, Thomas. 1966. *The Midwife and the Witch*, 145, 148. New Haven: Yale University Press.

Foucault, Michel. [1963] 1973. *Naissance de la clinique: une archéologie du regard medical [The Birth of the Clinic: An Archaeology of Medical Perception]*. London: Tavistock Publications.

Fox, Daniel. 1979. "The Segregation of Medical Ethics: A Problem in Modern Intellectual History." *Journal of Medicine and Philosophy*, 4: 81–97.

Fox, Daniel. 1988. "The Politics of Physicians' Responsibilities in Epidemics: A Note on History." *Hastings Center Report*, 18(2): 5–9.

Fox, Renée C., and Judith P. Swazey. 2009. *Observing Bioethics*. New York: Oxford University Press.

Frank, Johann Peter. 1779–1827. *System einer vollständigen medicinischen Polizei*. 9 vols. Mannheim: C. F. Schwann.

Franklin, Benjamin. 1813. *The Life of the Late Dr. Benjamin Franklin*. New York: Evert Duyckinck.

Franklin, Benjamin. 1818. *Memoirs of the Life and Writings of Benjamin Franklin*. Edited by William Franklin. Philadelphia: T. S. Manning.

Freedman, Benjamin. 1988. "Health Professions, Codes, and the Right to Refuse HIV Infectious Patients." *Hastings Center Report*, 18: S 20–S 26.

Friendly Thomsonian Botanic Society of the United States. [1837] 2000. "Test Resolution." In *The People's Doctors: Samuel Thomson and the American Botanical Movement, 1790–1860*, by John Haller. Carbondale: Southern Illinois University Press.

Gallinger, Jacob. [1900] 1995. "A Bill for the Regulation of Scientific Experiments upon Human Beings in the District of Columbia (S. 3242) (56th Cong. 1st sess.)." In *Subjected to Science: Human Experimentation in America Before the Second World War*, by Susan Lederer. Baltimore: Johns Hopkins University Press.

Garnet, R. [1649] 1995. "The Book of Oaths." In *Renaissance Woman: A Sourcebook: Constructions of Femininity in England*, edited by Kate Aughterson, 212–214. New York: Routledge.

Gaw, Allan. 2012. "Exposing Unethical Human Research: The Transatlantic Correspondence of Beecher and Pappworth." *Annals of Internal Medicine*, 156: 150–155.

Gilje, Paul, A. 1983. "Infant Abandonment in Early Nineteenth-Century New York City: Three Cases." *Signs*, 8(3): 580–590.

Gisborne, Thomas. 1794. *An Enquiry into the Duties of Men in the Higher and Middle Classes of Society in Great Britain Resulting from their Respective Stations, Professions and Employment*. London: Printed by J. Davis, for B. and J. White.

Glynn, Ian, and Jennifer Glynn. 2004. *The Life and Death of Smallpox*. New York: Cambridge University Press.

Goffman, Erving. 1958. "The Characteristics of Total Institutions." *Symposium on Preventive and Social Psychiatry*, 43–84. Washington D.C.: Walter Reed Army Institute of Research.

Goldfarb v. Virginia State Bar. 1975. 421 U.S. 773.

Goldner, Ellen J. 2001. "Arguing with Pictures: Race, Class and the Formation of Popular Abolitionism Through Uncle Tom's Cabin." *Journal of American & Comparative Cultures*, 24: 71–84.

Goodman, Nathan. 1934. *Benjamin Rush, Physician and Citizen, 1746–1813*, 132–133. Philadelphia: University of Pennsylvania Press.

Governors of the General Hospital at Bath. 1744. *A short vindication of the proceedings of the governors of the General Hospital at Bath, in relation to Mr. Archibald Cleland, late surgeon to the said hospital: wherein the several facts misrepresented in a pamphlet, call'd, An appeal to the publick, by Mr. Cleland, are fairly stated: to which is prefix'd, A short narrative of the proceedings*. Bath: James Leake.

Graham, D. W. 1886. "The Demand for Medically Educated Women." *Journal of the American Medical Association*, 6(18): 477–480.

Graham, Henry. 1899. *The Social Life of Scotland in the Eighteenth Century*, vol. 1. London: Adam and Charles Black.

Grant, Alexander. 1884. *The Story of the University of Edinburgh During Its First Three Hundred Years*, vol. II, 255. London: Longmans Green and Co.

Green, Alexa. 2010. "Working Ethics: William Beaumont, Alexis St. Martin, and Medical Research in Antebellum America." *Bulletin of the History of Medicine*, 84: 193–216.

Gregory, John. [1767–1768] 1998. "Lectures on the Practice of Physick, Sir Charles Blagden Notes." In *John Gregory's Writings on Medical Ethics and the Philosophy of Medicine*, edited by Laurence McCullough, 70. Dordrecht: Kluwer Academic Publishers.

Gregory, John. [1770] 1998. "Observations on the Duties and Offices of a Physician." In *John Gregory's Writings on Medical Ethics and the Philosophy of Medicine*, edited by Laurence McCullough, Dordrecht: Kluwer Academic Publishers.

Gregory, John. [1771] 1998. *Clinical Lectures by Dr. Gregory*, C36, 9–10. Royal College of Physicians of Edinburgh. In *John Gregory and the Invention of Professional Medical Ethics and the Profession of Medicine*, edited by Laurence McCullough, 249. Dordrecht: Kluwer Academic Publishers.

Gregory, John. 1772. *Lectures on the Duties and Offices of a Physician.* London: W. Straham and T. Cadell.

Gregory, John. [1772] 1998. *John Gregory's Writings on Medical Ethics and the Philosophy of Medicine*, edited by Laurence McCullough, 102–103, 170. Dordrecht: Kluwer Academic Publishers.

Gregory, John. 1776. *Clinical Lectures by Dr. Gregory*, lecture 1, 13. Royal College of Physicians of Edinburgh. Manuscript collection of the College of Physicians of Philadelphia.

Gregory, Samuel. 1850. *Letter to Ladies in Favor of Female Physicians.* New York: Fowler and Wells.

Grier, Katherine. 2006. *Pets in America: A History.* Chapel Hill: North Carolina University Press & Orlando (FL) Harcourt Books.

Gross, Samuel. 1879. "Obituary Notice of Isaac Hays, M.D." *American Journal of Medical Science, New series,* 78: 281–292.

Gruenewaldt, Otto von. 1854. "Untersuchungen über den Magensaft des Menschen." *Archiv für physiologische Heikunde,* 13: 460. Cited in "William Beaumont and the Ethics of Human Experimentation," by Ronald L. Numbers, 1979. *Journal of the History of Biology,* 12(1): 130–131.

Guerrini, Anita. 1987. "Archibald Pitcairne and Newtonian Medicine." *Medical History,* 31: 70–83.

Guerrini, Anita. 2006. "Alexander Monro Primus and the Moral Theatre of Anatomy." *The Eighteenth Century,* 47 (1): 1–18.

Haakonssen, Knud. 1996. "Enlightened Dissent: An Introduction." In *Enlightenment and Religion: Rational Dissent in Eighteenth-Century Britain*, edited by K. Haakonssen, 1. Cambridge: Cambridge University Press.

Haakonssen, Lisabeth. 1997. *Medicine and Morals in the Enlightenment: John Gregory, Thomas Percival, and Benjamin Rush*, 216–226. Amsterdam: Ridopi.

Haber, Samuel. 1991. *The Quest for Authority and Honor in the American Professions 1750–1900.* Chicago: University of Chicago Press.

Hahnemann, Samuel. 1810. *Organon der rationellen heilkunde.* Dresden: Arnold.

Haller, John S. 2000. *The People's Doctors: Samuel Thomson and the American Botanical Movement, 1790–1860.* Cabondale: Southern Illinois University Press.

Haller, John S. 2005. *A History of American Homeopathy: The Academic Years, 1820–1935.* Binghamton: The Haworth Press, Inc.

Hamilton, Alexander. [1804] 1965. Cited in Robert Baldick, 1965, *The Duel, A History of Duelling, 120.* New York: Clarkson N. Potter.

Hamilton, Frank H. 1884. *Conversations Between Drs. Warren and Putnam on the Subject of Medical Ethics.* New York: Bermingham and Company (originally published in the *Medical Gazette*).

Hamilton, John. 1889. "The Retirement of Dr. Davis." *Journal of the American Medical Association*, 12(1): 22.

Harkness, Jon. 2002. "Book Review." *Isis*, 93:732–733.

Harkness, Jon, Susan Lederer, and Daniel Wikler. 2001. "Laying Ethical Foundations for Clinical Research." *Bulletin of the World Health Organization*, 79(4): 365–2366.

Harley, David. 1990. "Historians as Demonologists: The Myth of the Midwife-Witch." *Social History of Medicine*, 3: 1–27.

Harley, David. 1990 "Honour and Propriety: The Structure of Professional Disputes in Eighteenth-Century English Medicine." In *The Medical Enlightenment of the Eighteenth Century*, edited by A. Cunningham and R. French. Cambridge, 138–164. Cambridge University Press.

Harris, E. Eliot. 1901. "Proposed Union of the N. Y. Associations and Societies." *Journal of the American Medical Association*, 35(23): 1545.

Harris, E. Eliot. 1902. "Report of the Committee on Medical Ethics." *Journal of the American Medical Association*, 38(25): 1649–1652.

Harris, E. Eliot. 1903. "Report of the Committee on Medical Ethics." *Journal of the American Medical Association*, 40(20): 1379, 1381.

Harris, Seale. 1950. *Woman's Surgeon: The Life of J. Marion Sims.* New York: The Macmillan Company.

Hartley, Leslie. 1953. *The Go-Between.* London: H. Hamilton.

Hays, Isaac. 1843. "Prospectus." *The Medical News and Library*, 1(1): 1. Philadelphia: Lea and Blanchard.

Hays, Isaac. 1843. "Homeopathic Fictions." *The Medical News and Library*, 1(1): 13. Philadelphia: Lea and Blanchard.

Hays, Isaac. 1843. "Victim to Homeopathy." *The Medical News and Library*, 1(3): 46. Philadelphia: Lea and Blanchard.

Hays, Isaac. 1847. "Medical reform." *The Medical News and Library*, 5(53): 49–54. Philadelphia: Lea and Blanchard.

Hays, Isaac. 1847. "Infinitesimal Morality." *The Medical News and Library*, 5(53): 62. Philadelphia: Lea and Blanchard.

Hays, Isaac. 1847. "Note to Convention." *Proceedings of the National Medical Conventions Held in New York, May, 1846, and in Philadelphia, May, 1847.* Philadelphia: Printed for the American Medical Association, T. K. & P. G. Collins, Printers.

Hays, Isaac. [1847] 1999. "Note to 1847 Convention." In *The American Medical Ethics Revolution*, edited by Robert Baker, Arthur Caplan, Linda Emanuel, and Stephen Latham, 315. Baltimore: Johns Hopkins University Press.

Hench, Philip Showalter. October 26, 1940. *Text of Speech: Dr. Jesse Lazear and his Contribution to the Conquest of Yellow Fever.* Archives of the Philip D. Hench Walter Reed Collection, University of Virginia http://yellowfever.lib.virginia.edu/reed/collection.html

Hilberman, Mark. 1975. "The Evolution of Intensive Care Units." *Critical Care Medicine,* 3(4): 159–165.

Hill, Andrew. "Thomas Aikenhead." http://www25.uua.org/uuhs/duub/articles/thomasaikenhead.html (accessed January 18, 2009).

History of Soft Drinks. http://www.essortment.com/history-soft-drinks-40721.html (accessed August 19, 2012).

Hoblyn, R. 1844. *A Dictionary of Terms Used in Medicine and the Collateral Sciences.* London: Gilbert and Rivington.

Hodge, Hugh [1839] 1854. *On Criminal Abortion; A Lecture Introductory to the Course on Obstetrics, and Diseases of Women and Children. University of Pennsylvania, Session 1854–5*, 7, 8, 12–13, 19. Philadelphia: T. K. and P. G. Collins.

Hodge, Hugh L. 1864. *The Principles and Practice of Obstetrics.* Philadelphia: Blanchard and Lea.

Hoeber, F. W. 2001. "Drama in the Courtroom, Theater in the Streets: Philadelphia's Irish Riot of 1831." *Pennsylvania Magazine of History and Biography,* 125(3): 199–232.

Hoffer, Peter C., and N. E. H. Hull. 1981. *Murdering Mothers: Infanticide in England and New England, 1558–1803*, 13–15, 128. New York: New York University Press.

Holmes, Chris. 1966. "Benjamin Rush and the Yellow Fever." *Bulletin of the History of Medicine,* 40: 246–260.

Holmes, Oliver Wendell. [1842] 2007. "Homeopathy and Its Kindred Delusions." In *Medical Essays.* Charleston: BiblioBazaar. [Reprint edition.]

Holmes, Oliver Wendell. 1842. *Homeopathy and its Kindred Delusions: Two Lectures Delivered Before the Boston Society for the Diffusion of Useful Knowledge.* Boston: William D. Ticknor.

Holmes, Oliver Wendell Sr. [1843][1855][1891] 2007. "The Contagiousness of Puerperal Fever." In Oliver Wendell Holmes Sr. [1843][1855][1891] 2007. *Medical Essays.* Charleston: BiblioBazaar [Reprint edition].

Holmes, Oliver Wendell Sr. [1860][1891] 2007. "Current and Counter-Currents in Medical Science." In Oliver Wendell Holmes Sr. [1843][1855][1891] 2007. *Medical Essays.* Charleston: BiblioBazaar [Reprint edition].

Holton, H. D. 1894. "Report of the Committee on Revision of the Code." *Journal of the American Medical Association,* 22(25): 950–951.

Holton, H.D., et al. 1894. "Code of Medical Ethics and Etiquette of the American Medical Association: Report of the Majority Committee on Revision of the Code of Ethics." *Journal of the American Medical Association,* 22(14): 508.

Holy Bible. 1611. The King James Translation. Accessed online: December 1, 2012 http://www.kingjamesbibleonline.org/Bible-Books/1611–KJV-Books.php.

Homberger, Julius. [1865] 1868. "Report of the Committee on the Relations of Specialists to the Medical Profession." In *Batpaxomyomaxia: A Fight on "Ethics,"* by Julius Homberger. Self published: New Orleans, 1869.

Homberger, Julius. 1869. *Batpaxomyomaxia: A Fight on "Ethics."* Self published: New Orleans, 1869. [from copy at the Francis A. Countway Library of the Harvard Medical School].

Hooker, Worthington. 1849. *Physician and Patient; or a Practical View of the Mutual Duties, Relations, and Interests of the Medical Profession and the Community.* New York: Baker and Scribner.

Hornsby, John A., and Richard E. Schmidt. 1913. *The Modern Hospital: Its Inspiration: Its Architecture: Its Equipment: Its Operation*, 281–282, 465. Philadelphia: W. B. Saunders Co.

Horsman, Reginald. 1996. *Frontier Doctor: William Beaumont, America's First Great Medical Scientist*, 71, 78. Columbia: University of Missouri Press.

Hosack, David to William Coleman, August 17, 1804. http://www.digitalhistory.uh.edu/learning_history/burr/burr_duel5.cfm (accessed January 1, 2010).

Houlbrooke, Ralph. 1998. *Death, Religion, and the Family in England 1450–1750*, 292–293. Oxford: Oxford University Press.

Howell, Thomas Bayly. 1817. *A Complete Collection of State Trials and Proceedings for High Treason and Other Crimes and Misdemeanors from the Earliest Period to the Year 1783, with Notes and Other Illustrations.* London: Longman, Hurst, Rees, Orme.

Huber, Samuel, and Matthew Wynia. 2004. "When Pestilence Prevails... Physician Responsibilities in Epidemics." *American Journal of Bioethics*, 4(1): W7.

Hunter, William. 1784. *Two Introductory Lectures Delivered by Dr. William Hunter, to His Last Course of Anatomical Lectures at this Theatre in Windmill-Street*, 72. London: J. Johnson.

Hurd, H. M. 1912. "The Records of the Baltimore Medico-Chirurgical Society." *Bulletin of the Medical and Chirurgical Society of Maryland*, 4: 57–58.

In Re Quinlan, In The Matter Of Karen Quinlan, An Alleged Incompetent. Supreme Court of New Jersey, 70 N.J. 10. 1976. 355 A.2d 647.

Inquirer. 1892. "Revision of the Code of Ethics." *Journal of the American Medical Association*, 19(27): 780; 1893, 20(3): 82.

International Association of Fire Fighters. "IAFF History." http://www.iaff.org/about/history/ourhistory.htm#1982 (accessed August 24, 2012).

International Federation of Social Workers. 2012. Ethics: Statement of Principles. http://ifsw.org/policies/statement-of-ethical-principles/ (accessed December 1, 2012).

Jackson, Mark. 1994. "Suspicious Infant Deaths: The Statute of 1624 and Medical Evidence at Coroner's Inquests." In *Legal Medicine in History*, edited by Michael Clark and Catherine Crawford, 67. Cambridge: Cambridge University Press.

Jackson, Samuel. 1850. *Review of the Memorial of Doctor John Bell to the Trustees of the University of Pennsylvania.* Philadelphia: B. Mifflin.

Jacobi, Abraham. 1882. "Inaugural Address." *Transactions MSSNY*, 10–12.

Jacobi, Abraham. 1883. "Requiescat In Pace," in, *An Ethical Symposium: Being A Series of Papers Concerning Medical Ethics and Etiquette from the Liberal Standpoint*, edited by Albert C. Post, William C. Ely, S. Oakley Vanderpole, et al., 156–175. New York: G. P. Putnam.

Jalland, Pat. 1996. *Death in the Victorian Family.* Oxford: Oxford University Press.

Journal of the American Medical Association Board of Trustees. 1895. "Report of the Board of Trustees." *Journal of the American Medical Association*, 24(20): 760.

Journal of the American Medical Association Editors. 1883. "Address on the Present Status and Future Tendencies of the Medical Profession in the United States, Delivered at the Annual Meeting of the American Association of Medical Editors in Cleveland, June 5, 1883." *Journal of the American Medical Association*, 1(2): 37.

Journal of the American Medical Association Editors. 1883. "Contract Practice Ethics." *Journal of the American Medical Association*, 1(8): 246.

Journal of the American Medical Association Editors. 1883. "Specialties, and Their Ethical Relations." *Journal of the American Medical Association*, 1(17): 511–512.

Journal of the American Medical Association Editors. 1885. "Domestic Correspondence." *Journal of the American Medical Association*, 5(16): 445.

Journal of the American Medical Association Editors. 1885. "The American Academy of Medicine." *Journal of the American Medical Association*, 5(20): 551–552.

Journal of the American Medical Association Editors. 1895. "Anonymous Publications." *Journal of the American Medical Association* 24(4): 141.

Journal of the American Medical Association Editors. 1886, "Book Reviews." *Journal of the American Medical Association*, 7(25): 697.

Journal of the American Medical Association Editors. 1886. "Gynecological Society of Boston." *Journal of the American Medical Association*, 7(19): 529–531.

Journal of the American Medical Association Editors. 1886. "Letter From London." *Journal of the American Medical Association*, 7(6): 166–167.

Journal of the American Medical Association Editors. 1886. "What Constitutes a Consultation." *Journal of the American Medical Association*, 7(4): 99–100.

Journal of the American Medical Association Editors. 1887. "Clergymen and Patent Medicines." *Journal of the American Medical Association*, 9(4): 118.

Journal of the American Medical Association Editors. 1887. "Criminal Abortions." *Journal of the American Medical Association*, 8(11): 298.

Journal of the American Medical Association Editors. 1887. "Indirect and Improper Advertising." *Journal of the American Medical Association*, 9(18); 9(22): 704.

Journal of the American Medical Association Editors. 1887. "Physicians Names in Newspaper Advertisements." *Journal of the American Medical Association*, 8(21): 575–576.

Journal of the American Medical Association Editors. 1887. "Railroad Rates." *Journal of the American Medical Association*, 8(22): 616.

Journal of the American Medical Association Editors. 1887. "Sects and Schools of Medicine." *Journal of the American Medical Association*, 9(23): 722–723.

Journal of the American Medical Association Editors. 1888. "A Question in Ethics." *Journal of the American Medical Association*, 10(3): 94.

Journal of the American Medical Association Editors. 1888. "Criminal Abortion and State Laws." *Journal of the American Medical Association*, 11(12): 428–429, 11(14): 502, 11(16): 573.

Journal of the American Medical Association Editors. 1888. "Doctors and Advertising." *Journal of the American Medical Association*, 16(8): 275–276;

Journal of the American Medical Association Editors. 1888. "Editorial Notes." *Journal of the American Medical Association*, 11(24): 850.

Journal of the American Medical Association Editors. 1888. "Professional Abortionists." *Journal of the American Medical Association*, 11(26): 912–913.

Journal of the American Medical Association Editors. 1888. "The Ethics of Marriage." *Journal of the American Medical Association*, 11(9): 309–311.

Journal of the American Medical Association Editors. 1888. "To Be Tried Under the Code." *Journal of the American Medical Association*, 16(21): 749–750.

Journal of the American Medical Association Editors. 1888. "Unethical Use of Physicians' Names." *Journal of the American Medical Association*, 10(10): 271; 15(19): 698–699.

Journal of the American Medical Association Editors. 1890. "Antivivisection Bitterness." *Journal of the American Medical Association*, 15(7): 268.

Journal of the American Medical Association Editors. 1891. "The Ethics of Experimentation Upon Living Animals." *Journal of the American Medical Association*, 16(7): 242.

Journal of the American Medical Association Editors. 1892. "Honesty in Experimental Research." *Journal of the American Medical Association*, 19(20): 592.

Journal of the American Medical Association Editors. 1895. "Anonymous Publications." *Journal of the American Medical Association*, 24(4): 141.

Journal of the American Medical Association Editors. 1900. "Report." *Journal of the American Medical Association*, 34: 1553, 1557, 1559.

James, William. [1875] 1987. "Vivisection." *Collected Papers of William James: Essays, Comments, and Reviews*, vol.15, 11. Cambridge: Harvard University Press.

James, William. [1909] 1987. "On Vivisection: Letter to the Secretary of the Vivisection Reform Society (Sidney Taber)." In *Collected Papers of William James: Essays, Comments, and Reviews*, vol. 15, 191. Cambridge: Harvard University Press.

Jewson. N. D. 1974. "Medical Knowledge and the Patronage System in Eighteenth-Century England." *Sociology* 8(3): 369–385.

Jewson, Nicholas. 1976. "The Disappearance of the Sick-Man from Medical Cosmology, 1770–1870." *Sociology*, 10:225–244.

Johnson, Samuel. [1755] 1818. *A Dictionary of the English Language*. Philadelphia: Moses Thomas.

Johnston, A. J. B. 1996. *Life and Religion at Louisbourg, 1713–1758*. Montreal: McGill-Queen's Press.

Joint Commission on the Accreditation of Healthcare Organizations. 1989. *Accreditation Manual*. Oakwood (IL): Joint Commission on the Accreditation of Healthcare Organizations.

Jones, Gorden. 1962. "Doctor John Mitchell's Yellow Fever Epidemics." *Virginia Magazine of History and Biography*, 70(1), part one (January): 43–48.

Jonsen, Albert. 1993. "The Birth of Bioethics." *Hastings Center Report*, 23(6), S1.

Jonsen, Albert. 1998. *The Birth of Bioethics*. New York: Oxford University Press.

Jonsen, Albert. 2005. "Origins and Future of the Belmont Report." In *Belmont Revisited: Ethical Principles for Research with Human Subjects*, edited by James Childress, Eric Meslin, and Harold Shapiro, 4. Washington, DC: Georgetown University Press.

Kaal Kadosh Micve Israel. 1824. *Constitution and Bylaws of the Kaal Kadosh Micve Israel of the City of Philadelphia*. Philadelphia: John Bioren. https://pantherfile.uwm.edu/corre/www/occasionalw/constitution.html (accessed February 2, 2011).

Kahn, R. J., and P. G. Kahn. 1997. "The Medical Repository: The First U.S. Medical Journal (1797–1824)." *New England Journal of Medicine*, 337: 1926–1930.

Kampmeier, Rudolph. 1972. "The Tuskegee Study of Untreated Syphilis." *Southern Medical Journal*, 65(10): 1247–1251. In *Tuskegee's Truths: Rethinking the Tuskegee Syphilis Study*, edited by Susan Reverby, 199–200. Chapel Hill and London: University of North Carolina Press.

Kant, Immanuel. [1798] 1998, 2004. "The Conflict of the Faculties." In "Kant, Immanuel, by Paul Guyer." In *Routledge Encyclopedia of Philosophy*, edited by E. Craig. London: Routledge. http://www.rep.routledge.com/article/DB047SECT9 (accessed August 11, 2012).

Kaplan, Martin. 1971. *Homeopathy in America*. Baltimore: Johns Hopkins University Press.

Kappa Lambda Society of Hippocrates. 1821. *Extracts from the Medical Ethics or a Code of Institutes and Precepts, Adapted to the Professional Conduct of Physicians & Surgeons in Private or General Practice by Thomas Percival, MD.* Lexington: T. Smith at the Reporter Office.

Kappa Lambda Society of Hippocrates. 1822–1835. *Minute Book of the Society*. Philadelphia: Library of the College of Physicians of Philadelphia.

Kappa Lambda Society. 1823. *Extracts from the Medical Ethics of Dr. Percival*. Philadelphia: Kappa Lambda.

Kappa Lambda Society. 1823. "Oath of Affirmation." *College of Physicians of Philadelphia. Manuscript collection of the College of Physicians of Philadelphia.*

Kass, Leon. 1990. "Practicing Ethics. Where's the Action?" *Hastings Center Report*, 20(1): 5–6.

Katz, Jay. [1984] 2002. *The Silent World of Physician and Patient*, 2. Baltimore: Johns Hopkins University Press.

Kaufman, M. 1971. *Homeopathy in America: The Rise and Fall of a Medical Heresy*. Baltimore: Johns Hopkins University Press.

Kaumheimer, G. J. 1894. "He Very Properly Calls Medicus to Order." *Journal of the American Medical Association*, 22(13): 480. (Similar letter in the same issue).

Keen, William. 1900. "The Ideal Physician." *Journal of the American Medical Association*, 34(25): 1592–1594.

Kelly, Walt. 1953. *Pogo Papers*. New York: Simon and Schuster.

Kiernan, V. G. 1988. *The Duel in European History: Honour and the Reign of Aristocracy*, 155–156. Oxford: Oxford University Press.

King, Lester. 1958. *Medical World of the Eighteenth Century*, 149–150. Chicago: University of Chicago Press.

Kipling, Rudyard. 1902. *The Elephant's Child*. http://www.poetryloverspage.com/poets/kipling/I_keep_six_honest.html (accessed May 25, 2012).

Koblenzer, P. J. 1982. "Edinburgh's Influence on Medicine in the New World." In *Proceedings of the Royal College of Physicians of Edinburgh Tercentenary Congress, 1981*, edited by R. Passmore, 143–158. Edinburgh: Royal College of Physicians of Edinburgh.

Kohn, Linda T., Janet M. Corrigan, and Molla S. Donaldson. 2000. *To Err Is Human*. Washington, DC: Institute of Medicine/National Academy Press.

Kollock, P. M. 1857. *History and Treatment of Vesicovaginal Fistula: A Report Read Before the Medical Society of the State of Georgia, at their Annual Meeting at Augusta, April 8th, 1857.* Augusta, GA: McCafferty's Office, J. Morris, Printer. Cited in Wall, L. Lewis. 2006. "The Medical Ethics of Dr. J. Marion Sims: A Fresh Look at the Historical Record." *Journal of Medical Ethics*, 32: 346–350.

Konold, Donald E. 1962. *A History of American Medical Ethics 1847–1912*. Madison: State Historical Society of Wisconsin.

Kopperman, Paul E. 2004. "'Venerate the Lancet': Benjamin Rush's Yellow Fever Therapy in Context." *Bulletin of the History of Medicine*, 78(3): 539–574.

Kuhn, Adam. [1793] 1794. "Letter to Benjamin Rush." In *An Account of the Bilious remitting Yellow Fever as it appeared in the CITY OF PHILADELPHIA in the year 1793*, by Benjamin Rush, 207–208. Philadelphia: Thomas Dobson.

Kuhn, Thomas. [1962] 1996. *The Structure of Scientific Revolutions*. Chicago: University of Chicago Press.

Kuhn, Thomas. 1970. "*The Structure of Scientific Revolutions*." In *International Encyclopedia of Unified Science*, vol. 2, no. 2. Chicago: University of Chicago Press.

"Laudable." 1828. *Webster's American Dictionary of the English Language*. http://www.1828-dictionary.com/d/search/word,laudable (accessed October 3, 2010).

Laennec, René-Théophile-Hyacinthe [1821] 1827. *A Treatise on the Diseases of the Chest and on Mediate Auscultation*, translated by Sir John Forbes, T. London, and G. Underwood. From French original (1819), *De l'Auscultation Médiate ou Traité du Diagnostic des Maladies des Poumons et du Coeur.* Paris: Brosson & Chaudé.

Lambert, Alexander, A. B. Cooke, James E. Moore et al. 1913. "Report of the Committee on the Secret Division of Fees, Taking of Commissions, and Contract Practice." AMA. 1913. *Minutes of the House of Delegates Proceedings of the Sixty-Fourth Annual Session, Minneapolis, Minn. June 16–20, 1913*, 12–15.

Lane, Levi C. 1885. *Shadows in the Ethics of the International Medical Congress*. San Francisco: A. L. Bancroft & Company.

Larkey, Sanford V. 1977. "The Hippocratic Oath in Elizabethan England," *Bulletin of the History of Medicine*, 4: 201–219. In *Legacies in Ethics and Medicine*, edited by Chester Burns, 218–236. New York: Science History Publications.

Lawrence, Christopher. 1988. "Alexander Monro Primus and the Edinburgh Manner of Anatomy." *Bulletin of the History of Medicine*, 62(2): 195–196.

Lawson, John Parker. 1843. *History of the Scottish Episcopal Church from the Revolution to the Present Time*, 164. Edinburgh: Gallie and Bayley.

Lazare, Aaron. 2005. *On Apology.* New York: Oxford University Press.

Leake, Chauncey. 1927. "Introduction," in *Medical Ethics by* Percival, Thomas, [1803] 1927, edited by Chauncey Leak. Baltimore: Williams & Wilkins.

Leape, Lucian L., and Donald M. Berwick. 2005. "Five Years After To Err Is Human: What Have We Learned?" *Journal of the American Medical Association*, 293(19): 2384–2390.

Leavitt, Judith. 1996. *Typhoid Mary, Captive to the Public's Health*. Boston: Beacon Press.

Lederer, Susan. [1995] 1997. *Subjected to Science: Human Experimentation in America Before the Second World War.* Baltimore: Johns Hopkins University Press.

Lederer, Susan. 2008. "Walter Reed and the Yellow Fever Experiments." In *The Oxford Textbook of Clinical Research Ethics*, edited by Ezekiel Emanuel, Christine Grady, Robert Crouch et al., 12–13. New York: Oxford University Press.

Leon, Estela Agramonte Rodriguez. 1940. *Letter and Notes from Estela Agramonte Rodriguez Leon to Philip Showalter Hench, October 10, 1940* and *Text of Speech: Dr. Jesse Lazear and His Contribution to the Conquest of Yellow Fever, by Philip Showalter Hench, October 26, 1940.* All items cited are available at the online archives of the Philip D. Hench Walter Reed Yellow Fever Collection, University of Virginia. http://yellowfever.lib.virginia.edu/reed/collection.html.

Levy, E. C., John F. Anderson, Charles V. Chapin, and H. W. Hill. 1912. "Report of the Committee on the Reporting of Typhoid Fever, American Public Health Association." *American Journal of Public Health,* April, 2(4): 275.

Lichterman, Boleslav. 2009. "Medical Ethics and Communism in the Soviet Union." In *The Cambridge World History of Medical Ethics*, edited by Robert B. Baker and Laurence B. McCullough, 661. New York: Cambridge University Press.

Lifton, Robert J. 1986. *The Nazi Doctors: Medical Killing and the Psychology of Genocide*, 207. New York: Basic Books.

Lombardo, Paul. 2008. *Three Generations, No Imbeciles: Eugenics, the Supreme Court and Buck v. Bell.* Baltimore: Johns Hopkins University Press.

Louis, Pierre-Charle-Alexandre A. [1835] 1836. *Researches Sur les Effets de la Saigneé dans Quelques Maladies Inflammatoires.* Paris: Librairie de l'Académia Royale de Medicine. Translated by C. G. Putnam in *Effects of Bloodletting on Some Inflammatory Diseases and of the Influence of Tartarized Antimony and Vesication in Pneumonitis.* Boston: Hillard, Gray, & Company. fhttp://www.jameslindlibrary.org/illustrating/records/recherches-sur-les-effets-de-la-saignee-dans-quelques-maladies/key_passages?page=2 (accessed January 3, 2011).

Luce, J., A. Birdman, and R. Lee. 1994. "A Brief History of Health Care Quality Assessment and Improvement in the United States." *Western Journal of Medicine*, 160: 263–268.

Luker, Kristin. 1984. *Abortion and the Politics of Motherhood*, 22. Berkeley: University of California Press.

M. D. 1871. "The American Medical Association." *National Medical Journal* (1870–1871), 1: 174–175, 178.

Maclean, Fitzroy, and Magnus Linklater. 1991. *Scotland, A Concise History.* New York and London, Thames & Hudson.

Maehle, Andreas-Holger. 1999. *Drugs on Trial: Experimental Pharmacology and Therapeutic Innovation in the Eighteenth Century.* Amsterdam: Ridopi.

Maehle, Andreas-Holger. 2009. *Doctors, Honour, and the Law: Medical Ethics in Imperial Germany.* Basingstoke: Palgrave-Macmillan.

Maehle, Andreas-Holger, and U. Tröhler. 2009. "The Discourses of Medical Practitioners in the Nineteenth- and Twentieth-Century Germany." In *The Cambridge World History of Medical Ethics*, edited by Robert B. Baker and Laurence B. McCullough, 432–438. New York: Cambridge University Press.

Maitland, Charles. 1722. *Mr. Maitland's Account of Inoculating the Small Pox*, 21. London: Printed for the author, by J. Downing and to be sold by J. Roberts, at the Oxford-Arms in Warwick-Lane. Retrieved from Harvard University Library. http://pds.lib.harvard.edu/pds/view/8072674.

Markham, H. C. 1888. "Foeticide and Its Prevention." *Journal of the American Medical Association*, 11(23): 805–806.

Marvin, Abijah P. 1892. *The Life and Times of COTTON MATHER; D.D., F.R.S. or A Boston Minister of Two Centuries Ago. 1663–1728*. Boston and Chicago: Congregational Sunday-School and Publishing Soceity.

Mary Mallon (Typhoid Mary). 1939, *American Journal of Public Health and the Nations Health*. January 29 (1): 66–68. doi:10.2105/AJPH.29.1.66 http://ajph.aphapublications.org/cgi/reprint/29/1/66?view=long&pmid=18014976 (accessed September 18, 2011).

Massachusetts Medical Society. 1881. *Records of Board of Trials, 1858–1881*, 2, 62. Manuscript collection of the Countway Medical Library.

Mather C., J. Dummer, and W. Tumain. 1722. *An Account of the Method and Success of Inoculating the Small-Pox in Boston in New England*. London: J. Peele.

Mather, Cotton, Zabdiel Boylston, and Samuel Gerrish. 1721. *Some Account of What Is Said of Inoculating or Transplanting the Small Pox*. Boston: S. Gerrish. http://pds.lib.harvard.edu/pds/view/7910093 (accessed May 8, 2010).

Matthews, Williams. W. 1827. W. W. (William) Matthews, American Fur Company [Mackinac, MI] to W. Beaumont [Green Bay, WI] regarding encounter with St. Martin at La Chalupe and request for reimbursement of expenses. August 13, 1827. William Beaumont Papers, Bernard Becker Medical Library, Washington University School of Medicine, St. Louis, Mo. http://beckerweb.wustl.edu/libdept/arb/findaid/PC001.html (visited February 4, 2012).

Matthews, W. William. August 18, 1827. "Letter from American Fur Company, Mackinac, Michigan to William Beaumont [Green Bay, WI] regarding reimbursement of Matthews' expenses and negotiations for employment of St. Martin and wife. August 18, 1827." Beaumont Papers, Bernard Becker Medical Library, Washington University School of Medicine, St. Louis, MO.

Mays, Jeff. 2011. "Councilwoman Wants to Remove Statue of Doctor Who Operated on Slaves." *DNAinfo*. http://www.dnainfo.com/20110214/harlem/east-harlem-councilwoman-wants-controversial-statue-removed.

McCaw, Walter. 1904. *Walter Reed—The Man, His Work, and the Appreciation Shown of the Results Accomplished by Him and His Associates on the Yellow Fever Commission*. Washington: Walter Reed Memorial Association.

McCullough, Laurence. *John Gregory and the Invention of Professional Medical Ethics and the Profession of Medicine*. Dordrecht: Kluwer Academic Publishers.

McDaniel II, W. B. 1958. "A Brief Sketch of the Rise of American Medical Societies." In *History of American Medicine: A Symposium*, edited by Felix Marti-Ibañez, 134. New York: MD Publications.

McGregor, Deborah Kuhn. 1998. *From Midwives to Medicine: The Birth of American Gynecology*, 51, 54. New Brunswick: Rutgers University Press.

McVickar, John. [1822] 1931. *A Domestic Narrative of the Life of Samuel Bard, M.D., LL.D.: Late President of the College of Physicians and Surgeons of the University of the State of New-York, &c*, 112–113. New York: The Literary Room.

Measuring Worth Website. http://www.measuringworth.com/uscompare/relativevalue.php (accessed February 13, 2012).

Medical Association of Washington. 1833, 1837. *Regulations and System of Ethics of the Medical Association of Washington*. Washington, DC: Medical Association of Washington, D. C.

Medical Examiner, The. 1839. "History of the New York Kappa Lambda Conspiracy." In *Essays Taken from the Medical Examiner*. New York: Stuart.

Medico-Chirurgical Society of Baltimore. 1832. *A System of Medical Ethics Adopted by the Medico-Chirurgical Society of Baltimore; Being the report of the Committee on Ethics and Published by Order of the Society*. Baltimore: James Lucas and E. K. Deaver.

Medicus. 1894. "The Advertising Question." *Journal of the American Medical Association*, 22(12): 438–439.

Meigs, C. D. 1854. *On the Nature, Signs, and Treatment of Childbirth Fevers; In Series of Letters Addressed to the Students of his Class*. Philadelphia: Blanchard and Lea.

Merck & Company. 1899. *Merck's Manual of the Material Medical Together with a Summary of Therapeutic Indications and a Classification of Medicaments: A ready-reference Pocket Book for the Practicing Physician*. New York: Merck & Company.

Meyer, Jesse. 1912. *The Life and Letters of Dr. William Beaumont: Including Hitherto Unpublished Data Concerning the Case of Alexis St. Martin*, 23, 57–60, 78, 148. St. Louis: C.V. Mosby Company.

Miller, Henry. 1859. "Presidential Address." *Transactions of the Thirteenth Annual American Medical Association Meeting in Louisville, Kentucky, 1859 XIII*, 57.

Miller, Thomas, and J. W. H. Lovejoy. 1870. "Majority Report of the Committee on Arrangements." In "The American Medical Association." *National Medical Journal* (1870–1871), 1: 173–174.

Milton, Thomas H. 1931. "Doctor Samuel Bard." *Columbia University Quarterly*, June: 112–130.

Mitchell, S., J. Manley, F. Pascalis, and C. Drake. 1821. "Letter of Editors." *The Medical Repository of Original Essays and Intelligence, Relative to Physic, Surgery, Chemistry and Natural Philosophy, with a Critical Analysis of Recent Publications on these Departments of Knowledge and their Auxiliary Branches, vol. 6*, 95–100. New York: William A. Mercein.

Mohr, James C. 1978. *Abortion in America: The Origins and Evolution of National Policy*, chapter three. Oxford: Oxford University Press.

Mohr, James C. 2000. "American Medical Malpractice Litigation in Historical Perspective." *Journal of the American Medical Association*, 283(13): 1731–1737.

Monro, Alexander. 1691. *Presbyterian Inquisition as it was Lately Practised Against the Professors of the College of Edinburgh, August and September, 1690, in which the Spirit of Presbytery and their Present Method of Procedure is Plainly Discovered, Matter of Fact by Undeniable Instances Cleared, and Libels Against Particular Persons Discussed*. London: J. Hindmarsh.

Monro *Primus*, Alexander. 1739. *Essay on Female Conduct Contained in Letters from a Father to his Daughter*, 342–343. Unpublished manuscript. National Library of Scotland Mss. #6658, 6659.

Monroe *Primus*, Alexander. [1739] 2004. "The Professor's Daughter: An Essay on Female Conduct contained In Letters from a Father to His Daughter." In *Conduct Literature for Women (1720–1770)*, edited by Pam Morris, vol. 2. London: Pickering & Chatto.

Montagu, Lady Mary. [1718] 1763. *Letters of the Right Honourable Lady M—y W—y M—e: Written During her Travels in Europe, Asia and Africa*, vol. II, Letter XXXIII, 61–63. http://archive.org/details/lettersofrighthoo1montiala (accessed May 16, 2013).

Moore, Wendy. 2005. *The Knife Man: The Extraordinary Life and Times of John Hunter, Father of Modern Surgery*. New York: Broadway Books/Random House.

Moran, John J. 19??. *Memoirs of A Human Guinea Pig*. Manuscript 8054–g War Department, Surgeon General's Office, Army Medical Museum and Library, Washington, D.C. Charlottesville: Philip D. Hench Walter Reed Collection, University of Virginia.

Morgan, John. [1765] 1965. *A Discourse Upon the Institution of Medical Schools in America*, 28–30. Philadelphia: University of Pennsylvania.

Morgan, William. 1827. *Illustrations of Masonry by One of the Fraternity who has Devoted Thirty Years to the Subject: "God said, let there be light, and there was light."* Batavia: David C. Miller.

Morghenstern, Leon. 2004. "Isaac Hays, MD, Nineteenth Century Pioneer in Ophthalmology." *Archives of Ophthalmology*, 122. www.archophthalmol.com (accessed March 31, 2011).

Morrice, A. A. G. 2002. "'Honour and Interests': Medical Ethics and the British Medical Association." In *Historical and Philosophical Perspectives on Biomedical Ethics: From Paternalism to Autonomy?*, edited by A. H Maehle and J. G. Kordesch, 11–36. Aldershot: Ashgate.

Morris, Pam, ed. 2004. *Conduct Literature for Women (1720–1770)*. London: Pickering & Chatto.

Mount Sinai Journal of Medicine Editors. 1989. [The HIV-AIDS issue]. Vol. 56.

MSCNY. 1794. *Minute Book of the Medical Society of the County of New York* (November 14, 1794). Library of the New York Academy of Medicine.

MSCNY. 1796. *Minute Book of the Medical Society of the County of New York* (February 9, 1796). Library of the New York Academy of Medicine.

MSCNY. 1797. *Minute Book of the Medical Society of the County of New York* (February 14, 1797). Library of the New York Academy of Medicine.

MSCNY. 1806. *Minute Book*. Library of the New York Academy of Medicine.

MSCNY. 1806. *Proceedings of the Medical Society of the County of New York*. Library of the New York Academy of Medicine.

MSCNY. 1808. *Proceedings of the Medical Society of the County of New York*. Library of the New York Academy of Medicine.

MSCNY. 1824. *Proceedings of the Medical Society of the County of New York* (August 9, 1824). Library of the New York Academy of Medicine.

MSCNY. 1825. *Proceedings of the Medical Society of the County of New York* (July 6–October 11, 1825). Library of the New York Academy of Medicine.

MSCNY. 1827. Committee on Quack Medicines. *Report of the Medical Society of the City of New-York, on Nostrums, or Secret Medicines.* New York: E. Conrad.

MSCNY. 1827. *Proceedings of the Medical Society of the County of New York* (July 16–August 20, 1827, 49–51). Library of the New York Academy of Medicine.

MSCNY. 1831. *Proceedings of the Medical Society of the County of New York* (December 12, 1831). Library of the New York Academy of Medicine.

MSCNY. 1832. *Minutes of the Comita Minora of the Medical Society of the County of New York* (December 5, 1832). Library of the New York Academy of Medicine.

MSCNY. 1864. *Report of the Delegates to the N. Y. State Medical Soc. For Feb. 3 & 4.* Library of the New York Academy of Medicine.

MSSNY. 1806. *Minutes of the Comita Minora of the Medical Society of the State of New York.* Founding meeting September 18, 1806. Library of the New York Academy of Medicine.

MSSNY. [1821] 1832. *Transactions of the Medical Society of the State of New York: From its Organization in 1807, up to and including 1831.* Albany: Printing House of Charles Van Benthuysen & Sons.

MSSNY. 1823. *A System of Medical Ethics, Published by the Order of the State Medical Society of New York.* New York: William Grattan.

MSSNY. 1868. *Transactions of the Medical Society of the State of New York from its Organization in 1807, Up to and Including 1831.* Albany: Charles van Benthuysen & Sons. Also reprinted in *History of the Medical Society of the State of New York*, by James J. Walsh, 1907, 90 and Appendix: By-laws. New York: Medical Society of the State of New York.

MSSNY. 1881. "Report of the Committee on Medical Ethics," *Transactions of the Medical Society of the State of New York.* Library of the New York Academy of Medicine.

Myerson, A., J. Ayer, T. Putnam, et al. 1936. *Eugenic Sterilization: A Reorientation of the Problem.* New York: The Macmillan Company.

National Commission for the Protection of Human Subjects of Biomedical and Behavioral Research. 1979. *The Belmont Report: Ethical Principles and Guidelines for the Protection of Human Subjects of Research.* http://ohsr.od.nih.gov/guidelines/belmont.html (accessed December 20, 2012).

Neal, Daniel. 1817. *The History of the Puritans or Protestant Non-Conformists, from the Death of Queen Elizabeth to the Beginning of the Civil War in the Year 1642*, edited by Joshua Toulmin vol. II, 38–39. Boston: Charles Ewer; Newburyport (MA); William B. Allen & Co.

Neuhauser, D. 2002. "Heroes and Martyrs of Quality and Safety: Ernest Amory Codman MD." *Quality Safety Health Care*, 11: 104–105.

New Jersey Medical Society. [1766] 1966. "Instruments of Association and Constitutions of the New Jersey Medical Society." In *The Healing Art: A History of the Medical Society of New Jersey*, edited by Fred B. Rogers and A. Reasoner Sayer, 309. Trenton: Medical Society of New Jersey.

New York City. 1731. *Laws, Statutes, Ordinances and Constitutions of the City of New York.* 27–29.

New York Times. October 21, 1894, "Sims Statue Unveiled." http://query.nytimes.com/mem/archivefree/pdf?res=F70C14F63E5515738DDDA80A94D8415B8485F0D3 (accessed August 12, 2011).

New York Times Editors. 1898. Cited in Malkin, Harold, 1993, "The Trials and Tribulations of George Miller Sternberg (1838–1915) America's First Bacteriologist." *Perspectives in Biology and Medicine*, 36 (4), 677.

New York Times. 1902. "Roosevelt to Physicians: Urges them Not to Neglect Duties of Citizenship—Rush Statue Dedicated: June 11, 1902."

New York Times. November 12, 1938. "Typhoid Mary' Dies of a Stroke at 68: Carrier of Disease, Blamed for 51 Cases and 3 Deaths, but She Was Held Immune. Services This Morning. Epidemic Is Traced."

New York Times. May 27, 2007. "I'd Like to Sell the World a Coke." http://www.nytimes.com/ref/business/20070527_COKE_GRAPHIC.html (accessed August 23, 2012).

Nickens, H. W. 1985. "A Case of Professional Exclusion in 1870: The Formation of the First Black Medical Society." *Journal of the American Medical Association*, 253(17): 2549–2552.

Nourse, Victoria. 2008. *In Reckless Hands: Skinner v. Oklahoma and the Near Triumph of American Eugenics*. New York: W. W. Norton & Co.

Numbers, Ronald L. 1979. "William Beaumont and the Ethics of Human Experimentation." *Journal of the History of Biology*, 12(1) 113–135.

Nuremberg Trials: The Doctors' Trial. http://law2.umkc.edu/faculty/projects/ftrials/nuremberg/nurembergdoctortrial.html#COUNT%20THREE (accessed July 16, 2012).

Nutton, Vivian. 1995. "What's in an Oath?" *Journal of the Royal College of Physicians of London*, 29(6): 518–524.

Nye, Robert A. 1993. *Masculinity and Honor Codes in Modern Day France*. Oxford: Oxford University Press.

Nye, Robert A. 2009. "The Discourses of Medical Practitioners in the Nineteenth- and Twentieth-century France." In *The Cambridge World History of Medical Ethics*, edited by Robert B. Baker and Laurence B. McCullough, 418–426. New York: Cambridge University Press.

Oath of Soviet Physicians. [1971] 2004. In *Encyclopedia of Bioethics*, vol. 3, 3rd ed. edited by Stephen Post, 2719. New York: Macmillan Reference.

Ojanuga, Durrenda. 1993. "The Medical Ethics of the "Father of Gynecology," Dr. J. Marion Sims." *Journal of Medical Ethics*, 19: 28–31, 30.

Orr, R. D., N. Pang, E. D. Pellegrino, and M. Siegler. 1997. "Use of the Hippocratic Oath: A Review of Twentieth Century Practice and a Content Analysis of Oaths Administered in Medical Schools in the U.S. and Canada in 1993." *Journal of Clinical Ethics*, 8(4): 377–388.

Osler, Sir William. [1897] 1898. *The Principles and Practice of Medicine*, 3rd ed., 183. New York: D. Appleton and Company.

Osler, Sir William. [1897] 1901. *The Principles and Practice of Medicine*, 4th ed., 183–184. New York: D. Appleton and Company. http://mcgovern.library.tmc.edu/data/www/html/people/osler/PPM4th/OP420011B.htm (accessed February 19, 2012).

Osler, Sir William. 1907. "The Evolution of the Idea of Experiment in Medicine." *Transactions of the Congress of American Physicians and Surgeons*, 7: 8.

Packard, Francis R. 1901. *The History of Medicine in the United States: A Collection of Facts and Documents Relating to the History of Medical Science in this Country, from the Earliest English Colonization to the Year 1800s*, 18, 23 158–164, 200, 210. Philadelphia: J. B. Lippincott.

Parker, Samuel. 1715. *An Essay Upon the Duty of Physicians and Patients, the Dignity of Medicine, and the Prudentials of Practice in Two Dialogues*. London: National Library of Medicine.

Parks, Ward. 1989. *Verbal Dueling in Heroic Narrative: The Homeric and Old English Traditions*. Princeton: Princeton University Press.

Parvin, Theophilus. 1890. "Casuistry in Obstetrics." *Journal of the American Medical Association*, 14(11): 371–373.

Pattison, F. L. 1987. *Granville Sharp Pattison: Anatomist and Antagonist (1791–1851)*. Tuscaloosa: University of Alabama Press.

"Peculiar." 1828. *Webster's American Dictionary of the English Language*. http://machaut.uchicago.edu/?resource=Webster%27s&word=peculiar&use1828=on (accessed May 11, 2013).

"Pecuniary." 1828. *Webster's American Dictionary of the English Language*. http://www.1828-dictionary.com/d/search/word,pecuniary (accessed October 3, 2010).

Pellegrino, Edmund. 2008. *The Philosophy of Medicine Reborn*. Notre Dame: University of Notre Dame Press.

Pence, Gregory. 2008. *Classic Cases in Medical Ethics: Accounts of the Cases that Shaped and Define Medical Ethics*. New York: McGraw Hill.

People v. Clarissa Davie. March 1818. New York City-Hall Recorder 3. 45–46.

Percival, Thomas. 1794. *Medical Jurisprudence or A Code of Ethics and Institutes, Adapted to the Professions of Physic and Surgery*. Manchester: S. Russell.

Percival, Thomas. 1803. *Medical Ethics: Or a Code of Institutes and Precepts, Adapted to the Professional Conduct of Physicians and Surgeons*. London: J. Johnson & R. Bickerstaff.

Percival, Thomas. [1803] 1985. *Medical Ethics; Or, A Code of Institutes or Precepts Adapted to the Professional Conduct of Physicians and Surgeons*, edited by Edmund. Pellegrino. Facsimile edition Birmingham (AL): The Classics of Medicine Library.

Pernick, Martin. 1982. "The Patient's Role in Medical Decision-Making: A Social History of Informed Consent in Medical Therapy." *The President's Commission for the Study of Ethical Problems in Medicine and Biomedical and Behavioral Research: Making Health Care Decisions*, 3, Appendices: Studies on the foundations of informed consent, 1–35.

Pernick, Martin. 1985. *A Calculus of Suffering: Pain, Professionalism, and Anesthesia in Nineteenth-Century America*. New York: Columbia University Press.

Pernick, Martin. 1996. *The Black Stork: Eugenics and the Death of "Defective" Babies in American Medicine and Motion Pictures Since 1905*. New York: Oxford University Press.

Peters, Richard, ed. 1845. *The Public Statutes at Large of the United States of America*, vol. 1, 23. Boston: Charles C. Little and James Brown.

Petrelli, Richard L. 1971. "The Regulation of French Midwifery During the Ancien Régime," *Journal of the History of Medicine and Allied Sciences*, 26(3): 276–292.

Phelps, James L. 1854. "Religion, as an Element in Medicine; or the Duties and Obligations of the Profession." *Western Journal of Medicine and Surgery,* June, 1: 462.

"Physician." 1828. *Webster's American Dictionary of the English Language.* www.1828-dictionary.com.

Pilcher, Lewis. 1883 "Codes of Medical Ethics." In *An Ethical Symposium: Being a Series of Papers Concerning Medical Ethics and Etiquette from Liberal Standpoint*, edited by Albert C. Post et al., 42–43, 52–53. New York: G. P. Putnam.

Pius XII. 1957. "Address to an International Congress of Anesthesiologists." Official Documents Pope Pius XII, November 24, 1957. *L' Osservatore Romano*, November 25–26. http://www.lifeissues.net/writers/doc/doc_31resuscitation.html (accessed April 28, 2011).

"Police." 1913. *Webster's American Dictionary of the English Language* http://www.1828-dictionary.com/d/search/word,police (October 3, 2010).

Pollard, A. F. 1910. "Edmund Bonner." *Encyclopedia Britannica*, 11th edition, vol. 4: 211.

Porter, Dorothy, and Roy Porter. 1989. *Patient's Progress: Doctors and Doctoring in Eighteenth-Century England.* Cambridge: Cambridge University Press.

Porter, Roy. 1989. "Death and doctors in Georgian England." In *Death, Ritual, and Bereavement*, edited by R. Houlbrooke, 77–94. London: Routledge.

Porter, Roy. 2001. *Enlightenment: Britain and the Creation of the Modern World.* London: Penguin Books.

Posner, E. 1975. "William Withering versus the Darwins." *History of Medicine,* 6(1): 51–57.

Post, Albert C., William C. Ely, S. Oakley Vanderpole, et al., eds. 1883. *An Ethical Symposium: Being A Series of Papers Concerning Medical Ethics and Etiquette from the Liberal Standpoint.* New York: G. P. Putnam.

Post, Alfred. 1883. "Reasons for Preferring a Larger Liberty in Consultations than that Which is Allowed by the Code of Ethics of the American Medical Association." In *An Ethical Symposium: Being a Series of Papers Concerning Medical Ethics and Etiquette from Liberal Standpoint*, edited by Albert C. Post et al., 1. New York: G. P. Putnam.

Powderly, Kathleen. 2000. "Patient consent and Negotiation in the Brooklyn Gynecological Practice of Alexander J. C. Skene: 1863–1900." *Journal of Medicine and Philosophy,* 1(25): 12–27.

Powell, John H. 1970. *Bring Out Your Dead: The Great Plague of Yellow Fever in Philadelphia in 1793.* New York: Arno Press of the New York Times.

Presad, Govind, Linden Elder, Laura Sedig, et al. 2008. "The Current State of Medical School Education in Bioethics, Health Law, and Health Economics." *Journal of Law and Medical Ethics,* 36(1): 4, 89–94.

President's Commission for the Study of Ethical Problems in Medicine and Biomedical and Behavioral Research. 1981. *Defining Death: Medical, Legal and Ethical Issues in the Determination of Death.* Washington, DC: U.S. Government Printing Office (81-600150).

President's Commission for the Study of Ethical Problems in Medicine and Biomedical and Behavioral Research. 1983. *Deciding to Forego Life-Sustaining Treatment: A Report on the Ethical, Medical and Legal Issues in Treatment Decisions*. Washington DC: U.S. Government Printing Office (83–600503).

Prince, Carl E. 1985. "The Great 'Riot Year': Jacksonian Democracy and Patterns of Violence in 1834." *Journal of the Early Republic*, 5(1): 1–19.

"Professional." 1828 *Webster's American Dictionary of the English Language*. http://machaut.uchicago.edu/websters (accessed May 11, 2013).

"Professional." 1919 *Webster's Revised Unabridged Dictionary* http://machaut.uchicago.edu/websters (accessed May 11, 2013).

Prosnitz, Mary Beth. 1983. "A Model Bill to Establish Hospital Ethics Committees." In *Deciding to Forego Life-Sustaining Treatment: A Report on the Ethical, Medical and Legal Issues in Treatment Decisions by the* President's Commission for the Study of Ethical Problems in Medicine and Biomedical and Behavioral Research. Washington, DC: U.S. Government Printing Office (83–600503).

"Punish." 1828. *Webster's American Dictionary of the English Language*. http://www.1828-dictionary.com/d/search/word,punish (accessed October 3, 2010).

Queens County (NY) Grand Jury. [1984] 1995. "Report of the Special January Third Additional 1983 Grand Jury Concerning 'Do Not Resuscitate Orders' At a Certain Hospital in Queens, Sup. Ct. Queens Co, February 8, 1984." In "Do Not Resuscitate Orders: The Proposed Legislation and Report of the New York State Taskforce on Life and the Law." In *Legislating Medical Ethics: A Study of the New York State Do-Not-Resuscitate Law*, edited by Robert Baker and Martin Strosberg. Dordrecht: Kluwer Academic Publishers.

Ramsey, Paul. 1970. *The Patient As Person: Explorations in Medical Ethics*. New Haven: Yale University.

Rancich, A.M., M. L. Pérez, C. Morales, and R. J. Gelpi. 2005. "Beneficence, Justice, and Lifelong Learning Expressed in Medical Oaths." *Journal of Continuing Education in the Health Professions*, 25(3): 211–220.

Reed, Walter, James Carroll, and Aristides Agramonte. 1901. "The Etiology of Yellow Fever. An Additional Note." *Journal of the American Medical Association*, 35 (7): 431–440. Later republished as Reed, Walter, James Carroll, and Aristides Agramonte. 1983. "The Etiology of Yellow Fever: An Additional Note." *Journal of the American Medical Association* 250(5): 649–658.

Reed, Walter. 1900. *Letter from Walter Reed to Jefferson Randolph Kean, September 25, 1900*, Philip D. Hench Walter Reed Yellow Fever Collection. Charlottesville: University of Virginia.

Reed, Walter. November 22, 1900. Letter from Walter Reed to Emilie Lawrence Reed, Philip D. Hench Walter Reed Collection. Charlottesville: University of Virginia.

Reich, Warren T. 1993. "How Bioethics Got Its Name." *Hastings Center Report*, 23: S6–S7.

Reich, Warren T. 1994. "The Word 'Bioethics': Its Birth and the Legacies of those Who Shaped It." *Kennedy Institute of Ethics Journal*, 4: 319–335.

Reich, Warren T. 1995. "The Word 'Bioethics': The Struggle Over its Earliest Meanings." *Kennedy Institute of Ethics Journal*, 5: 19–34.

Reiser, Stanley. 1978. *Medicine and the Reign of Technology.* Cambridge: Cambridge University Press.

Reyburn, R. R., J. G. Stephenson, A. T. Augusta, et al. [1870] 1967. "A Plea for Racial Equality." *The New Era* (Washington). January 27, 1870. In *The History of the Negro in Medicine*, edited by H. Morais 1st ed., 215–216. New York: Association for the Study of Negro Life and History and Publishers Company, Inc.

Richardson, Ruth. 2000. *Death, Dissection and the Destitute.* Chicago: University of Chicago Press.

Rogers, F. 1960. "Nicholas Romanyne, 1756–1817: Stormy Petrel of American Medical Education." *Journal of Medical Education*, 35(3): 258–263.

Rogers, Fred B., and A. Reasoner Sayer. 1965. *The Healing Art: A History of the Medical Society of New Jersey*, 17, 309. Trenton: Medical Society of New Jersey.

Rolls, Roger. 1984. "Archibald Cleland, c 1770–1771." *British Medical Journal*, 288: 1132–1134.

Roman, C. V. 1909. *Journal of the American Medical Association* 1(1): cover page. http://www.ncbi.nlm.nih.gov/pmc/articles/PMC2574061/pdf/jnma00212-0001.pdf

Romayne, Nicholas. 1809. "Anniversary Address to the Medical Society of the State of New York by the President." In *Transactions of the Medical Society of the State of New York from its Organization in 1807, Up to and Including 1831*, 32–33. Albany: Charles van Benthuysen & Sons.

Roosa, Daniel Bennett St. John. 1883. "Objections to the Code of Ethics and to the Disciplinary Authority of the American Medical Association." In *An Ethical Symposium: Being a Series of Papers Concerning Medical Ethics and Etiquette from Liberal Standpoint*, edited by Albert C. Post et al., 106. New York: G. P. Putnam.

Rosen, George. 1953. "Cameralism and the Concept of Medical Police." *Bulletin of the History of Medicine*, January–February, 27(1): 21–42.

Rosen, George, ed. 1974. "The Fate of the Concept of Medical Police, 1780–1890." In *From Medical Police to Social Medicine: Essays in the History of Health Care*, edited by George Rosen, 142–158. New York: Science History Publications.

Rosner, Lisa. 1991. *Medical Education in the Age of Improvement: Edinburgh Students and Apprentices, 1760–1826.* Edinburgh: Edinburgh University Press.

Rothman, David. 1991. *Strangers at the Bedside: A History of How Law And Bioethics Transformed Medical Decision Making.* New York: Basic Books.

Rothstein, William G. 1972. *American Physicians in the Nineteenth Century: From Sects to Science.* Baltimore: Johns Hopkins University Press.

Rowton, Joseph. 2009. "Sir Patrick Manson and Sir Ronald Ross' Struggle for the Malaria Breakthrough." *Historia Medicinae*, 2(1): 1–11.

Rudacille, Deborah. 2000. *The Scalpel and the Butterfly: The Conflict Between Animal Research and Animal Protection.* Berkeley: University of California Press.

Runes, Dagobert, ed. 1947. *The Selected Writings of Benjamin Rush.* New York: The Philosophical Library.

Ruschenberger, William. S. W. 1887. *An Account of the Institution and Progress of the College of Physicians of Philadelphia During a Hundred Years, From January 1787.* Philadelphia: William. J. Doran.

Ruschenberger, William. S.W. ed. 1887. *Transactions of the College of Physicians of Philadelphia: Centennial Volume.* Philadelphia: College of Physicians of Philadelphia, Dornan Printers.

Ruschenberger, William. S.W., ed. [1813] 1887. "Notice of Dr. Benjamin Rush." In *Transactions of the College of Physicians of Philadelphia.* Philadelphia: College of Physicians of Philadelphia.

Ruschenberger, William. S. W. 1891. *A Sketch of the Life of Dr. Gouverneur Emerson.* Philadelphia: MacCalla & Company.

Rush, Benjamin. [1773] 1997. *An Address to the Inhabitants of the British Settlements in America Upon Slave Keeping.* Boston: Langdon.

Rush, Benjamin. 1781. *The New Method of Inoculating for the Small Pox: Delivered in a Lecture in the University of Philadelphia, Feb. 20th 1781.* Philadelphia: Charles Cist.

Rush, Benjamin. 1786. *An Oration, Delivered before the American Philosophical Society, held in Philadelphia on the 27th of February, 1786; Concerning an Enquiry into the Influence of Physical Causes on the Moral Faculty.* Philadelphia: Charles Cist.

Rush, Benjamin. 1789. "An Enquiry into the Consistency of Oaths with Reason and Christianity," *Columbia Magazine,* 3 (February):104–108. Reprinted in Rush, Benjamin. (1798 and later editions). *Essays, Literary, Moral & Philosophical.* Philadelphia: Thomas and Samuel F. Bradford.

Rush, Benjamin. [1789] 1815. "Observations on the Duties of a Physician, and the Methods of Improving Medicine. Accommodated to the Present State of Society and Manners in the United States." Delivered at the University of Pennsylvania, February 7, 1789, at the conclusion of a course of lectures on chemistry and the practice of physic. Published at the Request of the Class. In, Benjamin Rush, *Medical Inquiries and Observations,* 4th edition, Philadelphia: M. Care., Vol. 1, pp. 251–264.

Rush, Benjamin. [1789] 1947. *Observations on the Duties of A Physician and the Methods of Improving Medicine, Accommodated to the Present State of Society and Manners in the United States. Delivered in the University of Pennsylvania, February 7, 1789, at the Conclusion of a Course of Lectures upon Chemistry and the Practice of Physic.* Published at the Request of the Class. Philadelphia: Prichard & Hall.

Rush, Benjamin. [1789] 1988. "An Inquiry into the Consistency of Oaths with Reason and Christianity." In *Essays Literary, Moral and Philosophical: Benjamin Rush,* edited by Michael Meranze, 73–78. Schenectady: Union College Press.

Rush, Benjamin. [1793] 1794. "Letter to Adam Kunh." In *An Account of the Bilious Remitting Yellow Fever as it Appeared in the CITY OF PHILADELPHIA in the Year 1793,* by Benjamin Rush, 211–212. Philadelphia: Thomas Dobson.

Rush, Benjamin. [1793] 1951. "Letter to Julia Rush. 10 September 1793." In *Letters of Benjamin Rush,* edited by L. H. Butterfield, vol. II, 657–658. Philadelphia: Princeton University Press for the American Philosophical Society.

Rush, Benjamin. [1793] 1951. "To His Fellow Citizens: Treatment for Yellow Fever. 12 September 1793." In *Letters of Benjamin Rush,* edited by L. H. Butterfield, vol. II: 660–661. Philadelphia: Princeton University Press for the American Philosophical Society.

Rush, Benjamin. [1793] 1951. "To John R. B. Rodgers: An Account of the Prevailing Epidemic. 3 October 1793." In *Letters of Benjamin Rush*, edited by L. H. Butterfield, vol. II: 697. Philadelphia: Princeton University Press for the American Philosophical Society.

Rush, Benjamin. [1793] 1951. "To Mrs. Rush. 11 September 1793." In *Letters of Benjamin Rush*, edited by L. H. Butterfield, vol. II: 659. Philadelphia: Princeton University Press for the American Philosophical Society.

Rush, Benjamin. [1793] 1951. "To the College of Physicians: The Use of the Lancet in Yellow Fever. 12 September 1793." In *Letters of Benjamin Rush*, edited by L. H. Butterfield, II: 661–662. Philadelphia: Princeton University Press for the American Philosophical Society.

Rush, Benjamin 1794. *An Account of the Bilious Remitting Yellow Fever, as it Appeared in the City of Philadelphia, in the Year 1791*. Philadelphia: Thomas Dobson.

Rush, Benjamin. [1796] 1979. Lectures on the Practice of Physic. MSS Library of the University of Pennsylvania. In *The Development of Modern Medicine*,edited by Richard Shryock. Madison: University of Wisconsin Press, 3.

Rush, Benjamin. [1801] 1811. "Lecture V, On the Vices and Virtues of Physicians." In *Sixteen Introductory Lectures, to Courses of Lectures upon the Institutes and Practice of Medicine, with a syllabus of the Latter… Delivered in the University of Pennsylvania*, edited by Benjamin Rush. Philadelphia: Bradford and Innskeep.

Rush, Benjamin. [1801] 1811. "Upon the Causes Which Have Retarded the Progress of Medicine and the Means of Promoting Its Certainty and Greater Usefulness." In *Sixteen Introductory Lectures, to Courses of Lectures upon the Institutes and Practice of Medicine, with a syllabus of the Latter… Delivered in the University of Pennsylvania*, edited by Benjamin Rush, 150–154. Philadelphia: Bradford and Innskeep.

Rush, Benjamin. [1803] 1811. "On the Pains and Pleasures of a Medical Life." In *Sixteen Introductory Lectures, to Courses of Lectures Upon the Institutes and Practice of Medicine, with a Syllabus of the Latter… Delivered in the University of Pennsylvania*, edited by Benjamin Rush, 212–213. Philadelphia: Bradford and Innskeep.

Rush, Benjamin. [1807] 1811. "On the Means of Acquiring Business and the Causes Which Prevent the Acquisition and Occasion the Loss of It in the Profession of Medicine." In *Sixteen Introductory Lectures, to courses of Lectures upon the Institutes and Practice of Medicine, with a Syllabus of the Latter… Delivered in the University of Pennsylvania*, edited by Benjamin Rush, 245. Philadelphia: Bradford and Innskeep.

Rush, Benjamin. [1808] 1811. "On the Duties of Patients to Their Physicians." In *Sixteen Introductory Lectures, to courses of Lectures upon the Institutes and Practice of Medicine, with a Syllabus of the Latter… Delivered in the University of Pennsylvania*, edited by Benjamin Rush. Philadelphia: Bradford and Innskeep, 336–337.

Rush, Benjamin. [1808] 1951. "Letter to John Adams. 24 August 1808." In *Letters of Benjamin Rush*, edited by L. H. Butterfield, vol. II: 975. Philadelphia: Princeton University Press for the American Philosophical Society.

Rush, Benjamin. 1809. "Outlines of the Phenomenon of Fever." In *Medical Inquiries & Observations*, edited by Matthew Carey, et al., 31. Philadelphia: Johnson and Warner.

Rush, Benjamin. 1811. *Sixteen Introductory Lectures, to Courses of Lectures Upon the Institutes and Practice of Medicine, with a Syllabus of the Latter…Delivered in the University of Pennsylvania.* Philadelphia: Bradford and Innskeep.

Rush, Benjamin. 1948. *The Autobiography of Benjamin Rush, His "Travels Through Life" Together with His "Commonplace Book" for 1789–1813*, edited by George Corner. Princeton: Princeton University Press for the American Philosophical Society.

Ryan, Michael. [1831] 2009. *A Manual of Jurisprudence, compiled from the best medical and legal works: comprising an account of: I. The Ethics of the Medical Profession II. The Charter and Statutes Relating to the Faculty; and III. All Medico-legal Questions, with the latest discussions. Being an Analysis of a Course of Lectures on Forensic Medicine Annually Delivered in London and intended as a compendium for the use of barristers, soliciters, magistrates, coroners, and medical practitioners.* London: Renshaw and Rush. Retrieved from Google Books. In *Michael Ryan's Writings on Medical Ethics*, edited by Howard Brody, Zahara Meghani, and Kimberly Greenwald. Dordrecht: Springer.

Ryan, Michael. 1831. Letter from Dr. Ryan. *Lancet*, 1: 222–224.

Ryan, Michael. 1832. *A Manual of Medical Jurisprudence, Compiled from the Best Medical and Legal Works; Being an Analysis of a Course of Lectures on Forensic Medicine, Annually Delivered in London*, 2nd ed., Philadelphia: Carrey and Lea.

Sade, Robert, and Karine Morin. 2001. "Principles of Medical Ethics: The Proposed Revision of 2001." *Journal of the South Carolina Medical Association*, 97(2): 72–75.

Sanders, David, and Jesse Dukeminier. 1968. "Medical Advance and Legal Lag: Hemodialysis and Kidney Transplantation." *UCLA Law Review*, 15: 366–380.

Sappol, M. 2002. *A Traffic of Dead Bodies: Anatomy and Embodied Social Identity in Nineteenth-century America.* Princeton: Princeton University Press.

Saundby, Robert. 1902. *Medical Ethics: A Guide to Professional Conduct.* London: Charles Griffin.

Saundby, Robert. 1907. *Medical Ethics: A Guide to Professional Conduct.* London: Charles Griffin.

Savitt, Todd. 2007. *Race and Medicine in Nineteenth and Early-twentieth Century America.* Kent: Kent State University Press.

Saxe, John Godfrey, "The Blind Men and the Elephant." http://www.dle.ufms.br/daniel/literature/23-Inter_War_Years.pdf (accessed August 19, 2012).

Schleiner, Winifred. 1995. *Medical Ethics in the Renaissance.* Washington, DC: Georgetown University Press.

Shattuck, Frederick 1910. Letter to George H. Simmons, MD, editor of *Journal of the American Medical Association*, "Report of Committee on Elaboration of the Principles of Ethics," AMA 1910. *Minutes of the House of Delegates Proceedings of the Sixty-First Annual Session in St. Louis*, 30.

Shippen, William Jr. January 31, 1765. *Pennsylvania Gazette.* Cited in *Midwifery in America, 1760–1860: A Study in Medicine and Morality*, by Jane Bauer, 1972, 45. Unpublished doctoral dissertation (Ph.D., History), Syracuse University, NY.

Shorter, Edward. 1991. *Women's Bodies: A Social History of Women's Encounter with Health, Ill Health, and Medicine.* New Brunswick: Transaction Publishers.

Shrady, G. F. 1872. *The Medical Record.* New York: W. Wood.

Shryock, Richard. 1967. *Medical Licensing in America, 1650–1965.* Baltimore: Johns Hopkins University Press.

Shryock, Richard. 1971. "The Medical Reputation of Benjamin Rush: Contrasts Over Two Centuries." *Bulletin of the History of Medicine* 45(6): 541, 507–552.

Shryock, Richard. 1979. *The Development of Modern Medicine.* Madison: University of Wisconsin Press.

Shultz, Suzanne M. 1992. *Body Snatching: The Robbing of Graves for the Education of Physicians in Early Nineteenth Century America.* Jefferson (NC) and London: MacFarland & Company Inc.

Shultz, Suzanne M. 2008. "The Kappa Lambda Society of Hippocrates: Historical Perspective on an Early Medical Professional Society." *Southern Medical Journal,* 101(4): 415–418.

Sibbald, Sir Robert. 1706. *In Hippocratis Legem, et in ejus Epistolam ad Thessalum Filium, Commentarii: in quibus Ostenditur, quae Medico Futuro, Necessaria Sunt.* Edinburgh: Symson.

Sill, Geoffrey. 1997. "Neurology and the Novel: Alexander Monro Primus and Secundus, Robinson Crusoe, and the Problem of Sensibility." *Literature and Medicine,* 16(2): 250–265.

Sims Statue Unveiled. 1894. *The New York Times,* October 21, 1894. http://query.nytimes.com/mem/archive-free/pdf?res=F70C14F63E5515738DDDA80A94D8415B8485F0D3 (accessed August 12, 2011).

Sims, J. Marion. [1858] 1990. "Silver Sutures in Surgery: The Anniversary Discourse Before the New York Academy of Medicine." In Lawrence Longo edition of *Silver Sutures in Surgery Together with Clinical Notes on Uterine Surgery.* Birmingham (AL): The Classics of Obstetrics & Gynecology Library. Reprint of the original published by the New York Academy of Medicine, 1858, New York: Samuel & William Wood.

Sims, J. Marion. 1852. "On the Treatment of Vesico-vaginal Fistula." *American Journal of the Medical Sciences,* 23: 59–87.

Sims, J. Marion. 1854. Two Cases of Vesico-Vaginal Fistula, Cured. *New York Medical Gazette and Journal of Health.* 5(1): 1. Note: A shortened version of this statement is given in Silver Sutures lecture, 52, and in *The Story of My Life,* 236.

Sims, J. Marion. [1858] 1990. *Silver Sutures in Surgery Together with Clinical Notes on Uterine Surgery.* New York: Samuel & William Wood.

Sims, J. Marion. [1866] 1990. "Clinical Notes on Uterine Surgery." In *Silver Sutures in Surgery together with Clinical Notes on Uterine Surgery.* Birmingham (Al): The Classics of Obstetrics & Gynecology Library. Reprint of the original of 1866, London: Robert Hardwicke.

Sims, J. Marion. 1870. Letter of Defense. April 4, 1870. Manuscript in Archives, New York Academy of Medicine Committee on Ethics, Scrapbook 1867–1884.

Sims, J. Marion. 1876. "Presidential Address," *AMA Transactions,* 27: 91–111.

Sims, J. Marion. [1884, 1885] 1898. *The Story of My Life,* edited by Harry Marion-Sims. New York: D. Appleton and Company.

Sloan, Douglas. 1971. *The Scottish Enlightenment and the American College Ideal*, 12–14. New York: Teacher's College Press, Columbia.

Smellie, William. 1754. *A Sett of ANATOMICAL TABLES, with Explanations, and an Abridgment, of the PRACTICE of MIDWIFERY, with a View to Illustrate a Treatise on that Subject and Collection of Cases.* London. http://www.nlm.nih.gov/exhibition/historicalanatomies/smellie_home.html (accessed September 15, 2008).

Smith, J. V. C. 1847. Unsigned. "Editorial." *The Boston Medical and Surgical Journal*, February 17, 1847, 35(3): 63–64.

Smith, Russell G. 1994. *Medical Discipline: The Professional Conduct Jurisdiction of the General Medical Council, 1858–1990.* Oxford and London: Clarendon Press.

Smith, Russell G. 1995. Legal Precedent and Medical Ethics: Some Problems Encountered by the General Medical Council in Relying Upon Precedent When Declaring Acceptable Standards of Professional Conduct. In *The Codification of Medical Morality: Historical and Philosophical Studies of the Formalization of Western Medical Morality in the Eighteenth and Nineteenth Centuries: Vol. 2: Anglo-American Medical Ethics and Medical Jurisprudence in the Nineteenth Century*, edited by R. Baker, 205–218. Dordrect: Kluwer Academic Publishers.

Smith, Thomas Southwood. 1827. *Use of the Dead to the Living.* Albany: Websters and Skinners.

Smith-Rosenberg, Carol. 1985. *Disorderly Conduct: Visions of Gender in Victorian America*, 217–244. New York: Oxford University Press.

Snyder, Charles. 1962. "Julius Homberger, M.D. 'A Mere Adventurer Whom Chance has Thrown Among Us.'" *Archives of Ophthalmology*, 69(6): 876–877.

Solis-Cohen, Solomon. 1892. "Shall Physicians Become Sales-agents for Patent Medicines?" *Journal of the American Medical Association*, 18(22): 682–683.

Solis-Cohen, Solomon. 1894. "As to 'Nostrum' Advertisements in the Journal." *Journal of the American Medical Association*, 22(3): 95–96.

Soper, George. 1907. "Work of a Chronic Typhoid Germ Distributor." *Journal of the American Medical Association*, 48(24): 2019–2022.

Spalding, James A. 1916. *Dr. Lyman Spalding: The Originator of the United States Pharmacopoeia.* Boston, MA: W. M. Leonard.

Starr, Paul. 1982. *The Social Transformation of American Medicine: The Rise of a Sovereign Profession and the Making of a Vast Industry.* New York: Basic Books.

Stebbins, Emma. 1879. *Charlotte Cushman: Her letters and Memories of Her Life Edited by Her Friend.* Boston: Houghton, Osgood and Company, The Riverside Press.

Steele, A. K. 1887. "The Medico-Legal Aspect of Criminal Abortion." *Journal of the American Medical Association*, 9(24): 762–764.

Sternberg, George. 1900. *Letter to Agramonte. Philip D. Hench Walter Reed Yellow Fever Collection.* Charlottesville: University of Virginia.

Sternberg, George. 1901. "The Transmission of Yellow Fever Mosquitos." *Popular Science Monthly*, 59: 225–241. Cited by Lederer, Susan, 2008, "Walter Reed and the Yellow Fever Experiments." In *The Oxford Textbook of Clinical Research Ethics*, edited by Ezekiel

Emanuel, Christine Grady, Robert Crouch et al., 9–17. New York: Oxford University Press.

Stevens, M. L. Tina. 2000. *Bioethics in America.* Baltimore: Johns Hopkins University Press.

Stewart, M. A. 2003. "Religion and Rational Theology." In *The Cambridge Companion to the Scottish Enlightenment*, edited by Alexander Broade, 34–35. Cambridge: Cambridge University Press.

Stillé, Alfred. 1871. "Address of Alfred Stillé M.D., President of the Association." *Transactions of the American Medical Association, 1871:* 91–96.

Stillé, Alfred. 1880. "Memoir of Isaac Hays, M. D." *Extracted from Transactions of the College of Physicians of Philadelphia, 3rd series,* 5. Philadelphia: College of Physicians of Philadelphia.

Stirling, W. 1904. The Hippocratic and Other Academic Oaths. *Medical Chronicle,* 4 (S7): 400–406.

Stock-Morton, Phyllis. 1996. "Control and Limitation of Midwives in Modern France: The Example of Marseille." *Journal of Women's History,* 8: 60–95.

Stookey, B. 1967. "Nicholas Romayne: First President of the College of Physicians and Surgeons, New York City." *Bulletin of the New York Academy of Medicine,* 43(7): 579–581.

Storer, David Humphreys. [1855] 1872. "Two Frequent Causes of Uterine Disease," *Journal of the Gynecological Society of Boston*, March. Cited in Dyer, Frederick, 1999, *The Lecture That Started The Successful Physicians' Crusade Against Abortion,* 6–7. http://www.abortionessay.com/files/humphreys.html (accessed February 12, 2011). Parts of the lecture are also available in Dyer, Frederick, 1999, *Champion of Women and the Unborn: Horatio Robinson Storer, M.D.,* 80–86. Canton: Science History Publications.

Storer, David Humphreys. 1866. "Presidential Address." *Transactions XVII,* 53–66.

Storer, Horatio R. 1865. "Prize Essay: The Criminality of and Physical Evils of Forced Abortions Being the Prize Essay to which the American Medical Association Awarded the Gold Medal for MDCCCLXV." *Transactions vol. XVI,* 722–733, 713, 724–736, 744–745.

Storer, Horatio R. 1866. *Why Not? A Book For Every Woman,* 65, 84–85. Boston: Lee and Shepard.

Storer, Horatio R. 1867. "Female Physicians." *Boston Medical and Surgical Journal,* 75: 191.

Storer, Horatio R. 1867. *Is it I? A Book for Every Man,* 72. Boston: Lee and Shepard.

Storer, Horatio R. 1868 "Advertisement." *Chicago Medical Examiner,* 9: 189–190.

Storer, Horatio. R. [1911] 1999. "Letter to Dr. Jas. J. Walsh, September 12, 1911." Cited in Dyer, Frederick, 1999, *Champion of Women and the Unborn: Horatio Robinson Storer, M.D.,* 483. Canton: Science History Publications.

Storer, Horatio R., Thomas Blatchford, and Hugh Hodge, et al. 1859. "Report on Criminal Abortion." *Transactions of the American Medical Association, XII,* 75–78.

Storer, Horatio R., and Franklin R. Heard. 1868. *Criminal Abortion: Its Nature, Its Evidence and Its Law.* Boston: Little Brown and Company.

Stowe, Harriet. [1852] 1853. *Uncle Tom's Cabin or Life among the Lowly*, Chapter XX, "Topsy," 266. Edinburgh: Adam and Charles Black. http://fax.libs.uga.edu/PS2954xU5/1f/uncle_toms_cabin.pdf (accessed August 13, 2012).

Struthers, Sir John. 1867. *Historical Sketch of the Edinburgh Anatomy School.* Edinburgh: Maclachlan and Stewart.

Styrap, Jukes. [1878] 1995. "A Code of Medical Ethics." In *The Codification of Medical Morality: Historical and Philosophical Studies of the Formalization of Western Medical Morality in the Eighteenth and Nineteenth Centuries: Vol. Two: Anglo-American Medical Ethics and Medical Jurisprudence in the Nineteenth Century*, edited by Robert Baker, 149–171. Dordrecht: Kluwer Academic Publishers.

Styrap, Jukes. [1878], [1886], [1895], 1899. *A Code of Medical Ethics: With Remarks on the Duties of Practitioners to their Patients, etc*… London: J. and A. Churchill, H. K. Lewis.

Subcommittee of the [New York State] Committee on Grievances. [1965] 1972. "Report." In *Experimentation with Human Beings*, edited by Jay Katz New York: Russell. Sage Foundation, 54.

Sullivan, Robert B. 1994. "Sanguine Practices: A Historic and Historiographic Reconstruction of Heroic Therapy in the Age of Rush." *Bulletin of the History of Medicine*, 68: 211–234.

Swaim, W. 1822, 1824. *A treatise on Swaim's panacea; Being a recent discovery for the cure of scrofula or king's evil, mercurial disease, deep-seated syphilis, rheumatism, and all disorders arising from a contaminated or impure state of the blood.* Philadelphia: Clark and Raser.

Taber, Sidney. 1906. *Illustrations of Human Vivisection.* Chicago: Vivisection Reform Society.

Taber, Sidney. 1907. *Reasonable Restriction vs. Absolute License in Vivisection.* Chicago: Vivisection Reform Society.

Taubenberger, Jeffrey, and David Morens. 2006. "1918 Influenza: The Mother of All Pandemics." *Emerging Infectious Diseases*, 12(1): 15–22.

Taylor, D. W. 1986. "The manuscript lectures of Alexander Monro Primus." *Medical History*, 30: 444–467.

Taylor, Telford. [1946] 1992. "Opening Statement of the Prosecution, December 9, 1946." In *The Nazi Doctors and the Nuremberg Code: Human Rights in Human Experimentation*, edited by George Annas and Michael Grogdin, 67. New York: Oxford University Press.

Teel, Karen. 1975. " The Physician's Dilemma: A Doctor's View—What the Law Should Be." *Baylor Law Review*, 27(1): 6–9.

Temkin, Owesi, C. Lilian Temkin. 1967. *Ancient Medicine: Selected Paper of Ludwig Edelstein.* New York: Oxford University Press.

Thalidomide Trust. "The Story of Thalidomide." http://www.thalidomidetrust.org/story (accessed August 23, 2012).

Thomas, Milton H. 1931 "Doctor Samuel Bard." *Columbia University Quarterly*, June: 112–130.

Thomasma, David, Thomasine Kushner, Gerrit Kimsma, et al. 1998. *Asking to Die: Inside the Dutch Debate About Euthanasia.* Dordrecht: Kluwer Academic Publishers.

Thompson, Roger. 1986. *Sex in Middlesex: Popular Mores in a Massachusetts County, 1649–1699*. Amherst: University of Massachusetts Press.

Thorton, John. 1967. "A Biographical Sketch of James Hobson Aveling (1828–1892) with a List of His Writings." In *English Midwives Their History and Prospects*, edited by John Thorton, xvi. London: Hugh L. Elliot Ltd.

Truman, John T. 1997. "The Ethics of Dr. Samuel Bard." *P & S Medical Review*, Fall 4(2): 29–32.

Turner, James. 1980. *Reckoning with the Beast: Animals, Pain and Humanity in the Victorian Mind*. Baltimore: Johns Hopkins University Press.

Tyler, Anne. 1985. *The Accidental Tourist*. New York: Alfred A. Knopf.

U.S. Constitution, Fourteenth Amendment. http://www.usconstitution.net/const.html#Am14 (accessed March 29, 2011).

U.S. Department of Health and Human Services. 1978. "The Belmont Report." Summary. http://www.hhs.gov/ohrp/archive/belmontArchive.html#histArchive2 (accessed July 13, 2012).

U.S. Senate Subcommittee on Government Research. 1968. Committee on Government Operations. *Hearings on S. J. Resolution 145*. 90th Congress, 2nd session. March 8–9, 21–22, 27–28, April 2, 1968.

U.S. Public Health Service. 1973. "Selections from the Final Report of the Tuskegee Syphilis Study Ad Hoc Advisory Panel." In *Tuskegee's Truths: Rethinking the Tuskegee Syphilis Study*, edited by Susan Reverby, 166, 172–173. Chapel Hill and London: University of North Carolina Press.

Ulrich, Laurel Thatcher. 1990. *A Midwife's Tale: The Life of Martha Ballard, Based on Her Diary, 1785–1812*. New York: Vintage Books.

Universities of Oxford and Cambridge Act of 1859. http://www.legislation.gov.uk/ukpga/Vict/22–23/19 (accessed December 21, 2012).

Vainio, Jari, and Felcity Cutts. 1998. "Untreated Yellow Fever May Have a Mortality Rate of Between 15% and 95%." In *Yellow Fever*, 62–65. Geneva: World Health Organization.

Vainio, Jari, and Felcity Cutts. 1998. "Appendix I: Examples of Historical Yellow Fever Epidemics." In *Yellow Fever*, 62–65. Geneva: World Health Organization.

Vanderpole, S. Oakley. 1883. "The Futility of a Formal Code of Ethics." In *An Ethical Symposium: Being a Series of Papers Concerning Medical Ethics and Etiquette from Liberal Standpoint*, edited by Albert C. Post et al., 26–41. New York: G. P. Putnam.

Vann Sprecher, T., and R. M. Karras. 2011. "The Midwife and the Church: Ecclesiastic Regulation of Midwives in Brie, 1499–1504." *Bulletin of the History of Medicine*, 85: 172.

Veatch, Robert. 2005. *Disrupted Dialogue: Medical Ethics and the Collapse of Physician-Humanist Communication (1770–1980)*. New York: Oxford University Press.

Von Baer, Karl Ernst. 1828–1837. *Entwickelungsgeschichte der Thiere: Beobachtung und Reflexion [Form and Function: A Contribution to the History of Animal Morphology]*. Königsberg: Bornträger.

Von Staden, Heinrich. 1996. "'In a Pure and Holy Way': Personal and Professional Conduct in the Hippocratic Oath." *Journal of the History of Medicine and Allied Sciences*, 51: 406–408.

Vonnegut, K. 1976. *Slapstick*, ch. 48. http://en.wikiquote.org/wiki/Kurt_Vonnegut (accessed April 10, 2010).

Wangensteen, Owen. [1968] 1991. "Testimony at U.S. Senate Subcommittee on Government Research, Committee on Government Operations." Cited in *Strangers at the Bedside: A History of How Law And Bioethics Transformed Medical Decision Making*, by David Rothman, 173. New York: Basic Books.

Wakely, T. 1824. "Dissection." *Lancet*, 1(17): 135–138. In Shultz, S. M., 1992, *Body Snatching: The Robbing of Graves for the Education of Physicians in Early Nineteenth Century America*. Jefferson and London: MacFarland & Company Inc.

Wall, L. Lewis. 2006. "Did J. Marion Sims Deliberately Addict His First Fistula Patients to Opium?" *Journal of the History of Medicine and Allied Sciences*, 62(3): 336–356.

Wall, L. Lewis. 2006. "The Medical Ethics of Dr. J. Marion Sims: A Fresh Look at the Historical Record." *Journal of Medical Ethics*, 32: 346–350.

Wallis, Patrick. 2011. "Debating a Duty to Treat: AIDS and the Professional Ethics of American Medicine." *Bulletin of the History of Medicine*, 85(4): 620–649.

Walsh, James J. 1906. "History of the Medical Society of the State of New York." *New York State Journal of Medicine*, 6(5): 219–220.

Walsh, James J. 1907. *History of the Medical Society of the State of New York*. New York: MSSNY.

Walsh, James. J. 1919. *History of Medicine in New York: Three Centuries of Medical Progress*, vol. 1. New York: National Americana Society, Inc.

Walter, Jennifer K., and Eran P. Klein. 2003. *The Story of Bioethics: From Seminal Works to Contemporary Explorations*. Washington, DC: Georgetown University Press.

Warner, John Harley. 1991. "Ideals of Science and Their Discontents in Late Nineteenth-Century American Medicine." *Isis*, 82(3): 454–478.

Warner, John Harley. 1999. "The 1880s Rebellion Against the AMA Code of Ethics: 'Scientific Democracy' and the Dissolution of Orthodoxy." In *The American Medical Ethics Revolution*, edited by R. Baker, A. Caplan, L. Emanuel, and S. Latham, 52–69. Baltimore: The Johns Hopkins University Press.

Warren, Edward. 1860. *The Life of John Collins Warren, M.D., Compiled Chiefly from His Autobiography and Journals, Vol. I.* Boston: Ticknor and Fields.

Washington, Harriet A. 2007. *Medical Apartheid: The Dark History of Medical Experimentation on Black Americans from Colonial Times to the Present*. New York: Doubleday.

Washington, Harriet A. Robert B. Baker, Ololade Olakanmi, Todd L. Savitt, Elizabeth A. Jacobs, Eddie Hoover, and Matthew K. Wynia, for the Writing Group on the History of African Americans and the Medical Profession. 2009. "Segregation, Civil Rights, and Health Disparities: The Legacy of African American Physicians and Organized Medicine, 1910–1968." *Journal of the National Medical Association*, 101(6): 513–527.

Watson, Sir Thomas. 1850. *Lectures on the Principles and Practice of Physic*, edited by Francis Condie, 25. Philadelphia: Lea and Blanchard.

Webster, Noah. 1828. *An American Dictionary of the English Language (1828)*, http://1828.mshaffer.com/ (accessed December 1, 2012).

Webster, Noah. 1913. *Webster's Revised Unabridged Dictionary.* http://1913.mshaffer.com/d/browse/letter (accessed December 1, 2012).

Webster, Noah. [1948] 1978. *Webster's New Collegiate Dictionary,* edited by Henry Woolf. Springfield: G. & C. Merriam Company.

Wenger, O. C. [1933] 2000. "Letter to R. A. Vonderlehr, July 21, 1933." In *Tuskegee's Truths: Rethinking the Tuskegee Syphilis Study,* edited by Susan Reverby, 85. Chapel Hill and London: University of North Carolina Press.

Whalley, Lawson, 1818. "A Vindication of the University of Edinburgh (As a School of Medicine), From the Aspersions of 'A Member of the University of Oxford.'" In *The Pamphleteer,* edited by Abraham John Valpy, vol. 13 (1818). New York Public Library.

Whalley, Lawson. [1823] 1826. "A Defense of the Literary and Scientific Institutions of Scotland for the Term 'Illegitimate,' in the Review of the 'Cambridge Tart.'" *The Edinburgh magazine, and literary miscellany, a new series of The Scots magazine,* January-June 1826 Vol. XVIII. Edinburgh: Archibald Constable and Company, 193–194.

Whewell, W. 1840. *The Philosophy of the Inductive Sciences, Founded Upon Their History.* London: John W. Parker.

Whewell, W. 1847. *The Philosophy of the Inductive Sciences, Founded Upon Their History.* London: John W. Parker.

Wiesner, Merry. 2004. "Early Modern Midwifery: A Case Study." In *Midwifery and the Medicalization of Childbirth: Comparative Perspectives,* edited by E. van Tiejlingen, G. Lowis, P. McCaffery, and M. Porter, 70–71. Hauppauge: Nova Science Publishers.

Wildes, Kevin. 1996. "Ordinary and Extraordinary Means and the Quality of Life." *Theological Studies,* 56: 500–512.

"Wight." 1828. *Webster's American Dictionary of the English Language.* http://www.1828-dictionary.com/d/search/word,wight (accessed October 3, 2010).

Williamson, William. 1966. "Life or Death—Whose Decisions?" *Journal of the American Medical Association,* 197(10): 793–795.

Wilson, James C. 1904. *An Address Delivered at the Unveiling of a Monument Erected by the American Medical Association to the Memory of Benjamin Rush, in Washington D. C. June 11, 1904.* Philadelphia: J. B. Lippincott Company.

Wilson, K., and J. Coval. "City of Unbrotherly Love: Violence in Nineteenth-century Philadelphia." In *Exploring Diversity in Pennsylvania History.* Philadelphia: Historical Society of Pennsylvania and the Batch Institute for Ethnic Studies. http://www.hsp.org/files/thephiladelphiariotsof1844.pdf (accessed November 11, 2010).

Winthrop, John. [1630–1649] 1908. "Journal." In *History of New England: Original Narratives of Early American History,* edited by James K. Hosmer, 317–318. Cited in Hoffer, Peter C. and N. E. H. Hull, 1981, *Murdering Mothers: Infanticide in England and New England, 1558–1803,* 42–43. New York: New York University Press.

Wittgenstein, Ludwig. 1955. G. E. M. Anscombe, trans. *Philosophical Investigations,* §109. Oxford: Blackwell.

Wittgenstein, Ludwig. 1961. *Tractatus Logico-Philosophicus,* translated by D. F Pears and B. F. McGuinnes. London: Routledge & Kegan Paul.

Wittgenstein, Ludwig. [1980] 1984. *Culture and Value*, translated by Peter Winch from *Vermischte Bemerkungen* (1977). Chicago: University of Chicago Press.

Wolpe, P. 1999. "Alternative Medicine and the AMA." In *The American Medical Ethics Revolution*, edited by R. Baker, A. Caplan, L. Emanuel, and S. Latham, 218–239. Baltimore: Johns Hopkins University Press.

Woodhouse, George, Robertson Ward, J. Morrison Hutcheson, Louis A. Buie, and Homer L. Pearson (chair). 1957. "Principles of Medical Ethics of the American Medical Association: Annotated: Prepared by the Judicial Council." Report JC 4234, 1966. Archives of the American Medical Association.

World Health Organization. 2010. "Ten Facts on Obstetric Fistula." http://www.who.int/features/factfiles/obstetric_fistula/en/.

World Medical Association. 1949. "Declaration of Geneva, preliminary publication." *World Medical Association Bulletin*, 1(1):13. Official publication in 1949 as "Serment de Geneve, Declaration of Geneva, Declaracion en Gemebra," *World Medical Association Bulletin*, 1(2):35–37.

Wright-St. Clair, R. E. 1964. *Doctors Monro.* London: Wellcome Historical Medical Library.

Young, J., R. Sumant, R. Wachter, C. Lee, et al. "'July Effect': Impact of the Academic Year-End Changeover on Patient Outcomes. A Systematic Review." *Annals of Internal Medicine*, http://www.annals.org/content/early/2011/07/11/0003-4819-155-5-201109060 00354.full#fn-group-1 (accessed July 21, 2011).

Young, James Havery. 1961. *The Toadstool Millionaires: A Social History of Patent Medicines in America Before Federal Regulation.* Princeton: Princeton University Press.

Younger, Stuart, David Jackson, Claudia Coulton, et al. 1983. "A National Survey of Hospital Ethics Committees." In *President's Commission for the Study of Ethical Problems in Medicine and Biomedical and Behavioral Research. Deciding to Forego Life-Sustaining Treatment: A Report on the Ethical, Medical and Legal Issues in Treatment Decisions.* Washington, DC: U.S. Government Printing Office (83-600503).

Zaibert, Leo. 2006. *Punishment and Retribution.* Aldershot: Ashgate Publishing Limited.

Zakrzewska, Marie Elizabeth. 1924. *A Woman's Quest: The Life of Marie E. Zakrzewska*, edited by Agnes C. Vietor. New York: D. Appleton.

INDEX

Printed in the USA/Agawam, MA
April 29, 2015

613826.004